D1383051

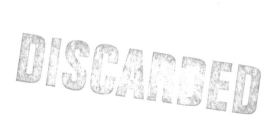

The Woman
Who Saved
the Children

The Woman
Who Saved
the Children

A Biography of Eglantyne Jebb
Founder of Save the Children

Clare Mulley

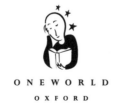

ONEWORLD

OXFORD

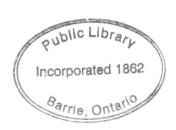

A Oneworld Book

Published by Oneworld Publications 2009

Copyright © Clare Mulley 2009

The right of Clare Mulley to be identified as the Author of this
work has been asserted by her in accordance with the Copyright,
Designs and Patents Act 1988

ISBN 978–1–85168–657–5

Typeset by Jayvee, Trivandrum, India
Cover design by Rose Cooper
Printed and bound in Great Britain by TJ International, Padstow

Oneworld Publications
185 Banbury Road
Oxford OX2 7AR
England
www.oneworld-publications.com

All author royalties donated to Save the Children,
registered charity in England and Wales (213890)
and Scotland (SC 039570)

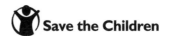

Save the Children

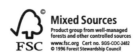

Mixed Sources
Product group from well-managed
forests and other controlled sources
www.fsc.org Cert no. SGS-COC-2482
© 1996 Forest Stewardship Council

Learn more about Oneworld. Join our mailing list to
find out about our latest titles and special offers at:

www.oneworld-publications.com

To my three wonderful daughters, Millicent Eglantyne, Florence Minerva and Hester Eve – symbols of universal human potential and very lively little girls in the here and now.

Contents

Foreword   ix

Acknowledgements   xi

Family Trees   xiii

Illustrations   xv

Cast of Characters   xix

1 Imagining Eglantyne, 2009–1876   1

2 Meeting the Family, 1876–1894   7

3 Unravelling Her Surroundings, 1895–1898   28

4 Testing the Maternal Impulse, 1898–1900   52

5 Happy Days, 1901–1902   70

6 Brief Studies in Social Questions, 1902–1910   92

7 Love Letters, 1907–1913   115

8 Relief in 'The Barbarous Balkans', 1913   140

9 Conversations with the Dead, 1914–1915   168

10 Surrounded by Action, 1914–1916   190

11 Found in Translation, 1917–1919   209

12 Save the Children, 1919   232

13 Hearts and Minds, 1919–1920   252

14 'Supranationalism', 1920–1923   273

15 The Rights of the Child, 1922–1925   300

16 Blue Plaques, 1920–2009   317

    Epilogue: Truths and Lives   331

    The International Save the Children Alliance   335

    Endnotes   336

    Bibliography   358

    Index   379

Foreword

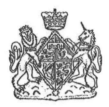

BUCKINGHAM PALACE

Eglantyne Jebb became the child's greatest champion in the aftermath of World War One. In 1919 she and her sister Dorothy founded an emergency relief fund for the starving children of Europe. The International Save the Children Alliance is now the world's largest independent organization for children, with staff working in partnership with thousands of local organizations, supported in different ways by millions of people, to improve the lives and life-chances of children in over 120 countries. But Eglantyne's legacy went even further when she drafted a pioneering statement of 5 children's rights and responsibilities in 1923, getting it adopted by the League of Nations the following year.

Eglantyne's achievement in putting children's welfare on the world's agenda ranks as one of the great triumphs of humanity and yet although celebrated around the world after her death, her own remarkable story is now almost forgotten. Published to coincide with the 90th anniversary of Save the Children, and the 20th anniversary of the UN Convention on the Rights of the Child, this biography restores that balance, showing just how important a contribution one person with the right combination of imagination and determination can make.

Eglantyne's memory lives on today with Save the Children working around the world to address children's basic needs, such as education and health. But much remains to be done: 75 million children do not go to school and one mother dies in childbirth every minute of every day. Thank you for supporting Save the Children by your interest in this book about a remarkable lady.

Her Royal Highness The Princess Royal
President, Save the Children UK

Acknowledgements

Thank you very, very much indeed to Ian Wolter for everything, and the key editorial team, Kate, Gill and Derek Mulley. This book could not have been written without the very kind support of Lionel and Corinna Jebb, Ben Buxton and the Buxton family, Susannah Burn, Philippa Hill, Nicholas Humphrey, Charlotte Humphrey, Robert Dimsdale, Nicholas Dimsdale, Dickie Hughes and David Marshall – thank you all for your great generosity. Sincere thanks are also due to the archivists and experts at the Save the Children Fund; the Library at the League of Nations Archives Collections, the United Nations Office at Geneva; the State Archives of Geneva, Switzerland where the UISE (International Union of Save the Children) papers are kept; the Principal and Fellows of Lady Margaret Hall, Oxford; Newnham College, Cambridge; and King's College Cambridge where the Keynes papers are kept; the Master Fellows and Scholars of Churchill College, Cambridge, and the staff of the Churchill Archive Centre where the A.V. Hill papers are kept; the William Ready Division of Archives and Research Collections, McMaster University Library, Hamilton, Ontario where the C.K. Ogden papers are kept; the British Library manuscripts and newspaper archives; *The Times* archives; the Labour History Archive at the People's History Museum; the Women's Library; the Corporation of London Records Office; the President and Council of the Royal College of Surgeons of England; The Royal Society of Medicine; The Wellcome Institute; The National Gallery Libraries and Archive Department; and the Met Office, National Meteorological Archive;

as well as Dr Michael Tunbridge, former President of the British Thyroid Association and author of M.P.J. Vanderpump and W.M.G. Tunbridge, *Thyroid Disease: The Facts*, 4th edition (OUP 2008); and Sam Dimmock, Programme Director – 'Get ready for Geneva' at the Child Rights Association of England for specialist advice. Also to my agent Andrew Lownie for believing in a book on a charitably minded 'spinster in a brown cardigan', and finally to my friends Rodney Breen, Dido Davies, Nicole DeSouza, Sheila Gower-Isaac; Lisa O'Connell, Jude Rudolf, Alison Pavier, Anna Rawlinson and Lucy Ward. Thank you.

Family Trees

Shropshire Jebbs referred to in this book

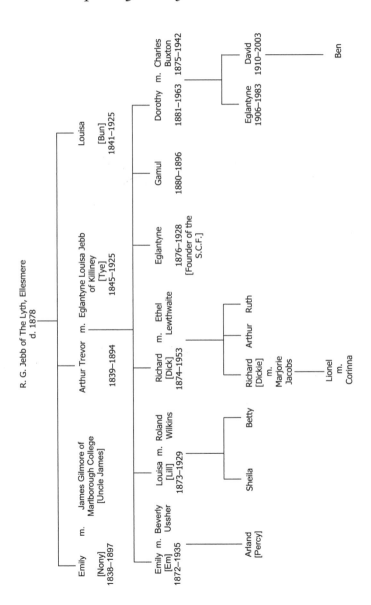

R. G. Jebb of The Lyth, Ellesmere
d. 1878

Emily [Nony] 1838–1897 m. James Gilmore of Marlborough College [Uncle James]

Arthur Trevor 1839–1894 m. Eglantyne Louisa Jebb of Killiney [Tye] 1845–1925

Louisa [Bun] 1841–1925

Emily [Em] 1872–1935 m. Beverly Ussher

Louisa [Lill] 1873–1929 m. Roland Wilkins

Richard [Dick] 1874–1953 m. Ethel Lewthwaite

Eglantyne 1876–1928 [Founder of the S.C.F.]

Gamul 1880–1896

Dorothy 1881–1963 m. Charles Buxton 1875–1942

Arland [Percy]

Sheila

Betty

Richard [Dickie] m. Marjorie Jacobs

Arthur

Ruth

Lionel m. Corinna

Eglantyne 1906–1983

David 1910–2003

Ben

Anglo-Irish Jebbs referred to in this book

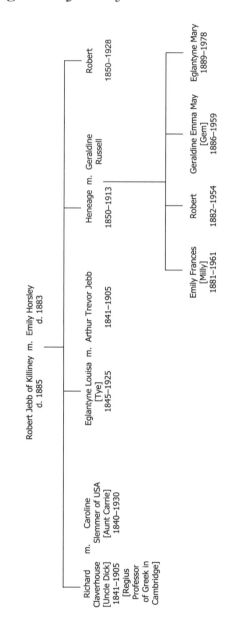

Robert Jebb of Killiney m. Emily Horsley
d. 1885   d. 1883

Richard Claverhouse [Uncle Dick] 1841–1905 [Regius Professor of Greek in Cambridge] m. Caroline Slemmer of USA [Aunt Carrie] 1840–1930

Eglantyne Louisa [Tye] 1845–1925 m. Artthur Trevor Jebb 1841–1905

Heneage 1850–1913 m. Geraldine Russell

Robert 1850–1928

Emily Frances [Milly] 1881–1961

Robert 1882–1954

Geraldine Emma May [Gem] 1886–1959

Eglantyne Mary 1889–1978

Illustrations

Plates

Plate 1   Arthur Jebb with, from left: Em, Dorothy, Gamul and Eglantyne, *c.*1889

Plate 2   Tye with parasol, and all six of her children, from left: Lill, Em, Dick with rifle, Gamul with butterfly net, Eglantyne and Dorothy, August 1890

Plate 3   Adults from left: Aunt Nony, Uncle James and Aunt Bun, with children: Eglantyne, Gamul, Dorothy and Lill, at The Lyth, 1889

Plate 4   'The Covey of Partridges': Dorothy, Eglantyne and Gamul, *c.*1888

Plate 5   Eglantyne as an Oxford student, *c.*1896

Plate 6   Eglantyne with her fellow Stockwell teacher trainees, 1899. Eglantyne is seated with her hands in her lap, third row from the back, fourth in the row

Plate 7   Eglantyne during what Dorothy scornfully called her 'worldly period', Cambridge, 1904

Plate 8   Marcus Dimsdale, about ten years after Eglantyne knew him, *c.*1913

Plate 9   Eglantyne and Tye in the Tyrol, *c.*1904–1908

Plate 10 Tom Buxton (Charlie's nephew) and Eglantyne, standing behind Dorothy and Charlie at their home in Bovey Tracey, Devon, where Charlie was MP, December 1910. Charlie had grown a moustache to try to impress potential voters.

Plate 11 Eglantyne and Margaret, possibly in the Tyrol, 1911

Plate 12 Margaret and AV Hill the year they married, 1913

Plate 13 A Macedonian family stabbed while at work, from Victoria de Bunsen's *Macedonian Massacres: Photos from Macedonia*, c.1907. © British Library Board. All Rights Reserved (8027.a.29)

Plate 14 Fliers from Eglantyne's Macedonian Relief Fund fundraising and publicity tour, 1913

Plate 15 Lill as Director of the Agricultural Organisation Society (AOS), in her Women's Land Army armband, c.1916

Plate 16 The leaflet, showing a starving Austrian infant, that Eglantyne was arrested for distributing in Trafalgar Square, May 1919. The word 'suppressed!' is pencilled in Eglantyne's writing in the top right hand corner

Plate 17 *Daily Herald*, 16 May 1919, featuring Eglantyne and Barbara Ayrton Gould outside their Mansion House court case, as well as the leaflets and poster they were arrested for distributing

Plate 18 19 May 1919, Eglantyne and her sister Dorothy launched the Save the Children Fund at a public meeting in the Albert Hall, which was packed to overflowing

Plate 19 Save the Children's HQ in Golden Square, Soho, 1919. Staff and volunteers worked with leftover barrack room furniture and old shoe boxes. Eglantyne never wasted a penny that could be used for a child, and former workers recalled her retrieving errant pins from the office floor

Plate 20 'The Most Awful Spectacle in History'; Save the Children fundraising advert, *The Times*, 4 March 1920

Plate 21 Eglantyne in Save the Children had and armband, *c.*1920

Plate 22 Fridtjof Nansen on his arrival in London at Victoria Station with Eglantyne, Lord Weatherdale (on left) and Ethel Snowdon, 1921

Plate 23 Eglantyne at her Save the Children desk, *c.*1922

Plate 24 Dorothy and Charlie Buxton, 1922

Plate 25 Bosnian Serb children as featured in the Bulletin of the Save the Children International Union (UISE), 10 March 1920

Plate 26 When news reached Britain of the famine in Russia, Save the Children was one of the first organisations to appeal on behalf of the six million children there who were suffering. By the autumn of 1921 they were running feeding programmes for up to 300,000 children every day

Plate 27 Facsimile of the Declaration of Geneva, signed by Eglantyne and international dignitaries, *c.*1924

Plate 28 Eglantyne, *c.*1928

Plate 29 Eglantyne's grave in Geneva, December 1928

Sketches

Chapter 1, p. 1   Self-portrait of Eglantyne losing important papers from her folder, Cambridge *c*.1906

Chapter 2, p. 7   'Visitors round corner of verandah. Exodus of inhabitants.' The Jebb children escape from The Lyth when dull visitors call, *c*.1895

Chapter 3, p. 28   Eglantyne's doodles of a sports day at Lady Margaret Hall, and of herself trailing in the wake of her college friend Dorothy Kempe, 1896. Reproduced by kind permission of the Principal and Fellows of Lady Margaret Hall

Chapter 5, p. 70   Eglantyne and Lill horse-riding around the margin of one of Eglantyne's letters to her aunt Nony, 1891

Chapter 6, p. 92   Eglantyne, relishing the 'austere domination' of her ideals, draws herself in black and laden down with papers, while walking against the tide of fashionable Cambridge society, *c*.1906

Chapter 7, p. 115   Eglantyne in her tobogganing clothes, drawn to amuse Margaret in a letter from Switzerland, 1910, and pencil portrait of Margaret Keynes by Gwen Darwin, later famous as the artist Gwen Raverat, August 1910

Chapter 9, p. 168   A childhood sketch by Dorothy entitled, 'The Phantoms of Eglantyne's Brain'

Chapter 10, p. 190   Eglantyne propped up on a couch, drawn by Tye, undated

Chapter 14, p. 273   The Save the Children International Union (UISE) logo, 1920

Cast of Principal
Characters

LADY ABERDEEN (1857–1939): President of the International Council of Women from 1893; member of the Association of Save the Children; Patron of the NSPCC.

GUSTAVE ADOR (1845–1928): Swiss politician; President of the Swiss Confederation 1919; President of the International Red Cross; member of the Honorary Committee of the Save the Children International Union 1920.

MOSA ANDERSON (1891–1978): Translator for 'Notes from the Foreign Press', replacing Dorothy as Editor in c.1919. Later Charlie and Noel Buxton's secretary; member of the Save the Children Council 1933–1967.

HIS HOLINESS, POPE BENEDICT XV (1854–1922): Pope 1914–1922. Benedict XV declared the neutrality of the Holy See at the start the First World War, supported a negotiated settlement, and later contributed so generously to aid and reconstruction appeals that funds had to be borrowed for his own funeral. Eglantyne dubbed him the 'Children's Pope'.

ARTHUR C. BENSON (1862–1925): Essayist, poet and journalist. Son of the Archbishop of Canterbury, Arthur Benson was close friends with Marcus Dimsdale at Cambridge, where he was a distinguished academic and later Master of Magdalene College. His best-known writing is the words to 'Land of Hope and Glory'.

LADY SARA BLOMFIELD (1859–1939): Humanitarian, writer, prominent member of the British Baha'i movement in the 1920s, and early Council Member of the British Save the Children Fund.

CHARLES RODEN BUXTON (1875–1942): Humanitarian, politician and scholar. Great grandson of Sir Thomas Fowell Buxton who brought the bill to emancipate slaves in 1833. Charlie married Eglantyne's sister Dorothy in 1904. First a

Liberal, then from 1917 a Labour MP. He survived a Turkish assassination attempt during a diplomatic mission in 1914. Having campaigned for a negotiated peace, he joined the Society of Friends in 1917, and after the war wrote with great insight about the risks of a one-sided exploitation of victory. He supported Save the Children, but saw his own contribution as primarily political. Among other, later roles he served as Secretary to the British Labour Delegation to Russia in 1920, and a member of the British Delegation to the League of Nations in 1924 helping secure endorsement for the Declaration of the Rights of the Child. He died in 1942, aged sixty-seven, still with a Turkish bullet in his lung.

DOROTHY FRANCES BUXTON, née JEBB (1881–1963): Eglantyne's younger sister, and co-founder of Save the Children. Joined the Women's International League for Peace and Freedom in 1915. Active in the Liberal Party until she joined Labour in 1917, the same year she joined the Society of Friends. Her 'Notes from the Foreign Press' inspired the Fight the Famine Council in 1918, leading to the launch of the Save the Children Fund in 1919. As well as writing several books, in 1935 she interviewed Göring, later Second-in-Command of the Third Reich, to urge restraint in the treatment of civilians, and during the Second World War she fought for the welfare of German prisoners of war and the refugees who fled to Britain from the Nazis. Her children described her as a 'devoted but bad mother'. Dorothy died in 1963, a vibrant and campaigning eighty-two-year-old.

NOEL EDWARD NOEL-BUXTON (1869–1948): Charlie's brother, high-profile Liberal, and later Labour MP, and philanthropist. Founded the Macedonian Relief Fund with Charlie in 1913, survived an assassination attempt during a diplomatic mission to Bulgaria in 1914. Treasurer of the Fight the Famine Council in 1919; President of Save the Children 1930–1948.

ÉTIENNE CLOUZOT (1881–1944): Chief of the Secretariat of the International Red Cross; General Secretary of the Save the Children International Union from 1920; member of the Save the Children Council 1922–1931. Eglantyne's ally in drafting and promoting the Declaration of the Rights of the Child.

LADY KATHLEEN COURTNEY (1881–1973): Honorary Secretary of the National Union of Women's Suffrage Societies in 1911, and leading figure in the Women's International League for Peace and Freedom, and Serbian Relief Fund. A contemporary of Eglantyne's at Lady Margaret Hall, and member of the Fight the Famine Council in 1918 when her brother-in-law, Lord Parmoor, became its President. Later an active supporter of Save the Children, and important figure in the League of Nations Union.

ARCHBISHOP RANDALL DAVIDSON (1848–1930): Archbishop of Canterbury 1903–1928. Davidson initially rejected a call to support Save the Children in 1919, but later helped to co-ordinate the international church appeal and became an influential supporter of the Fund.

VICTORIA DE BUNSEN, née BUXTON (1874–1953): Sister of Charles and Noel Buxton, and Lill's Newnham College friend and travelling companion through Asia Minor in 1902. Visited the Balkans in 1907, publishing an essay on the developing regional conflict. An active supporter of the Fight the Famine Council and Save the Children.

ELSBETH DIMSDALE, née PHILIPPS (*c.*1872–1949): Daughter of the Reverend Canon Sir James Erasmus Philipps, twelfth Baronet and Prebendary of Salisbury Cathedral. Left Oxford with first-class honours the year Eglantyne went up, and became the first woman to hold a research fellowship at Cambridge where she founded the Women's University Club. Married Marcus Dimsdale in 1902. Later worked for the Ministry of Health, and undertook considerable voluntary work with Cambridge County Council and Poor Law Board. Following the death of her baby in 1912 she co-founded the Papworth Tuberculosis Colony, the Cambridge Midwifery and Nursing Association, and threw herself into a campaign to eliminate TB from the milk supply, work for which she was later awarded the CBE.

MARCUS SOUTHWELL DIMSDALE (1860–1919): Second son of the sixth Baron Dimsdale, distinguished classical scholar and Fellow of King's College, Cambridge. Eglantyne fell in love with Marcus at the turn of the century, but he married Elsbeth Philipps in 1902.

DR FRÉDÉRIC FERRIÈRE: Swiss doctor and long-serving delegate of the International Red Cross, whose 1918 reports from Vienna inspired Eglantyne and Dorothy. Founding board member of the Save the Children International Union in 1920.

SUZANNE FERRIÈRE: Frédéric Ferrière's niece, Assistant Secretary to the International Save the Children Union committee, and Eglantyne's close friend and 'international sister' in Geneva. Dedicated her life to the protection of civilians, helping to draw up the influential draft Tokyo Convention, and becoming one of the three women to sit on the International Committee of the Red Cross during the Second World War.

DOROTHY GARDINER, née KEMPE (1873–1957): Eglantyne's closest college friend, author and active supporter of the settlement movement. She and Eglantyne lost touch after 1913 when Dorothy married Thory Gage Gardiner, later Canon of Canterbury.

JAMES GILMORE (UNCLE JAMES): Eglantyne's uncle, married to her father's sister Nony. Maths master at Marlborough College, Wiltshire.

LEWIS BERNARD GOLDEN (1878–1954): Russian-born British business-man, correspondent for the *Daily Mail*, and officer at the British Ministry of Information. First Secretary General of the British Save the Children Fund 1919–1937.

BARBARA BODICHON AYRTON GOULD (*c.*1886–1950): Secretary of the Women's International League for Peace and Freedom. Labour politician 1939–1950.

JANE HARRISON (1850–1928): Cambridge Classics scholar, feminist, Dorothy's friend and tutor, and a friend of Margaret Keynes and her set on the edge of the Bloomsbury Group.

ARCHIBALD VIVIAN HILL (AV) (1886–1977): Physiologist who, when just thirty-seven, shared the 1922 Nobel Prize in Physiology and Medicine. AV mar-ried Margaret Keynes in 1913, ending her and Eglantyne's intimate friendship. Succeeding indirectly from Eglantyne's uncle Richard, AV became MP for Cambridge and Oxford Universities, and played a crucial humanitarian role in arranging sanctuary for Jewish scientists in the years before the Second World War. Margaret and AV's four children, and many of their grandchildren, also became distinguished academics.

MARGARET HILL, née KEYNES (1885–1970): Cambridge social worker. Eglantyne's 'dearest and best' friend between 1906 and Margaret's marriage to AV Hill in 1913. Her brother was the economist John Maynard Keynes, and Marcus Dimsdale was a distant cousin. After the First World War Margaret became a local Poor Law Guardian, Alderman of her Borough Council and President of the National Council of Women. Her role in pioneering affordable residential care for the elderly left homeless after the Second World War earned her a CBE in 1957. She died in 1970 after a life of compassionate public service. As her biographer commented, Margaret 'inherited much of her temperament, and her particular abilities from her mother, but she took her first inspiration from the life of Eglantyne'.[1]

MAUD HOLGATE: Bursar at Lady Margaret Hall, Oxford, and lifelong friend of Eglantyne's.

ARTHUR TREVOR JEBB (1839–1894): Eglantyne's father, conservative country landowner, barrister and sensitive soul who was passionate about history, rural affairs, the written word and his six children.

CAROLINE JEBB (AUNT CARRIE), née SLEMMER (1840–1930): Vivacious American widow who married Eglantyne's uncle, Richard Claverhouse Jebb, helping establish them among the Cambridge elite in the 1870s. Also famous as Gwen Raverat's 'Aunt Cara' in her family memoirs, *Period Piece.*

DOROTHY JEBB, see Dorothy Frances Buxton.

EGLANTYNE JEBB (1876–1928): Champion of children's welfare and rights. Co-founder of the Fight the Famine Council 1918 and Save the Children 1919; founder of the Save the Children International Union 1920; author of the Declaration of Children's Rights 1922, as endorsed by the League of Nations 1924.

EGLANTYNE LOUISA JEBB (TYE) (1845–1925): Eglantyne's inspirational mother, and founder of the Home Arts and Industries Association.

EMILY JEBB (AUNT NONY) (1838–1897): Arthur Jebb's older sister. Married James Gilmore, maths master at Marlborough College, Wiltshire.

EMILY JEBB (EM), see Emily Ussher.

(ARTHUR) GAMUL JEBB (1879–1896): Eglantyne's younger brother, died while at boarding school aged just sixteen.

GERALDINE EMMA MAY JEBB (GEM JEBB) (1886–1959): Eglantyne's favourite cousin, daughter of Tye's younger brother Heneage. Eglantyne took on the history and literature education of Gem and her younger sister Eglantyne Mary Jebb in 1903. Gem became Principal of Bedford College, and Eglantyne Mary the Principal of the Froebel Institute.

LOUISA JEBB (AUNT BUN) (1841–1925): Arthur's younger sister, and Eglantyne's more radical aunt. A strident, agnostic Liberal, Bun was a firm supporter of women's rights and franchise, and inspired and supported many of the Jebb children's early dreams and activities.

LOUISA JEBB (LILL), see Louisa Wilkins.

SIR RICHARD CLAVERHOUSE JEBB (1841–1905): Tye's elder brother. One of the elite Cambridge 'Apostles', appointed Chair of Greek in 1889, and gained international respect as the leading Greek scholar of his day. Elected

Conservative MP for the University in 1891, a post retained through three elections, which he used to support women's higher education and suffrage. Received his Knighthood in 1900.

RICHARD JEBB (DICK) (1874–1953): Eglantyne's elder brother. An authority on Empire and Colonial Nationalism, publishing several influential books and a column in the *Morning Post*. Withdrew from public life when defeated as a Reform candidate in the 1910 General Election. His grandson, Lionel Jebb, continues to live at The Lyth with his wife Corinna.

TYE JEBB, see Eglantyne Louisa Jebb.

FRIEDA JONES: Fictional heroine of Eglantyne's only completed social novel, *The Ring Fence*, started around 1908. Frieda's experience of settlement work, love of riding, guilty enjoyment of socialising, and passionate support for farming co-operatives and social justice in general, was based on Eglantyne.

FLORENCE ADA KEYNES (1861–1958): Daughter of the Reverend John Brown of Bunyan's Chapel, she married the Cambridge economist John Neville Keynes, and had three children, John Maynard, Margaret and Geoffrey. A leading Cambridge social worker, both as a Poor Law Guardian and with the Charities Organisation Society, she provided Eglantyne with her first great social projects: producing a register of Cambridge charities, and running a pioneering boys' employment registry. Later the first female Councillor of Cambridge Borough Council, and its Mayor in 1932.

JOHN MAYNARD KEYNES (1883–1946): Margaret's elder brother, pioneering economist and British Deputy Chancellor representing Britain at the Paris peace talks. Having supported the movement towards a negotiated peace, Keynes proposed lifting the post-war economic blockade and providing loans for European economic reconstruction. He lent his support to the Fight the Famine Council among other organisations, and his 1919 *The Economic Consequences of the Peace* became the classic criticism of the European peace treaty.

MARGARET NEVILLE KEYNES, see Margaret Hill.

HENRIETTA LESLIE: Suffragette and journalist with the militant anti-war paper the *Daily Herald*. Translator for 'Notes from the Foreign Press' during the First World War, she became Save the Children's first community fundraising co-ordinator.

WILLIAM ANDREW MACKENZIE (1870–1942): Artist, journalist, writer of detective stories, the Pope's representative on the British Save the Children Council, and the Save the Children International Union's Treasurer, and Secretary General 1920–1939. He became Eglantyne's great friend, staunchest professional ally, and the executor of her will.

MARY PALEY MARSHALL (1850–1944): Social economist and lecturer, married to the leading economist Alfred Marshall, her former tutor at Newnham College, Cambridge. A friend of Florence Keynes to whom she introduced Eglantyne in 1902.

GEORGE MEWES: *Daily Mirror* cameraman who filmed the Russian famine and Save the Children's feeding centres in 1921. The pioneering footage was shown at fundraising events and in cinemas across Britain as part of the charitable sector's first comprehensive multi-media marketing campaign.

DR HECTOR MUNRO (1870–1949): Founder of the Munro Motor Ambulance Corps attached to the Belgian army in 1914, afterwards joining the Army Medical Corps. Awarded three war medals. Surgeon, consultant in psychotherapy and pioneer of 'nature-cure' methods in medicine, socialist and supporter of women's rights. Returning to his Harley Street clinic after the war, he counted George Bernard Shaw and G.K. Chesterton among his paying patients, as well as running free evening clinics.

GILBERT MURRAY (1866–1957): Classical scholar, friend of C.K. Ogden, and supporter of the 'Notes from the Foreign Press' during the First World War. Member of the Fight the Famine Council, and Save the Children association. He played a key role helping to found Oxfam after the Second World War.

FRIDTJOF NANSEN (1861–1930): Norwegian Arctic explorer and scientific researcher; Ambassador to the UK 1906–1908; High Commissioner for the Repatriation of Russian Refugees, lending his name to the 'Nansen passport'; League of Nations High Commissioner for Famine Relief in Russia 1921–1923. Received the Nobel Peace Prize in 1922.

C.K. OGDEN (1889–1957): Linguist, philosopher, writer. Before the First World War Charles Kay Ogden was a second-hand bookseller and editor of the intellectual university weekly, the *Cambridge Magazine*, in which he published Dorothy's 'Notes from the Foreign Press' from October 1915 until the Armistice.

SIR CHARLES ALFRED CRIPPS, LORD PARMOOR (1852–1941): Conservative, then Labour, MP; President of the Fight the Famine Council in 1919; later an influential supporter of the League of Nations and the international Save the Children movement. He married Marian Ellis in July 1919.

MARIAN CRIPPS, LADY PARMOOR, née ELLIS (1878– 1952): Philanthropist and political activist. Leading member of the Society of Friends; President of the Women's International League for Peace and Freedom. Marian joined Eglantyne to serve as the two Honorary Secretaries of the Fight the Famine Council in 1918. She married Lord Parmoor in July 1919.

EMMELINE PETHICK-LAWRENCE (1867–1954): Campaigner for women's suffrage and peace, initially with the Women's Social and Political Union, and later with the Women's International League. Emmeline was sympathetic to Save the Children, but doubted significant funds could be raised.

COLONEL HENRY LIONEL PILKINGTON (*c.*1857–1914): Decorated Boer War army officer who met Eglantyne when he became Secretary of the Agricultural Organisation Society in 1914.

JAMES RAMSAY MACDONALD (1886–1937): British politician and twice Prime Minister in 1924 and 1931. He supported the 'Notes from the Foreign Press' during the First World War, became a member of the Fight the Famine Council in 1918, and firm supporter of Save the Children thereafter. In 1924 he supported the League of Nations' endorsement of The Declaration of the Rights of the Child.

GWEN RAVERAT, née DARWIN (1885–1957): English wood engraver and author. Charles Darwin's grand-daughter, and Eglantyne's distant cousin through the marriage of her aunt Caroline Slemmer to Eglantyne's uncle, Richard Claverhouse Jebb. Gwen and Eglantyne were Cambridge friends for some years, Gwen producing the rent map for Eglantyne's social survey of the city in 1906. Married the French artist Jacques Raverat in 1911.

MAUDE ROYDEN (1876–1956): Suffragist and Christian pacifist until the Second World War. A contemporary of Eglantyne's at Oxford, Maude supported the settlement movement, and became an active campaigner for peace, aid, reconstruction and women's rights, through the Union of Democratic Control; the Women's International League for Peace and Freedom – of which she became founding Vice President in 1915; the Fight the Famine Council; and Save the Children.

EVELYN SHARP (1869–1955): Author, journalist and suffragist. Refused a passport to attend the 1915 conference of the International Committee of Women for Permanent Peace, but covered Eglantyne's 1919 trial and became a committed supporter of Save the Children.

CHARLOTTE TOYNBEE (1840–1931): Oxford social worker, and widow of Arnold Toynbee, the economics historian whose commitment to breaking down class barriers inspired the settlement movement. Devoted to the welfare of children in National Schools, Charlotte encouraged Eglantyne's ambitions to teach, and they remained good friends thereafter.

EMILY USSHER, née JEBB (EM) (1872–1935): Eglantyne's eldest sister who moved to Ireland on marrying Beverly Ussher. Em wrote a number of books including a popular novel about the fight for Irish independence published in 1921. Her son, Percy, became the respected author and critic Arland Ussher.

LORD WEARDALE (1847–1923): Liberal politician, pacifist, philanthropist and the first Chair of the British Save the Children Fund 1919–1923.

LOUISA WILKINS (LILL) née JEBB (1873–1929): Eglantyne's elder sister. Governor of the Agricultural Organisation Society, and founder of what became the Women's Land Army, for which she received an OBE. She turned down the offer to become Director of the women's branch of the Board of Agriculture. Having separated from her husband, Roland Wilkins, she lived with her two daughters until she died of cancer, a few months after Eglantyne, in early 1929.

ELIZABETH WORDSWORTH (1840–1932): Founding Principal of Lady Margaret Hall, Oxford, which Eglantyne attended 1895–1898. A great niece of the romantic poet William Wordsworth, her own niece, Ruth, became one of Eglantyne's lifelong friends.

RUTH WORDSWORTH: One of Eglantyne's closest college friends, Ruth stayed in regular contact with Eglantyne throughout her life.

Chapter 1

Imagining Eglantyne,
2009–1876

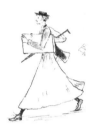

The world is not ungenerous,
but unimaginative and very busy.

Eglantyne Jebb, 1920

'To succeed in life, we must give life,' Eglantyne Jebb wrote as she searched for the way to give her life meaning. But Eglantyne did not 'give life' in the literal sense by becoming a mother. Despite social expectations she never married and she was not fond of children, the 'little wretches' as she called them, 'the Dreadful Idea of closer acquaintance never entered my head'. Eglantyne chose to give her life to the pursuit of children's welfare and human rights from a strategic distance. In doing so she helped to save the lives of millions of children left starving in Europe and Russia after the First World War. She also permanently changed the way the world considers and acts towards children. Her legacy, found both in the work of Save the Children, the world's largest independent

Self-portrait of Eglantyne losing important papers from her folder, Cambridge, c.1906

international children's development agency, and the recognition of children's rights as enshrined in the United Nations Convention on the Rights of the Child, now helps to protect the lives and support the life chances of millions of children around the world. This is giving life on a big scale, and yet despite helping to shape the modern world so dramatically through the lives of our children and the relationships between our generations, Eglantyne is all but forgotten today.

The biographer also gives life indirectly, if in a much more modest way. I first came across Eglantyne when working as a struggling corporate-fundraiser for Save the Children. The difficulty with raising funds was not with the charity's UK and international programmes, which being both innovative and effective screamed out for support. The problem was that so many people had stopped listening. The proliferation of children's charities and international development agencies repeatedly approaching the same donors meant that the concept of 'giving fatigue' was itself getting rather tired. Feeling somewhat brow-beaten after a few unsuccessful weeks of proposal writing I found my faith in human nature restored by a reassuring line that Eglantyne had written eighty years earlier: 'the world is not ungenerous, but unimaginative and very busy'. That's it, exactly. Her words had a startling immediacy for me, and soon an uncanny ability to make even the most recalcitrant potential donors reconsider their priorities and spare a moment to be generous. Eglantyne's genius was to catch people's imagination, enabling them both to empathise with the human issue, and believe that they could contribute personally to a meaningful solution. She was, in short, inspirational. It was therefore surprising how absent she now seemed to be from the organisation aside from a paragraph on the website; a meeting room name; one photo on an office wall; an archive fact sheet; and her Smith Corona Portable typewriter, 'such a bad one' she had once moaned, now permanently parked in the archive.

The photograph must have been a Save the Children publicity shot; it fits the bill so perfectly. Eglantyne looks sober and handsome, if slightly uncomfortable, sitting posed at her desk. Except for a few way-ward strands, her white hair is pulled back and pinned up, her lace collar sits softly over her smart dark jacket, and she gazes calmly down at her work, pen in hand. It must have been a wet morning; the shadow of rain is clearly cast on to the window-shutters and the light streaming in is diffused, lending a softness to the image which emphasises the femininity of this dignified campaigner for children's welfare. Despite her concern for children's rights, there is no touch of the suffragettes here. This photo hung above my manager's desk: two admirable women sitting behind dignified piles of papers. My manager also epitomised the consummate feminine professional; a wonderful fundraiser, she was utterly organised, appropriately witty and marvellously persuasive with the great and the good. Most of us thought she was pretty much perfect, if anything perhaps slightly too perfect. Was she a modern reflection of this feminine, dedicated Eglantyne?

Inevitably a degree of distortion takes place when a single photograph comes to represent a whole life, a whole person, so it was good to see the pleasingly eccentric fact sheet, 'Thirty-four things you didn't know about Eglantyne Jebb', compiled by Save the Children's archivist. Like all good lists this one demonstrated a certain eccentricity in its composition as well as in its contents. Eglantyne, I learned, was 'extremely warlike' when a child, and as an adult often forgot where she was going and left her luggage behind on trains. She was a 'shy furtive beauty' who loved rock-climbing and dancing, wrote bad romantic novels, endured failed romantic hopes, and was not, at least at first, that great a fundraiser. Hurray: a flawed heroine after all. I began to feel a growing sense of empathy, affection and curiosity.

Later I found another image of Eglantyne to stick above my own desk. It is a self-portrait in pen and ink, a small scratchy picture that she once sketched on the edge of a letter to a friend. Eglantyne here is a woman in motion, head up, eyes forward, striding down a street. Two feet in sensible shoes, although with trailing laces, appear at either end of her long plain skirt, pulling it into a taut triangle as she powers ahead. Her hair is still up, but here pinned under a flat black Edwardian hat, a bit new woman, nothing too fashionable but perfectly acceptable. A long thin umbrella is tucked under her long thin arm along with a huge sheath of papers from which several sheets fly loose to drift unnoticed in her wake. It is not well drawn, but the better for that; it is Eglantyne knowingly, happily, imperfect. It is tempting to take this self-portrait as the real picture, but of course the truth is that there is not a single picture of anyone. Almost certainly, the more an image appeals to, or reflects, the observer, the less likely it is to represent the whole contradicting set of human truths that makes people so intriguing.

In 2001, showing remarkably less dedication to the cause than Eglantyne, who never had children, I stopped working to have a baby; now seemed a good time to idly find out more about this perfect–imperfect woman. Just two years after Eglantyne's death her younger sister Dorothy co-authored the first biographical sketch of Eglantyne in her history of the early years of Save the Children. The book was called *The White Flame* after the nickname Eglantyne earned from admiring colleagues and supporters for her intense passion for her work towards the end of her life, and the quote on the title page read: 'Her greatness was the greatness of the spirit.'[1] All in it is a short and not impersonal portrait. A few other personal memoirs, some profiles in obscure anthologies as a Shropshire History Maker or a contender for canonisation, and a respectful biography, the wonderfully titled *Rebel Daughter of a Country House*, written by an aid worker who knew the Jebb family, soon followed.[2] Eglantyne has since made a good press hook for several Save the Children anniversaries and, in some ways a thoroughly modern woman, she now has an online *Oxford Dictionary of National Biography* entry and her own page on Wikipedia.

A digest of these various biographical sources provides a useful chronology, presenting Eglantyne's life as short but full of endeavour and achievement. Fiercely intelligent and passionate about her social mission, Eglantyne experimented bravely with career and voluntary work. Defying the law and often the more conservative ideas of her own colleagues and supporters she evolved the temporary Save the Children grant-giving 'Fund' into a permanent and pioneering development agency. Full of charm and charisma she won over the Pope and the miners, the British aristocracy and the Bolshevik government, the prosecution at her trial for distributing information not cleared by government censors, and the fledgling League of Nations in Geneva. Publicly she was a huge success; her achievement in promoting both Save the Children and the applied concept of children's universal human rights is undeniable. But personally the story is less clear. A compulsive writer, she failed to publish any of her novels and sometimes seemed to blur the distinction between reality and fantasy. Like all female students of that era she was not allowed to graduate, and she lasted less than a year in both of her paid jobs. She was repeatedly disappointed in love, quickly lost her health and more than once seemed to lose her mental grip.

This suggests some intriguing questions: What motivated Eglantyne? An intelligent and strikingly beautiful woman, why had she never married? Did she want children of her own, and was the fact that she was never a mother relevant to her passion for her cause? Or was her interest in children impersonal, and if so why? Were her regular illnesses, her emotional highs and lows, and the vivid imagination that was vital to her visionary work, in any way linked? And why did she often seem to wear such dour clothes? Who was this inspirational spinster in a brown cardigan and what, exactly, was going on in her head? The various published 'lives' of Eglantyne tend to focus on what she did rather than who she was, her 'doing' rather than her 'being'. When her being was considered she was often presented, dead unmarried and childless at the age of just fifty-two, as having martyred herself for her cause. 'She offered herself up as a sacrifice for her ideals,' Ramsay MacDonald, the then British Prime Minister, eulogised in a speech to mark Save the Children's tenth anniversary. Even her obituaries carried this theme, presenting

Eglantyne as a 'saint', 'humanity's conscience', and as having 'lived on a different plane from ordinary mortals'. But the trailing laces and bad novels suggest she lived on the just the same plane as the rest of us. I suddenly wanted to release Eglantyne from the 'tyranny of achievement'.

But just as I gained the time to find out more about Eglantyne by leaving work, I began to lose my sense of empathy by having a baby. Worse, I began to feel the antithesis of Eglantyne, who never had children and dedicated her life to the cause. This was irritating. Many modern biographers confess to a natural sense of connection with their subject. I compared my life to Eglantyne's and found some happy similarities; we were both well educated and middle class, and not at first particularly gifted fundraisers. On the flip-side Eglantyne was an independent single woman who never had children, seemed to suffer from some kind of bipolar disorder, dabbled with spiritualism, became an opportunist human rights monitor and developed an international social movement of global significance. I was a stressed new mum. On the face of it there was not much to work on. However the seeming contradictions in Eglantyne's life did strike a chord: here was a not obviously maternal woman giving up her freedom to devote herself to promoting children's welfare. Ironically I was sneaking away from childcare to gain the time to work on my own project. I was almost an anti-Eglantyne, a sort of Ms Hyde to her Dr Jebb. I took some comfort in the romantic biographer Richard Holmes' belief that 'the true biographical process begins precisely at the moment … when this naïve form of love and identification breaks down. The moment of personal disillusionment is the moment of impersonal, objective recreation.'

Holmes, like many other respected biographers, deliberately set out to find his subjects, in his case first retracing the steps of Robert Louis Stevenson through southern France in 'an act of deliberate psychological trespass'. I decided that it was time to go out and find Eglantyne.

Chapter 2

Meeting the Family, 1876–1894

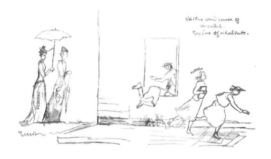

They gravely sit on their old rickety chairs,
and talk of poetry, articles, letters, affairs.

Eglantyne Jebb, 1888

Visiting Eglantyne's Shropshire home, the rather romantic Lyth, 'always seemed like walking into a novel' a guest once commented in the 1880s, 'such interesting people staying there and such interesting things going on'. Eglantyne's Aunt Carrie agreed. 'None of the places in novels are near the station, and no more was ours,' she wrote on first visiting The Lyth. 'We drove for a mile through the most beautiful country I have seen in England, full of lakes with distant hills, and then up a grand avenue of trees, until we came out on a lawn drive, and so to the front door.' Little had changed when I arrived over a hundred years later. Eglantyne's great nephew, Lionel Jebb, kindly met me at Oswestry station, dressed in

'Visitors round corner of verandah. Exodus of inhabitants.' The Jebb children escape from The Lyth when dull visitors call, c.1895

his shooting outfit, dogs barking at his heels, and drove us all back the beautiful mile to Ellesmere and The Lyth. The house was built in the colonial villa style by a West Indian planter in the early 1800s and bought by Eglantyne's paternal great grandfather, a Salopian landowner, in 1838.[1] A spacious two storeys, The Lyth's luxurious dimensions are accentuated by long verandas front and back, and a stretch of tall windows opening to the ground that lead out to landscaped gardens. The verandas were 'festooned by clematis and every rose then blowing', Eglantyne's eldest sister Em later wrote nostalgically about her childhood home, and 'the green lawns ... merge with sunk fences into park-like timbered field'. The clematis and rose were over when I arrived, but pots of geraniums, tiger lilies and tall agapanthus decorated the verandas, and immaculate lawns still led down to the park beyond where sheep were grazing in the late morning haze. It was an idyllic setting for an Edwardian childhood, that short moment when upper-class girls were free to roam house and gardens with their brothers but rarely allowed out to school.

As Lionel showed me round the house, half home, half fire-hazard, I began to feel like a fictional biographer in a post-modern satire. Assorted owls, hawks and herons observed our progress from glass cases, venerable ancestors peered down from gilt-frames, and a poster-sized photograph in the downstairs loo showed Lionel leaning dangerously into a hedge in 1830s costume, dressed for a party as the first Jebb to live at The Lyth. We eventually arrived, through lofty outer and inner halls, at the magnificent morning room where Lionel had stacked about twenty large boxes containing the family archive, or at least that part of it pertaining to Eglantyne. Here, surrounded by extraordinary hand-block-printed French wallpaper depicting rather frolicking scenes of 'airily clad virgins and noble Romans in helmets' – a design which would later reappear on the bedroom walls of one of Eglantyne's fictional heroines – I set to work poring over great bundles of letters, diaries and journals, photographs and press-clippings.

Born in 1876, Eglantyne grew up in an active and intellectual household. As a child she created her special place among her five siblings as the family storyteller, otherwise joining in the general melee as they melted lead soldiers to make bullets, milked cows to make cheese, collected butterflies, flew kites, read Scott and rode horses. Drawings by the Jebb children showed them piling out of the dining-room on to the veranda when tedious visitors called, diaries and letters had them staging battles in the gardens and passing the hours on wet afternoons writing poems about illustrious and romantic ancestors. 'You should see me,' Eglantyne wrote to a friend, 'sitting on a table on account of the mice, surrounded by a pile of books and all the ghosts clanking around.'

Eglantyne's father, Arthur Jebb, whom she characterised as 'a barrister, distressed landlord and father, Liberal-Unionist and grand old Tory', and her mother, Tye, founder of the 'Home Arts and Industries Association', were Anglican Conservatives who instilled a strong social conscience and commitment to public service in their children. The son of a wealthy landowner and grandson of the Mayor of Oswestry, Oxford-educated Arthur was an influential member of the Shropshire gentry. But he was also a gentle and some-what self-effacing intellectual; 'sensitive as a woman', his eldest daughter once commented.[2] Arthur's grandmother had been a pupil of the great portrait painter George Romney and his mother had inherited her artistic, poetic and deeply religious sensitivities. Although she died young his mother had a great influence on Arthur, who grew up with a love of literature and culture; interests that did not always sit easily with his position of country squire. As a young man Arthur found himself and his two sisters, Nony and Bun, the subjects of some gentle satire in the popular novel *Gracechurch* by John Ayscough.[3] 'Melancholy Launcelot', as Arthur was monikered, 'had been the old man's pride, and was now his special irritation. He did not care much for radical politics – only just enough to prevent his being popular with the Tory squires around and their sons: nor was he horsey, or doggy.' It was a sufficiently accurate picture to cause some mild local embarrassment, but Arthur accepted it gracefully enough for a copy of *Gracechurch* to find its way into the library at The Lyth.

Arthur's strong sense of family connection to Shropshire, and to Wales where he also owned farms, stimulated a life-long interest in local history, place names and folklore, and his traditional ideas about social responsibility focused him on the livelihoods of his tenants and the welfare of the local community more widely. He was a sympathetic landlord who refused to raise rents in bad years, and often when he went rent collecting in Wales he would come back with plenty of game from his shoots, but rhymes of his own in place of the rents he was due. Given that 'good hearts' was a term for empty pockets, one such verse ran rather sweetly:

'Silver and gold we are not rich in'
Said Mary dancing in the kitchen,
'But be it always understood,
In spite of all, our hearts are good.'

Arthur's family were Low Church Anglicans, and Arthur chose to pursue an active but secular role in the Shropshire community, serving as a government schools inspector among other civic positions, as well as helping to found the Ellesmere Literary and Debating Society, which was mainly a political forum discussing everything from state socialism to the Liquor Tariff. The children were encouraged to accompany their father to these meetings, where they would hear both Arthur and his more radical younger sister Bun speaking to local people of all classes, although the children themselves had strict instructions only to open their mouths if debate showed signs of flagging. Arthur was also a barrister, and he acted as a conscientious volunteer advocate helping to resolve disputes and grievances, and as a general champion of local lost causes. He once appealed as far as the Home Secretary to secure the release of three local boys imprisoned for stealing a fishing-net from the lake at Ellesmere. Told by the local magistrate that 'property had its rights', Arthur's delight at securing the release of the boys made a strong impression on his own children. Whether by choice or duty these many activities comfortably filled Arthur's days, enabling him to happily plan the books he would write if only someone had the 'kindness to lock him up in gaol', without his ever actually having to set to work on them.[4]

In 1871 Arthur married Eglantyne Louisa Jebb, his distant cousin from an Anglo-Irish branch of the family, and brought her back from beautiful Killiney Bay to live at The Lyth. Arthur and Tye, as his young wife was affectionately known, were well matched in both interests and disposition. Tye's father was a QC of the Irish bench, her grandfather had been a prominent judge, and she counted Sir Joshua Jebb, reformer of convict prisons; John Jebb, Bishop of Limerick and pioneer of the Oxford Movement; and Sir Richard Jebb, court doctor to George III, among her many illustrious ancestors. It was a well-connected, intellectual and affectionate family, although not overly prosperous. They kept a small library, printing press, amateur carpentry-shop, pony, maid and two romantic maiden aunts who had once scorned and been scorned in a series of marriage proposals – some of the few women that gain mention in the family records. Arthur first met Tye when as a fifteen-year-old she joined a family visit to The Lyth, a house that she romantically recorded seemed to be 'apparelled in celestial light'. Over the next ten years Tye blossomed into a pretty and accomplished young lady, taking art classes and dabbling in poetry, while her three brothers, Richard, the oldest and closest to his sister, and the younger twins, Heneage and Bob, mostly excelled at school and college. Warm-hearted, attractive and entertaining company, Tye soon earned the nickname the 'Rose of Killarney' and was quite in demand, but she turned down several suitors and waved aside the whole idea of romance by claiming she would only be persuaded to marry for the chance to change her ugly last name. Perhaps she was already teasing

Arthur Jebb with this sally, as aged twenty-five she accepted his proposal without demur. For his part Arthur was already devoted to his bride to be: 'I want nothing save to dwell on Tye in solitary corners of the earth,' he wrote to her, ostensibly to make suggestions for wedding presents.

With his country house inheritance and £3,000 a year, Arthur was a good catch for Tye, but theirs was also a deeply loving relationship in which traditional roles reflected their natural inclinations and helped to cement their partnership. 'I am domestic to the last degree,' Tye wrote home contentedly soon after her wedding, her happiness in turn reinforcing her belief in the natural order of gender relations. Tye was fascinated by the public debate that was taking place around women's roles and responsibilities. Under the mantle of social mothering, women from Mary Carpenter, who founded the Ragged School Movement in 1844, to Octavia Hill, who helped set up the Charities Organisation Society in 1869, were pushing the boundaries of women's public authority on the basis of their 'natural' maternal competencies and their ability to extend the values of care, nurturance and morality from the private family to society as a whole. But there was also a backlash to this development, vigorously led by Britain's first professional female journalist, Eliza Lynn Linton. Without any irony Linton condemned women's deviation from the traditional, domestic ideal in a series of articles and pamphlets criticising progressive middle-class women and those she called 'Modern Mothers'. Soon Tye was confidently joining in this debate, arguing in a temperance journal that a 'woman's right ... to live a life worth living, demands that she shall live as a help "meet" to man, using her special faculties and endowments to perform that part of the world's work as is fitted to woman rather than man'. For Tye this began with family.

Tye and Arthur produced a child a year over the next three years. Emily arrived promptly in February 1872, quickly followed the next summer by Louisa, known as Lill. Both girls' names were conveniently prominent on both sides of the family. 'Richard Jebb' conveniently prominent on both sides of the family. 'Richard Jebb' was such a common family name that he appears in the family histories as though a single character reincarnated in different guises through several centuries, which made naming Dick, who arrived in the autumn of 1874, equally easy. Tye 'seems not a bit the worse', Arthur wrote to his sister Nony after Dick's birth, 'quite the reverse – only her eyes a little more liquid than usual, and a softly whispered "Aren't you pleased, husband?"' No children the next year, and then the last three arrived, all also taking traditional family names, starting with Eglantyne, born on an exceptionally cold day on 25 August 1876. Eglantyne was to be in a rather isolated position caught in age between the three elder ones, and after a short gap, two little ones; (Arthur) Gamul born in 1879, and Dorothy in 1881, who completed the set. Eglantyne and Gamul were unusual names even in the 1880s, but both were traditional among the Jebbs. Eglantyne was of course Tye's name, and recurs up the Irish Jebb family tree. It is also the name of the fragrant but prickly briar rose, and it proved so appropriate for this pretty new daughter, with her English rose complexion, golden-red hair, sky-blue eyes and slightly wild and unruly behaviour, that Eglantyne's friends were often later struck by its aptness when they made the transition from knowing her formally as Miss Jebb to affectionately as Dear Eglantyne.[5] Gamul was an ancestral surname in the family, most famous for Sir Francis Gamul, who, family myth recorded, stood beside King Charles I watching defeat at Chester. The King's beautifully embroidered white leather gloves were later given to Sir Francis, and still lie in a glass-topped cabinet in The Lyth morning room, among other heirlooms with similarly romantic providence. This evidence of family heritage, both preserved under glass and living in their own names, inspired rather than intimidated the children. At The Lyth, Em later wrote, 'the past lay very near the present and … the future was ours for the making'.

Both Tye and Arthur were devoted parents, and Arthur's letters to his wife were filled with quotes from Wordsworth and George

Eliot pronouncing on the joys of parenthood beside which he scrawled with proud complicity, 'easy things to understand, precious'. Arthur understood his parental role as to inculcate a sense of self-respect and social responsibility within his six children, and he brought them up to understand that 'of those who lived in beautiful places much was required'. But he was also an affectionate father, reading aloud to the children and listening with delight to their own stories. A keen lover of language and literature, he contributed many romantic poems about lost love and fair ladies on horseback, mostly written tongue-in-cheek, to their evening recitals, and when away from home he always wrote to the children as well as to Tye, thanking them for their own letters which he found 'sweeter than sugar, and more full of matter than walnuts'. Even Arthur's tickings-off would sometimes be delivered in rhyme to the children, often causing greater remorse than a more traditional dressing down would have achieved, such as when Gamul lost his elder brother's volunteer equipment:

Can I forget that bayonet
Lost in its sheath upon the heath,
Which my father
Angry rather,
Paid in account, a huge amount!

Arthur greatly encouraged his children's love for literature and books of all sorts. The Lyth had a vast library which was ceremonially dusted on the veranda every spring, but many of the titles were obscure theology and law texts which the children rather impiously suspected their grandfather had ordered by the foot, as 'appropriate for a gentleman's library'. Despite the best efforts of an old Scottish nurse with an ingrained suspicion of literature, who would whisk any book, however innocent, away from her wards with the exclamation 'drop them lies', it was impossible not to grow up reading at The Lyth. Jane Austen, Charlotte Yonge and Charles Dickens all competed with Scott's novels and poems for the children's affections. 'Books, books, books! No single room without them,' Em recalled, and although the library only really appealed to Eglantyne, all the children absorbed a love of literature and later became published authors in their own fields.

Eglantyne was the main family scribbler, and the one whom everyone else suspected would become the great poet. Like many imaginative children she would often escape from the happy but hectic chaos of her large family into her own dreams. Tye would sometimes scold her for retreating into her own world too much, prompting Arthur to nickname her 'Scatter-brained Eglantyne':

Moving about in worlds unknown,
Entirely ignorant of her own.

Many of Eglantyne's daydreams made it on to paper as stories and poems. 'They were a family of sisters,' one narrative begins in rather Austen-like tone, 'all blessed with long noses, large eyes and opinions.'[6] However most of Eglantyne's tales were of chivalry, inspired by family anecdotes and her beloved Walter Scott. The heroines in these stories of self-sacrifice, brave knights and lonely castles all had names like Elizabeth Redspot, not only conveying romantic status but clearly marking them as incarnations of herself by reference to her own flaming auburn hair. Always sensitive to suggestions of her own self-importance however, she would quickly counter any teasing by earnestly declaring, 'my brother says I think myself a saint, but it isn't true'.

Age nine, having heard of her grandfather's work establishing the local Volunteers and learnt Tennyson's 'The Charge of the Light Brigade' by heart in the schoolroom, Eglantyne became possessed with a passion for soldiering. She now invested the whole family with military titles and duties to match. Hours were spent planting flags near the potting sheds, waging battles in the gardens – often attacking the long-suffering gardener and the boot-boy – and preparing elaborate maps of the world they were to conquer, all with constitutions drawn up, lists of lands to be won and rights to be defended. The children's tall and stately French–Alsatian governess, Heddie Kastler, herself seething with the invasion and abuse of Alsace-Lorraine by Germany after the 1870 war, became Eglantyne's appointed 'Queen of Blueland', and Eglantyne served as one of her Dukes. Heddie probably helped to fuel some of Eglantyne's ardour for all things military when she spoke to her wards about the cruel Prussian occupation of her country, giving them their first insight into the sufferings of minorities. 'I'd like to be a war correspondent and watch the battle from the hilltop,' Eglantyne wrote, but throughout her life verse came more easily to Eglantyne than prose. Her childhood image of a land of promise marked with 'flags unfurl'd' was a constant metaphor in her poems, reflected even in her 'land of a hundred flags', written forty years later about her hopes for a peaceful world in the last years of her life.[7]

Sometimes, to entertain Gamul and Dorothy, Eglantyne also invented more childlike stories like 'The Mischief Pot' that ran for several episodes in the family magazine, *The Briarland Recorder*. The mischief pot was a sort of Pandora's Box that unleashed bad behaviour on the 'goody little girls and boys' of the world, both exonerating naughty children from responsibility for their actions and playing with Eglantyne's not entirely uncomfortable feeling that imagination was somehow associated with naughtiness:

> 'At last! At last!' Feebly murmured the old magician, scratching his head with delight over a musty volume, repeating nervously and slowly: 'To make this mixture called Mischief, take 1 Tablespoon of naughtiness, 16 doses of idleness and 1½ drops of imagination (wicked) …'

Having drunk tea laced with this brew, children, Eglantyne revealed gleefully, 'were late for school, tore their clothes, spilt the ink, spoilt their books, got their feet wet with running through puddles …

climbed, broke hedges and literally all of a sudden, as it seems, became a terrible nuisance to their parents'. It was clearly a familiar picture of childhood mayhem. *The Briarland Recorder* produced its first issue in 1889 from a disused bedroom. Eglantyne described the preliminary meeting in verse:

Though the meeting house is dingy and full of dust,
And the audience are rude for with laughter they bust,
And the Editor Red on his fingers has ink
And Young often giggles and does not often think
And though the apartment ill comfort does afford,
Long may the Recorder live to record.
As they gravely sit on their old rickety chairs,
And talk of poetry, articles, letters, affairs,
Hurrah for the Pen, the writer's good sword!
So long may the Recorder live to record.

The 'Editor Red', elsewhere listed as R.E.D. Hare, was of course a thirteen-year-old Eglantyne, and Young was Dorothy, now eight. Over the next three years Eglantyne contributed numerous articles, poems and pen-and-ink sketches to the magazine, mostly poking fun at the family, while Gamul wrote on natural history, and everyone else submitted whatever they were coerced to produce, such as poems or even obituaries for the hens, pigs and geese who died 'from indigestion, deeply lamented', on the farm.

The three youngest children were particularly close, enjoying a childhood almost too good to be true. Gamul and Dorothy had dark brown hair and eyes 'like ripe chestnuts', while Eglantyne's eyes were a bright speedwell blue, and were often set off by the regular flush in her cheeks as well as the rich colour of her hair. When she was not riding her pony, Eglantyne would invent and lead many of the younger children's games. Em remembered that 'every tree in our gardens became a castle, every black peaty pool the haunt of

Grendel … every dark, mysterious wood became some haunt of witch or gnome or knight'. Gamul and Dorothy were an eager audience, and Eglantyne entertained them from morning to night with creations of her tireless imagination until they became collectively known as the 'covey of partridges', huddled together, lapping up Eglantyne's wonderful, and often terrible, stories. 'Oh … don't kill all the little children!' Lill once heard Dorothy beg Eglantyne.

As she grew up however Eglantyne increasingly began to need some daily solitude. At fifteen she was still reading Scott, but romantic fiction was now supplemented by copies of journals like *Atlanta* and *The Strand Magazine*, sent by remote aunts, which Eglantyne would pounce on and drag up a yew tree to read in privacy in the gardens. Riding also gave her the solitude she craved, though sometimes she would also join a hunt, or race her older siblings as they chased each other through the narrow openings between the trees on Ellesmere common where it fringed the mere, dodging the low branches of larches surrounding the glade of a neighbour's park. 'I do like a gallop with a kick in the middle,' a seventeen-year-old Eglantyne wrote to Em.

She was less happy on her own in the schoolroom at home however, since by the time Eglantyne started lessons the elder three had nearly finished, and Gamul and Dorothy were still in the nursery. Tye's thoughts on education were firmly rooted in religious instruction, supported by traditional ideas about what constituted a young lady's accomplishments; primarily drawing. 'Very well attempted,' she started her damning faint praise of a watercolour self-portrait by a sixteen-year-old Eglantyne, 'and except that the hands and feet are too small – and the nose too long, there is little to find fault with.' French, German and the piano were overseen by the governess – the last a particularly painful subject for the children, all of whom had inherited their father's tone deafness. The rest of their education was left to their aunt Bun, who lived with them at The Lyth.

Unmarried, unconventional and rather masculine, Bun, as Arthur's younger sister was known, provided an alternative role model for the Jebb children, slightly more at odds with social norms. Bun could not be more different from her rather sensitive and conservative brother. True they were both intellectuals with strong moral principles and were never happier than when engaging in the debates of the day, but the positions they took must have made for interesting evenings at The Lyth. Politically Bun was an ardent Liberal. An early enthusiast for Darwin she was personally agnostic, although always respectful of others' religious beliefs. She was also an active advocate of women's rights, including greater access to higher education and female suffrage. She herself had been one of the pioneering students at Cambridge's new Newnham College for women in the 1870s, and was later encouraged to apply as Principal of Alexandra College in Dublin, although she was too honest to do so as she did not feel able to subscribe to the religious tenets the post demanded. The novelist John Ayscough described Bun as having 'handsome features of decisive cast, a clever, hard mouth, and alert, penetrating eyes of unrestrained capacity for seeing the weak points in things and people'. She was certainly strikingly handsome and had a commanding presence. Short wavy white hair framed her strong face, and she wore double-breasted jackets with a man's linen collar, and practical skirts cut unfashionably high above the ankle. The severity of this outfit was only sometimes relieved by a silver brooch representing a greyhound's head given by her father, as like all the Jebbs she loved to ride and hunt. Bun's appearance reflected her determined rationalism and independence of character; it was a defiance of the Victorian standards by which femininity was so much valued and emphasised. 'Man Jebb' was her affectionate nickname in the town.

Bun was in charge of The Lyth with its twelve long-serving staff and the working farm estate until Tye arrived, and she stayed on thereafter. Although opposites in many ways she and Tye quickly became close, each welcoming the support of the other. Bun's great practical abilities with anything from carpentry to metalwork would soon make her a great asset to Tye when her interest in art and design found a valuable outlet in social work. Until then Bun was very involved in the children, counting fingers and toes as the babies arrived and in many ways acting as a second mother to them as they grew. 'Those were wonderful days', Tye later wrote warmly to her sister-in-law, 'when we together mothered six, a happy dual arrangement for them and for myself, my dearest and best of pals.'

Tye and Bun made an excellent team. Naturally conservative, Tye felt responsible for promoting the traditional moral code and the children's Anglican religious training. Bun felt free to indulge her less conventional ideas on a good upbringing. In some ways this meant that she was stricter than Tye, especially with regard to the girls' attendance at lessons. But she also insisted on an education outside of the classroom, giving the children a healthy respect for independence along with new bicycles, and forever taking them to explore Roman ruins, castles and factories. She was, Em later recalled

> the companion of pranks, the inspirer of dreams … the instigator of many ideas and of most doings which led the highly individualised six of us into endless achievement and adventure. A disused back bedroom was her workshop, where she introduced those who had a wish to carpentry, wood and metal turning, glass cutting and glazing; and she taught us besides how to make things like boomerangs, kites, popguns, bows and arrows, toboggans … stilts, fishing-nets, and – supreme joy, because so dangerous – over her bedroom fire, to melt lead and cast bullets.

Bun's aim was to bring the children up with a healthy curiosity about the world and the confidence to trust their own judgements. When they were little this might mean taking them bathing in the mere in summer, or ice-skating in winter, and even taking Dick trespassing to an unsurpassed trout-fishing spot when he should have been in school; when they grew up it meant supporting their plans to go to college or travel the world, however unconventional or dangerous these ambitions might appear.

The six Jebb children had to rely very much on each other and their aunt for their entertainment because there were few young visitors to the rather cold lamp-lit house. In many ways, despite their maids and other luxuries, life at The Lyth was austere. The round skylight in the inner hall leaked whenever it rained, regularly sending the family running for hip-baths, milk pails and pudding bowls, the wind blew freely through loose windows, and the kitchen and attics were infested with rats which could be heard at all times of night and day. For the children, typical days would start by breaking the ice in their basins to wash, followed by prayers and breakfast at half seven before the schoolroom routine began. All the children preferred farm chores, such as feeding the hens, to work in the schoolroom. Once they were thirteen the girls, and any boys home from school, were promoted to late dinners in evening dress, but were still all in bed by ten.

Weekends held greater diversions when the elder children, including Eglantyne, would often ride to hounds with Arthur or go fishing with Bun. At thirteen Gamul had got the naturalist bug and when back from school he was never happier than when netting butterflies with his father, joining Bun's expeditions to a local gravel pit to search for fossils, or roping in Eglantyne to help make a pond for frogs and newts. Patiently assisted by Em who was a budding botanist and Lill who was interested in geology as well as everything related to the farm, he had soon set up a small natural history museum at The Lyth to display his finds. Dorothy, who idolised Gamul, trailed around behind him, quickly catching his love of all things natural. Soon she could emulate birdsong well enough to call birds to her, and she started bringing both them and field-mice back to The Lyth to study. 'Dorothy is a funny little thing,' Eglantyne wrote affectionately. 'She has brought seven mice from the fields and is keeping them under glass and she goes about with chickens in her pocket.' Two years later Gamul was classifying moths with visitors from geological expeditions, and in Eglantyne's view, both he and his little sister had become rather tediously 'monopolised by natural history'. Of more interest to Eglantyne were the local Shakespeare readings in the surrounding country houses, with minor parts allotted to the children. These were sometimes re-enacted at home where Eglantyne would often steal the show, once savouring the chance as Elizabeth I to box the ears of her big brother Dick, playing Essex. The family would also go to country house parties to dance quadrilles, lancers, waltzes and polkas, as well as the more gentle country-dances that everyone could join in. Eglantyne went to her first party in 1889 when she was thirteen, dancing almost all the dances until they left around midnight when she was magnificently sick out of the carriage window. Dancing and horse-riding remained her greatest pleasures for many years, as both gave her some physical freedom and a pleasing sense of spiritual harmony with the world around her. 'To dance', she later wrote, 'was to share … a joy like that of a disembodied life, the sense of effort gone, the pleasure of movement remaining … a sensation which was an emotion.'

In winter The Lyth could be freezing. In 1890 Arthur wrote that they were having 'an old fashioned Christmas with ice upon the water in our bedroom jugs, and snow upon the ground'. Christmas by then had been celebrated at The Lyth in a pretty much unbroken tradition for over half a century. A meal of beef, goose, plum pudding and mince pies was provided for the staff and their families in the servants' hall, followed by an evening of songs and dancing to a fiddle. At some point 'the family' would come in. Arthur would make a speech and the children handed out presents, mostly repaired toys and home-made clothes. Eglantyne, with her golden-red hair, would be dressed as a fairy-godmother on these occasions, but later told her sisters that she had always been embarrassed by the patronage. More fun were the Christmas plays put on in the servants' hall. Somehow Eglantyne always seemed to get the darker roles in these productions and, as always, she relished the opportunity to be legitimately subversive. In 1892 she was the witch in 'Jack the Giant Killer', complete with pointed hat, shawl and 'lots of clanking chains and bracelets', and she managed to reduce several children in the audience to tears when she told how the giant ate little boys. Finally bell-ringing served as the prelude to stockings next morning, crammed with presents from each to all, often including large boxes of brightly painted lead soldiers to inspire more military games on the nursery floor.

Eglantyne loved The Lyth because out of the schoolroom it meant freedom. But she had a melancholic impression of Shropshire whose views she liked best when 'there was no rain, nor wind, nor softly gleaming sun. But that sad grey which seemed to suit the fields.' Like her brothers and sisters, she preferred the wilder landscapes of Wales. Frequent holidays were spent at the family's rather cold Welsh stone farmhouse, the imposing Tydraw in Denbigshire, among what Eglantyne described as those 'blue hills beyond the green'. Tydraw means 'the home over there', and the farm provided an early Welsh holiday home where the family indulged in a romantic simple life, as demarcated by only the two maids and an 'absence of puddings' despite a larder well stocked with hares, rabbits, pheasants, grouse and partridge.

Many as they were, the children were not the sole focus on Tye's time and attention. Tye was a loving and involved mother, but she was not expected to care for the children alone, and a succession of nurses and governesses filed through The Lyth. Soon after Dorothy was born Tye developed a project of her own to give her life greater meaning. A few years after she had arrived at The Lyth she had come across a boy on the estate crying from weariness and frustration as he worked six days a week removing stones from the fields. This dreary task had been his occupation for the last few years and there was no prospect of change. Shocked by this waste of life, Tye determined to provide more opportunities for the estate cottagers. Inspired by the example of Charles Leland, who was reviving rural crafts in

Philadelphia, she quickly set up free wood carving workshops in the servants' hall, soon followed by basket-making, chair-caning, carpentry, mosaic-making and painting. The elder Jebb children joined in these activities, enjoying the creativity while they gained an insight into lives outside their privileged family and social circle, and witnessed a compassionate idea being organised into a movement of real social value.[8]

Tye's scheme rapidly spread into Wiltshire, Wales, and her home estates in Killiney. In 1885, showing some flair for organisation, she roped in Walter Besant, the celebrated English author and historian, as Honorary Treasurer, and the local dignitary Lord Brownlow of Ellesmere as Patron of her fledgling movement. She staged the first of what she now called 'The Home Arts and Industries Association' exhibitions at Brownlow's fashionable London address in Carlton House Terrace, where, she noted with understandable satisfaction, 'some pale-faced London boys' went round the stands, 'pointing out with pride what they themselves had done'. This is 'all your doing, dear Mrs Jebb', Besant told Tye that year, praise which she proudly recorded in her diary.

In effect Tye was an early social entrepreneur harnessing a profit-making opportunity to create social capital. Classes were open to all but her real focus was on the younger generation like the boy from the fields who eventually became a professional cabinet-maker.[9] Her rather maternal vision was for 'a network of women's work, brightened by women's faith and love and hope, which shall spread abroad until it embraces within its folds every child'. Above all she hoped that self-improvement would foster a better society; 'happier lives and lighter hearts, tidier children, cleaner cottages, and a better moral tone all round'. In this way the Home Arts was a mechanism for cultural philanthropy that not only helped to promote citizenship, employment and the arts among the deserving poor, it was a rewarding way for Tye to discharge her own social duty and stake her personal, feminine, claim to citizenship.

By 1887 Tye was energetically promoting the association in pamphlets, through the regional press and at conferences around the country. Three years later the 'Home Arts' had achieved a truly national reach, with nearly five hundred classes throughout the country, attracting support from celebrities like William Morris who sent a length of printed cloth for an exhibition in Bethnal Green, and the popular Victorian artist George Frederic Watts who praised the movement in *The Times*. Soon the association ran a permanent office and annual exhibitions in London's Royal Albert Hall which were attended by both Princess Victoria, the eldest daughter of the Queen, and Princess Alexandra, who started a project at Sandringham.

Tye now officially gave up her commitment to the association on the grounds of exhaustion. However she continued to organise free classes at Ellesmere and Tydraw, giving over her afternoons until the light failed – on principle she refused to teach by candlelight. Although Arthur brusquely dismissed minor colds and ailments, Tye had been brought up to be almost obsessively concerned about her and her family's health. The robust American widow Carrie Slemmer, who married Tye's elder brother Richard, often teased him about this family trait. 'Such nervous people about their healths I never saw,' Carrie wrote, 'they are certainly not a family of soldiers … In that family the mole-hills are so very high, one hardly knows what to believe when anyone is said to be ill.' Tye was just forty-two, and would live until she was eighty, but ten years of childbirth and the subsequent promotion of a national social movement had depleted her energy reserves and she preferred to spend the rest of her life out of the limelight, and indeed often on the sofa, in turn supporting and being supported by her high-achieving children. The Tye best remembered by Eglantyne and Dorothy was 'often ailing yet always tender, sympathetic, [and] boundlessly ambitious for her children'.

Eglantyne would later share both Tye's boundless ambition and her severe bouts of exhaustion. But above all she inherited her parents' keen sense of social justice and personal social responsibility. When she was just eight, although her world was still mostly confined to nursery and schoolroom, Eglantyne already had an uncomfortable sense of social inequality, causing her the somewhat mysterious experiences she called her 'happy pains': 'I don't know all my complaints, only one … a complaint which does for everything,' she told her eldest sister Em. 'The world is wrong.' As a teenager this early impression of injustice was confirmed by her sensitive observation of local society, from the resentful look in the eyes of a working woman forced into a hedge when Eglantyne passed riding, to the story of a local magnate who had water laid to the kennels for his dogs but had not bothered to extend the pipes a short way further to his cottages.

Soon Eglantyne was writing the first of several social novels, none of which were to make it into print and sadly few parts of which survive as manuscripts. *The Rebel* directly challenged social assumptions in a way that few young people in Eglantyne's privileged position would have noticed or questioned. Her eldest sister Em later wondered at what she called Eglantyne's 'precocious sympathies', but Dorothy had a similar, if somewhat less defined, feeling that things needed to change. 'I have an object in life,' she pronounced aged sixteen to Lill, 'let me see, I forget what it is now – but I have written it down,' and she fumbled amongst the papers in her pocket. 'Oh, what a bore – I wrote it in pencil and it's all rubbed out – I shall have to think it all out again.'

Growing up in an atmosphere of social service at The Lyth was the perfect incubation for an Edwardian female social pioneer, but it ended abruptly when Arthur Jebb suddenly died of pneumonia on a cold and foggy day in early December 1894 aged only fifty-five. Tye and the whole family were devastated. Speaking at an Ellesmere meeting that Arthur himself had been due to address, his college friend, the MP Stanley Leighton, pronounced that Arthur's legacy was showing others how 'to discuss with candour difficult problems, and to use courtesy to our fellows in controversy'. It was a legacy that all his children would benefit from, along with their mother's efficient example of practical social work and their aunt's intelligent questioning of the world around them. Brought up in a house where a humane sympathy, if not radical politics, was the dominant perspective, it is perhaps not surprising that all of the Jebb children later sought their own ways to contribute to enhancing more equitable social relations, but none more effectively than Eglantyne.

Chapter 3

Unravelling Her Surroundings, 1895–1898

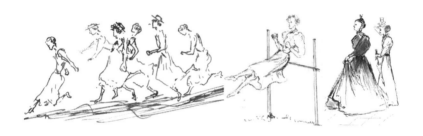

Dorothy … has been studying 'insect pests'. She calls these investigations, 'unravelling her surroundings', by which I see she is doing in the natural world what I try in vain to do in the human.

Eglantyne Jebb, 1896

With the death of Arthur, the last years of the nineteenth century were a period of great change for the Jebb family. The children were growing up and leaving home, and the happy dynamic of The Lyth, full of children, stories, butterfly nets and riding boots, began to seem like a nostalgic memory. Em, now twenty-two, was back at home after six months studying portrait painting and improving her German at Dresden, but in 1893 Lill had left to take a pioneering Agricultural Diploma at Newnham, one of the two women's colleges at Cambridge, and Dick had gone up to study

Eglantyne's doodles of a sports day at Lady Margaret Hall, and of herself trailing in the wake of her college friend Dorothy Kempe, 1896. Reproduced by kind permission of the Principal and Fellows of Lady Margaret Hall

Classics at Oxford. Eglantyne was still at home, but now eighteen she was plotting her escape to Oxford's Lady Margaret Hall to read history, for which she was qualified as much by her parents' social position as by her early education. Gamul was already following in Dick's footsteps, boarding at Marlborough College in Wiltshire, a forward-looking boys' school with a reputation for scholarship. Only Dorothy, who was just thirteen when her father died, was still in the schoolroom at home, dutifully learning languages, painting and music, and adding to her and Gamul's collection of birds, butterflies and beetles.

Eglantyne went up to Oxford in the autumn of 1895, just after her nineteenth birthday. She told her new friends that she possessed a 'hereditary mania for books', and had come to college simply because she had exhausted home supplies. In fact she had faced considerable parental resistance to her plans. Arthur had vehemently opposed the idea of any of his daughters going to college and particularly resisted Eglantyne's desire to take a degree course, fearing it might turn his beautiful teenage daughter, 'radiant with her bright red hair and exquisite complexion', into an unmarriageable bluestocking. Perhaps he was thinking of his sister Bun's track record of Newnham success followed by apparently unrepentant spinsterhood. 'If a girl were marked with small-pox and had good abilities, if she were short-sighted as to make spectacles a perpetual necessity and had great common sense, if she were obliged hereafter to gain her livelihood as a teacher at some sad seminary, there might be something to be said for Cambridge,' Arthur told Tye. 'Otherwise a ladies' college seems to me only a ladies' school with all its evils intensified.'

Arthur's concerns were not uncommon. Few parents were supportive of sending their girls to expensive colleges which at best seemed superfluous and at worst might transform them from dutiful daughters into independent new women. But after Arthur's death Bun's enthusiastic lobbying won Tye round to the idea. Bun had already paved the way for Em's six months at Dresden, and paid for Lill's Agricultural Diploma on the basis that she would return to run the home farm and dairy at The Lyth. She also offered to help pay for Dick's world tour in preparation for his proposed career in politics. But Eglantyne was the first daughter to want to undertake a degree course, and she was eternally grateful to Bun for championing her corner and eventually paying for it to happen. 'I wish you knew how much your educational £. s. d. has already been to me,' she wrote tactfully to her aunt during her first term. 'When I first heard of your helping in our educational expenses, I began to take an interest in living, as opposed to dreaming, and for many years it considerably added to my stock of cheerfulness … It must be a horrid thing to feel a dreadful door with "No Road" posted on it across your life and I'm sure your offer prevented me from raising many a one by my vivid imagination.'

Oxford's Lady Margaret Hall, named after Lady Margaret Beaufort, the pious but scholarly mother of Henry VII, had been founded in 1878 by Elizabeth Wordsworth, a great niece of the romantic poet. Somerville Hall followed a year later, named after the pioneering scientist and mathematician Mary Somerville. The choice of the colleges' eponymous patrons clearly reflected their distinct identities; LMH, as it was popularly known, was as traditional and religious as Somerville was progressive and political. Once she had plumped for Oxford rather than Cambridge, there was never any question as to which college Eglantyne, with her traditional Anglican upbringing, would be going.

Miss Wordsworth was still the Principal when Eglantyne arrived at LMH in 1895. Although a pioneer of women's access to higher education, her aim was not to promote a revolution in social relations, but 'to turn out girls so that they will be capable of making homes happy'. She ran the college like a large upper-class family, greatly reassuring concerned parents like Tye. Nonetheless Miss Wordsworth was an inspiring example of what women could achieve. Deeply religious, she was also intelligent, witty, determined and unaffected to the point of being considered slightly eccentric. As she valued an independent mind Eglantyne soon became one of her favourites. For her part

Eglantyne was rather romantically drawn to her Principal, with whom she would discuss Browning and Austen, and pay house calls on various Oxford luminaries. 'Miss W says she does not think. Her thoughts rush into her head all of a sudden,' Eglantyne babbled to friends. 'That is what it is to have genius.' She was perhaps more deeply impressed however by Miss Pearson, the college's Vice Principal, and an archetypical blue-stocking; short, square and slightly lame with unfashionably masculine clothes, and fiercely intelligent and well read. Miss Pearson took a huge interest in her young students, and would often stay up late discussing history, literature and the social issues of the day with Eglantyne and her friends. These were wonderful evenings, and later Eglantyne claimed that during them Miss Pearson taught her more than almost anybody in her life.

LMH had grown rapidly under Elizabeth Wordsworth; more rapidly than the Principal, with her desire to head a manageable family of students, wished. By Eglantyne's day there were about forty students, overflowing from the Old Hall into the 'Wordsworth hostel' across the road, and Eglantyne was among the first girls to share an ordinary north Oxford villa, at number 3 Crick Road. At first Eglantyne was quite dismissive of her house-mates, the 'Crickets' as they dubbed themselves: 'all look the one more noodlish than the other', she wrote to Bun. But before long she had formed close friendships, particularly with Dorothy Kempe, soon an intimate confidante, and Ruth Wordsworth, the niece of the Principal, who between them kept hundreds of Eglantyne's letters. Collectively the 'Crickets' were under the supervision of Mary Talbot, an academic with a strong social conscience, and a close friend of Gertrude Bell who had left LMH five years earlier.[1] Under Miss Talbot's sympathetic eye they enjoyed more personal freedom than most of their friends on campus – but none of the female students enjoyed the same independence and opportunities as their male counterparts.

Only two years before Eglantyne arrived at LMH women had to be chaperoned to lectures and could not join a university society, or cycle on Sundays. They could still not cross a college quad alone and had to be in by ten at night unless granted special leave. Tripos exams had only been open to Oxford women since 1881, and women were still awarded special certificates in place of recognised degrees. Eglantyne was not convinced that women should be granted university degrees, fearing that 'it would probably prevent forever the possible development of a separate and perhaps better system of our own ...', but she was fascinated by the debate. 'What annoys me so intensely', she let off steam to Dorothy Kempe, is that 'they talk as if we were actually ousting the men, or only going to lectures in order to imitate *them!* When our presence cannot and does not affect them in the slightest degree I do not think that they ought to be "dog in the manger" about our taking a share (not away from them) in educational advantages which cannot be had elsewhere and means so very much to us.'[2]

Nevertheless at the end of the nineteenth century college did offer unprecedented freedom for young women from upper-class homes, most of whom would never have dreamed of appearing in public alone and were well accustomed to chaperones and evening curfews. At LMH the girls had access to the highest standards of academic lectures, libraries and tutors. Furthermore they could manage their own days and enjoy unquestioned hours of privacy instead of having to be, and appear to be, busy with domestic tasks, charity or often tedious social rounds. But Eglantyne, used to the relative freedoms of The Lyth, was not on balance over-impressed. Presented with a copy of the rules on her arrival she sat down on her trunk and considered whether she should leave immediately or 'stay long enough to break all the rules and be sent down'. She stayed, but not quietly.

Eglantyne was determined to make the most of all the opportunities that LMH presented. Above all she wanted to learn. 'Cleverness is good,' she blithely reassured her sister Dorothy who at fifteen was worrying that her own ambitions to go to Newnham College, Cambridge, might be based on personal vanity. 'There is I think nothing wrong in hoping that this good gift may have been bestowed on us to use in God's service,' Eglantyne continued. 'It is perhaps a sacred duty to try and be as clever as we can.' It was a fine sentiment, but one that she sometimes found hard to live up to. After her limited home-schooling, college work, particularly maths, proved quite a challenge. Sometimes, she moaned to friends, her mind felt 'like a bicycle being ridden over a cartload of stones with a burst tyre', and the poems she scrawled when she should have been studying provide a cheerful record of her patchy efforts to apply herself:

> My lamp was lit, my fire was red
> And Euclid open lay;
> 'I really should work hard,' I said
> Nor waste my time away
> For over my defenceless head
> A sword does daily dangle,
> Prelims are hanging by a thread,
> And at a fated angle …
> I hope that [Euclid] is somewhere,
> His evil deeds repenting!
> Yea – dust and ashes seem too fair
> For one whose life was spent in
> Fresh tortures angular and square
> For unborn men intending
> And yet – bisections made *no* clearer,
> By indignations venting,
> And still prelims draw nearer, nearer,
> With foot-steps unrelenting.[3]

History seminars were more rewarding, although her poem 'To My History Lecturer' shows that even these, and the attitude she thought she spied among her male lecturers, were not beyond her mocking pen:

> I never wrote a poem before
> To such a thing as 'Man'!
> (Your sex indeed blue-stockings must
> Contemptuously scan.)

And so perhaps 'tis very wrong
To pen these lines unwise,
But 'tis your spectacles I like
And *not*, you know, your eyes.[4]

The Oxford history course covered a wide curriculum. Eglantyne studied Roman and Greek Classics, Greek and Stoic philosophy, architecture, archaeology, anthropology, psychology, abstract metaphysics, politics and economics among other disciplines. Pure history, which she referred to as 'the experience of the world', was her favourite subject; she devoured Voltaire and Rousseau, and found herself 'wildly indignant' at Carlyle. In romantic moods she took her inspiration from the very fabric of the university: 'the home of men who have known through the past centuries things that I wish to find … It is a comfort to tread the pavements that they trod,' she wrote to Dorothy, 'to see the towers of the university against the sunset as they saw them and to see the colleges they lived in bathed in the soft sun. It is unreal sometimes as a dream. I seem to feel them walk beside me, to hear their voices, to have their hands in mine.' Eglantyne was in her element; surrounded by historic colleges, helpful ghosts and, above all, books. 'To know, to know, to know! I go into the Bodleian as into a church …' she continued to her sister, while to her new college friends she bragged of possessing 'a devouring passion for Books just because they are BOOKS'. Even in the holidays books took centre stage, with 'reading parties' organised in the ancient market towns of Tavistock and Dorking, when mornings would be spent reading and sociable afternoons walking and riding.

Eglantyne also threw herself into the extra-curriculum activities at Oxford, most predictably the university debates. The Oxford Women's Inter-Collegiate Debating Society, founded less than ten years earlier, already had an impressive body of alumnae including Margery Fry, Eleanor Rathbone and Maude Royden.[5] Having spent years on the wings of the Ellesmere Debating Society, Eglantyne now jumped at the chance to take centre stage in this prestigious club. Her maiden speech, opposing the motion that the study of history destroys our confidence in human nature, could not have better played to her strengths. Soon she was elected the radical President of the society, and bored by dry academic discussions she implored the speakers to 'be more flippant'. When this failed she proposed and carried 'wildly anarchical' changes to the society's constitution. 'The bomb has gone off in the debating society' she proudly claimed, although many of her amendments were later quashed when Somerville students successfully plotted a vote of censure on her.

Apart from study and college societies, life at LMH was focused around drama and dancing, the hockey pitch and the river; all activities that Eglantyne threw herself into with gusto. The chilly LMH archive contains none of her course work or papers, but many of her quick ink sketches survive there, including numerous programmes for the Crick Road students' evening entertainments, all rather subversively presented by dancing imps complete with wings and pointed horns, prancing bespectacled horses and agile witches. Although her housemates are all well represented on these programmes, Eglantyne's initials appear only once, against the unlikely role of Mr Collins in a scene from Jane Austen's *Pride and Prejudice*, for which she earned particular praise for her 'delicious' rendering of the 'love scene'. Other sketches capture the archaic-looking antics of an LMH sports day: a high jump successfully navigated despite the added bulk of flowing skirts, petticoats and leg-of-mutton sleeves, and a vigorous downhill sprint also seemingly unhampered by high collars, hair-pins and straw hats. Eglantyne had always loved outdoor sports and quickly took up fencing and hockey, although with rather more enthusiasm than ability. 'I find that people show a very elementary side of their nature when they play hockey, one feels as if one were touching the original man!' she enthused to Dorothy Kempe. 'As for *my* play, there is only one thing wrong with it, namely that I never hit the ball ...' She was more adept on the water, partly owing to rowing lessons from her brother Dick, a frequent visitor from New College. Soon she was a qualified member of the LMH boat club, regularly filling punts and canoes with cushions and pushing off from their boat-house on the Cherwell, and later doing her bit by giving lessons in sculling to the freshers.

When she needed to escape college life, Eglantyne would cycle into the countryside, alone or just with her closest friends. The invention of pneumatic rubber bicycle tyres by John Dunlop in 1888, to prevent his son getting a sore bottom on his rides to school, had revolutionised cycling, but bikes were still fairly unwieldy and Eglantyne's excursions were not without mishap. Occasionally 'going downhill at my usual rate' she would career off her bike or, as she told it, 'my bicycle and I found that the road was between us'. And once she and Dorothy Kempe were threatened with a police summons after being caught cycling in the moonlight with their lamps out. But more often Eglantyne would ride out alone for twenty miles or more, sometimes before breakfast, quite a test of endurance on a bicycle with no free wheel.

Dick also invited Eglantyne over to his college where she caused quite a sensation over dinners in his rooms, and dancing all night and into the morning at the New College Ball. 'A college ball seems unlike any other', she laughed, 'for it is so very juvenile, and therefore has got some more real enjoyment floating about in it.' In fact she usually stunned observers one way or another, whether dressed as a 'scholar gipsy' for a fancy dress ball, or 'quite dazzling in black evening gown' at a more formal hall function. She 'could, when she chose to behave and dress as such, be a dazzlingly lovely woman', Ruth Wordsworth wrote.

All in, Eglantyne shone at college that first term, effortlessly attracting admirers with her lively mind, quick wit and classic Edwardian looks. Slim and tall, with delicate features and copper-red hair, in Ruth's adoring eyes she was 'the very ideal of a Burne-Jones beauty', and soon half of LMH was under her spell. 'Never was there a more charming girlish figure', Lilias Milroy gushed, remembering Eglantyne strolling through the quads, and Ruth described her coming up from boating on the Cher 'dressed in green, with golden-red curly hair and a complexion seldom found outside a novel'. Although generally careless about her appearance and horrified by the idea of personal vanity, Eglantyne clearly knew how to show herself off to best effect. But friends could always make her 'blush vividly' by pointing out, for example, that 'her choice of forget-me-not blue hat band and tie, the exact shade of her eyes and so exactly right with her goldy-red tendrils of hair and wild-rose complexion, made it impossible to believe she was impervious to considerations of what suited her'. The only photograph of Eglantyne at this time, a formal studio shot in which the sweeping satin dress rather wears the woman, is in fact all self-consciousness. With her wild beauty well hidden behind convention, Eglantyne looks dutifully at the camera with an expression caught somewhere between embarrassment and amusement. However a watercolour of the same pose betrays that her dress was still forget-me-not blue.

The bubble burst just halfway through her second term. In March 1896 Eglantyne heard that her younger brother Gamul had caught pneumonia at his Marlborough boarding school. At sixteen Gamul was already distinguished by his clear mind and passionate interest in the natural sciences. Praising his 'energetic work and singular independence of thought' his schoolmasters expected him to win a scholarship to Oxbridge to study medicine, and everyone believed he was looking at a brilliant career as a doctor. In March Gamul's house-master wrote to let Tye know that her son had caught a chill. She and Bun immediately set off for Marlborough, bringing an expensive London doctor with them. Within a few days the doctor was reporting that although 'not hopeless', Gamul had descended into a 'condition of the greatest danger'. On 10 March Tye must have feared the worst because she wrote to prepare her children: 'I want you all to rest in the peace giving assurance that he is in the hands of a Loving Father, and that whether He takes him or leaves him here, we may perfectly trust Him to do what is loving and merciful.'

Dorothy, Gamul's closest sister in terms of age and interests, knew that he was ill, but she had not taken in the gravity of the situation. All the family had been together at The Lyth over Christmas, and she and Gamul had celebrated the new year by vigorously pruning back the gooseberry and currant bushes in kitchen garden. Dorothy had continued her daily routines while her mother went to Marlborough, and was buying stamps at Ellesmere post office when she was casually told the worst by the young man behind the wire screen who had just taken Tye's telegram: 'All over, funeral Tydraw.' Eglantyne heard the news the same day by telegram to LMH, and immediately set off for home.

Gamul's funeral took place on 14 March at Rhiwas Church near Tydraw where his father, Arthur, had been buried just two years before. It was a bright, sunny day, which, Tye tried to console herself, 'seemed what our darling would have wished to have'. The coffin was covered in wreaths, some almost bridal, Tye felt in the nearest she allowed herself to anger or remorse, others of local heather and daffodils. After placing the family flowers on the coffin, Tye took comfort in receiving Holy Communion. 'It has been a lovely day,' she wrote stoically that evening. 'These early deaths have their sad side for us, but not for them,' the Canon Reginald Smith reflected in his sermon at Marlborough College the following day. 'We doubt not that those whom God calls home thus early will find a larger life than ours, in which all the promise which had begun to blossom here will bear its full harvest under happier conditions than ours.' Tye certainly fervently believed this and although she could not know why Gamul had been 'taken' from them, she was consoled by her faith that they would be reunited in another life.

Em, the eldest of the Jebb children, immediately set about supporting her mother and family with efficient as well as loving concern, even sending daily letters to Arthur's elder sister, Nony, whose husband was the maths master at Gamul's school. 'I don't like such a lot of England being between us just now', Em wrote, 'but after all it is only the bodies not the spirits which are apart.' Like Tye, Em tried to focus on celebrating Gamul's life. 'The more one thinks of it the more one feels lucky, thoroughly lucky, in having such a memory as that of Gam to carry about and cheer oneself with all one's life,' she told her aunt. 'I know I shall feel more and more like that though at present one is so numb and stupid ... The others are very brave, Dora especially.'

Heartbroken Dorothy was the least able to come to terms with Gamul's sudden death. Desperately trying to make sense of the senseless, she blamed her parents for jinxing him with an unlucky name. 'Gamul had been a family name in the past: as it happened these boys died young,' she later wrote bitterly, 'but neither of our parents were superstitious, and had no anxiety.' Far from it in fact: on a visit to Scotland in 1888 when Gamul was eight years old, Arthur had read that the name Gamul was derived from Gamall, an Icelandic word meaning 'old', 'the dear old boy', he had written cheerfully. But Gamul would never be old. More than anyone else, though, Dorothy blamed herself. She alone had known about what she now referred to as Gamul's 'dangerous habit' of wearing only one shirt in summer, a habit which it seemed he had continued during the winter months. Dorothy would carry an acute sense of responsibility throughout her life for not having intervened; at least by informing the Marlborough matron who could have insisted on the extra vest.

While home from college Eglantyne took Dorothy out for long walks, and together they drew comfort from seeing the first signs of spring returning to the countryside: 'there is a philosophy in it which is beyond us all', she bravely concluded. But in the evenings she wrote to Dorothy Kempe about her 'chaos of thoughts'. 'I feel that I'd better not see anyone,' she warned her friend, 'because I have a lot before me and must keep myself strong to do battle. Don't grieve too much about me, but let us trust in God. Pray that I may be the means by which my family may be strengthened. Pray especially for my younger sister; that will help.'

Tye soon sent Dorothy to visit her Irish Uncle Heneage, where she threw herself into a detailed study of mosses. When she returned she brought her young cousin Milly with her, who stayed at The Lyth as a rather bossed-about playmate for the rest of the year. Dorothy now devoted herself to following up Gamul's interests. With poor Milly in tow, she mainly added to Gamul's collection of beetles, later remembering how 'such a thing as a dead rabbit became a most attractive object for the sake of those handsome burying beetles of which few people are aware'. Tye had been considering sending her to the prestigious Wycombe Abbey School in Buckinghamshire, but she was increasingly concerned about her daughter, and also uneasy about the school's situation, 'at the bottom of a valley … a slummy little town too near its gates, and a large expanse of water, on a level with the house close at hand'. It was enough to persuade her against the idea; she was not going to risk losing another child, and instead she engaged an English governess to continue tutoring Dorothy at home.

Like Dorothy, Eglantyne also internalised her grief. Although she naturally turned to poetry to make sense of most of her thoughts and feelings, she seemed unable to lessen the pain of Gamul's death even by writing privately about him. The closest she managed was in another letter to Dorothy Kempe towards the end of the year, comforting her about her own brother's illness. 'I often wonder how it is that love, the first principle of existence is *yet* so thwarted,' Eglantyne wrote. 'We love our relations so, yet either we grow apart, or they go away, or they die. (Forgive me "ranting"!) Surely, one thinks, these things must work themselves straight, eventually somewhere, somehow, and love be satisfied unto the full …'

Time passed. Tye quietly tended her garden, Lill returned to Cambridge, Dick and Eglantyne to their separate Oxford colleges.

Occasionally Tye would mention a visit to Gamul's grave and how well the plants were doing, but otherwise his name did not come up in the frequent family letters. Life moved on, but Gamul was not forgotten by any of the family. As I researched different areas of this biography, Gamul kept turning up in unexpected places. On one of my regular sweeps of secondhand bookshops I came across a volume called *Observation Lessons on Plant Life: A Guide to Teachers*, co-authored by Dorothy and Em and published in 1903. Inside the front cover was a pencil inscription, 'From one of the authoresses, Sept 23 1904, Read, mark, learn and inwardly digest!' It looked like Em's writing, though the sentiment could have come equally from either of them. However the book contained another secret inside – a dedication to the memory of Gamul:

> Little Brother, sunny nature lover, you left us years ago; since then we have missed you in the fields, and the woods are more silent than they used to be. But we have found comfort in these humble studies, and should they help others to love the country as we loved it, then we should have fitly dedicated them to your bright spirit.

A few months later a small green notebook dated 1962 surfaced among Dorothy's many papers, containing a set of handwritten narratives headed 'Psychic Experiences'. The central one of these gave her own account of the days after Gamul's death. Acutely conscious of her brother's loss to the world as a doctor, Dorothy had determined to make her own contribution to society in Gamul's place. 'With this in mind, I was praying one night with great intensity when I felt as if I was slipping out of my body,' Dorothy looked back with remarkable clarity after more than sixty years. 'Unfortunately I was a timid child, and ... I struggled back into normal consciousness ...' Dorothy was convinced that she had had a spiritual experience, and in a sense Gamul did remain with her, as a constant inspiration, throughout her life. 'I did it all for Gamul' she pencilled on some papers relating to her life's work just before she died.

Perhaps Dorothy mentioned her 'psychic experience' to Eglantyne. Either way Eglantyne came to believe that Gamul haunted her dreams, both in the years just after his death, and again twenty years on as a generation of young men were losing their lives in the First World War. Spiritualism experienced a significant resurgence in Britain during the war years, and it would have been quite acceptable for Eglantyne to have held such beliefs. In a record of her own 'Dreams and Psychical Experiences' hidden among the family papers at The Lyth, Eglantyne recorded in June 1918 that she 'woke early this morning from unrecollected dreams of Gamul. I was most anxious to recollect whether he had died or not ... I couldn't remember. If he had not died, I would have set off instantly – that very day – to Marlborough, to see if I couldn't do anything to help him in regard to his health.' Like Dorothy, Eglantyne felt she had somehow failed Gamul, but 'this self-reproach must certainly refer to what happened since he died', she now commented:

> because I do not reproach myself in regard to our relations while he was on earth. But it is rather strange, now I think of it, how often I have dreamt about him as someone who had been growing apart from his contemporaries, huddled away in a corner somewhere and forgotten. More than once it has come to me with a kind of shock, 'Dear me! He is my brother!' And I had quite forgotten that I had him! And I've done nothing for him in all these years. Is it too late? But the fact of his being dead has made me assume, when I woke up again, that I couldn't do anything for him.

'It is clear anyhow', she concluded, 'that last night there came in my sleep an intense, concentrated desire to be of service to him.' Many years later Eglantyne told Em how at times Gamul still sometimes seemed to be standing beside her, reminding her of her pledge to public service.

Eternally young, Gamul had become Eglantyne and Dorothy's tragic Peter Pan; an emblem of the potential of youth, the value of life, and of their own commitment to live lives of social worth. 'I used to think that it was an easy way to satisfy all my ambitions and desires – just to read,' Eglantyne reflected when she was back at college. 'I have found out too late that this is a mistake ... One has to bring something more ... something which can only be acquired by living oneself.' Libraries and parties were no longer enough, Eglantyne needed to apply herself to some useful purpose.

Eglantyne's college friends noticed the change in her immediately; she was not exactly cold but much more focused, and there was a new reserve in place of the old vivacity. No longer relishing the attention that she still effortlessly attracted, Eglantyne would now often slip away to spend time studying, or simply walking, alone. 'Something a little mysterious, a little wayward in her constantly attracted, in spite of herself, friends for whom ... she had frankly little use,' Dorothy Kempe realised, while Lilias Milroy commented, 'I would not say she made friends but she gladly received their affection ... she had reserves all the time: she could on occasion be ruthless – almost brutal.' When pushed even loyal Ruth Wordsworth had to admit that, though always thoughtful with the unhappy or awkward, Eglantyne could also be cruelly snubbing, and Mildred Preston, who had been on the receiving end of Eglantyne's new abruptness, agreed: 'She was not an easy person to know. She had a way of picking your brains and pressing for views on this and that and then brooding over what you had said, then when she had assimilated it she might find a discrepancy or a weak point in your argument and point this out to you in a way that might have been devastating to friendship, if she had not invariably seen the funny side and laughed with you.' Eglantyne did not intend to be mean, 'fundamentally she was extraordinarily tender-hearted', Lilias excused her. It was simply that after Gamul's death she both realised the precious brevity of life, and made an unconscious mental shift away from investing in vulnerable individual relationships in favour of focusing on people in general; their collective ideas and insights. 'No individual friendship could … satisfy [or] absorb' her, Dorothy Kempe now recognised modestly, and Lilias similarly understood that 'mankind in general fired her imagination more than individuals'. As a result Eglantyne quickly gained a reputation for 'aloofness' along with that for her brilliance and beauty, and her supervisor, Mary Talbot, oscillated between fearing that she exerted too much influence over her often disciple-like friends, and that she would become a recluse given her 'hermit spirit'.

Perhaps partly for this reason, at the start of their second year Eglantyne and the other 'Crickets' were moved into the vacant rooms in the LMH halls. In an ostentatious rejection of material values Eglantyne immediately threw all of the furniture, including the carpet, out of her room – although the LMH bursar, Maud Holgate, suggested that this was in fact a deliberate strategy to keep unwanted guests at bay. 'I want to read. I am much more interested in William III than in visitors,' Eglantyne certainly grumbled to Dorothy Kempe. 'I am tired of them before they have come.' Either way it was a display that quickly gained Eglantyne legendary status at LMH, and was later referred to as her 'mad attack' by one of her friends, and as her having 'gone socialist' by another. But as well as being a reaction to anything that seemed vain and unnecessary after Gamul's death, Eglantyne's asceticism was inspired by her reading of Henry Thoreau, whose famous book *Walden*, extolling the virtues of the simple life, she greatly admired. 'Lill has been reading Walden at my instigation and now she wants to live in a hut in a wood, and have no servants and no furniture and nothing unnecessary, two skirts however on account of the rain,' Eglantyne wrote to Dorothy Kempe in a mock huff. 'She is telling me all my own ideas, as though they were quite new to me.' Critics of Thoreau however cynically observed that he was 'indolent rather than simple; what spoilt his simplicity was that he was forever hoping that he would be observed and admired'. A similar criticism might be made of Eglantyne's rather public exhibition of her own developing moral conscience. She was soon persuaded to move her furniture back on aesthetic grounds; beauty having an important role to play even in an equitable and non-materialist society. 'Questions concerned with luxury and expenditure are so difficult,' she sighed.

All the LMH students came from privileged homes, mainly vicarages and country houses much like The Lyth, and nearly all, like Eglantyne, were from essentially Tory families. 'Well of course everyone is a Conservative' the author Winifred Peck would voice the general consensus at LMH five years later: 'no one decent could be a Liberal.' But at Oxford the girls were exposed to new ideas and alternative philosophies, often for the first time. Eglantyne loved the past, but she did not want to live there and she was rather put out when her tutor described her writing as 'eighteenth century'. 'He meant it as a compliment, but why eighteenth century?' she balked, 'I should rather have it nineteenth cent, or better still twentieth.' Having resolved to 'equip herself to be of service', she now chose to supplement her history courses with contemporary moral and political philosophy, particularly the theories of Henry Sidgwick and Alfred Marshall. 'I am reading Sedgwick's *[sic]* "History of Ethics",' she wrote to Dorothy Kempe proudly one holiday, 'it is a subject which I am desperately ignorant about, still it is a consolation to find that my individual speculations have made me feel quite at home in it.' Sidgwick advanced the classical utilitarian doctrine of Jeremy Bentham and John Stuart Mill, advocating the greatest good for the greatest number, an idea that appealed strongly to Eglantyne. Marshall was interested in the social and economic problems that had accompanied Britain's transition from an agrarian to an urban, industrial society. Soon Eglantyne was writing to her aunt Nony that political science was 'the nicest branch of the history schools!' and at the end of the year she was even, she persuaded herself, 'getting very fond of' political economy.

Eglantyne supplemented her lectures by going to college events to hear Canon Gore, Henry Scott Holland and William Morris addressing the inaugural meeting of the Oxford Socialist Society. But her attempts to unravel her surroundings were not contained by college boundaries. Sometimes trailing reluctant friends, she went 'slumming' around the less affluent parts of Oxford like the alleys by the canal, quietly seeing for herself how the other half lived. Over the holidays she looked round National Schools for working-class children, and a 'pitiful little hospital for dying babies' in Shropshire, and during the Easter break of her second year she spent a week at the University Settlement in London's Bethnal Green. Settlements were houses bought to provide socially conscientious university students with the opportunity to live and work in working-class neighbourhoods, ostensibly providing an inspiration by their very presence as well as practical support through running youth clubs and vocational training. Initially a project led by male students, female undergraduates soon set up their own settlements, and by the 1890s short stays at London settlements had become almost fashionable among Oxford's women. At Bethnal Green Eglantyne spent her days at working people's clubs, and her evenings out dancing with East End factory girls with whom she 'felt instantly in touch'. However although she declared that her stay at Bethnal Green was one of the happiest weeks of her life, and she later supported Dorothy Kempe's plans for a new LMH settlement in Wandsworth, Eglantyne was not attracted to a vocation in settlement work herself. Not long later she would make Frieda Jones, her fictional alter ego and heroine of her only finished social novel, *The Ring Fence*, ruin her health by working long hours in a London settlement, and her description of 'the ugliness and dreariness of the slums' shows she held no illusions about the romance of poverty or settlement work. 'There was something about the place which suggested a painful effort to find happiness in drudgery,' Eglantyne wrote of Frieda's settlement, 'an effort which had failed.' Nonetheless Eglantyne was impressed by the settlement movement, commenting in a 1906 social report that the 'idea of the settlement was to bring the well-to-do educated to make their homes among the poor, and as neighbours to establish friendly and natural relations with them. This was going to the root of the matter and must remain the ideal.' Settlements had introduced Eglantyne to the idea of 'breaking down class barriers' and to the broader importance of active social participation that was later to become a key part of her social philosophy.

At the end of her second year Eglantyne was keen to quit college and apply herself to some useful work in the real world but her tutors persuaded her to stay the course. 'College begins to cast its shadow before,' she scribbled irritably to Dorothy Kempe as this final year loomed. 'I place my hope in the freshers. Really if there is still predominant the dress and tea-party set who have photographs of actors on their chimney pieces and are devoted admirers of Burne-Jones' pictures, when I go back next term I shall plant a bomb in the chapel.' The new intake did not impress and soon Eglantyne was railing against the 'curiously unplastic ideal' of the English girl. 'I am inclined to think that we like many kinds of men because there are many uses for them,' she vented her frustration in her diary. 'For girls til lately there has only been one use. The ideal domestic character has been made ideal for the whole female sex ... dainty ornaments of the drawing room.' She tried her best to tease out some original ideas and responses from the first years at rather patronising cocoa parties in her room, but soon reported dismally, 'it is no good – one cannot call forth one vital spark'. Eglantyne did not resort to direct action, but she never forgot the intensity of her frustrations, and later enjoyed making her fictional Frieda Jones be described by her conservative future lover as 'the sort of woman I detest. Pretends to be so sweet and gentle, and all the time you know that underneath she's a raging fanatic. The kind of person you'd expect to carry a bomb into St Paul's.' It is perhaps with some irony, then, that Eglantyne is commemorated at Oxford today with a glass chandelier in the LMH chapel, commissioned by her former college friends.

Eglantyne now strayed even further from her set history course. She had already begun to explore the issues surrounding poverty, and now she began to examine her faith more critically, especially where she felt these two interests intersected. This mainly involved attending events like Christian Social Science conferences at which she claimed to gain a wholesome sense of her own ignorance. She passed the time by discretely drawing caricatures of the speakers, and later she was not entirely upset to find 'I must have dropped – just like me – two of the most unflattering likenesses in the Congress Hall – two archdeacons, and they had got their names written beneath.' She also went to various Christian Socialist meetings, and undertook fact-finding visits to a Church Congress, and a Salvation Army rally which she described bluntly as 'one of the most curious sights I have ever seen'.

The more organised a church group or faith, the less it appealed to her. Tye had just been through a similar but more intense crisis in her faith. After Gamul's death she had joined the Catholic Apostolic Church, a small sect that believed in the return of the Apostles and imminent second coming, but which also respected personal spirituality, giving Tye the comfort that she could not find in the formalities of the established Church. Em called Tye's conversion 'catastrophic', but Lill, practical to her finger-tips, accepted the emotional appeal of this kind of mysticism, and Eglantyne was even more open-minded, sympathetically writing to her mother from college that 'we cannot expect to walk by the same paths to the goals which we have in common … yes, I am very glad that you are going to join, and I hope that it will bring you great peace'.

Eglantyne was soon so attracted to mysticism, with its fluid idea around people having a direct awareness of spiritual truth and a personal relationship with divine reality, or God, that she rejected a college course on Christian Foreign Missions in favour of some independent work on the mystic perspective and practice across different faiths. This mainly entailed a detailed study of the revealed texts of the Vedas, the primary text of Hinduism which also influences Buddhism, Jainism and Sikhism, but also took in the philosophy of the Greek Stoic Epictetus, and the visions of the seventeenth-century German mystic Jakob Böhme. Soon she began to experience her own modest impressions of the universal, spiritual, oneness of the world. 'The world was all gold and dancing ... It confused me and made one feel vague as in a dream,' she wrote to Dorothy Kempe during an October break in 1897. 'Every turn on the lane seemed to promise to take one straight into the infinite! Everything was changed.' Later she described the transcendental experience of spiritual awakening as 'the feeling of being lifted out of a dark cell and set in some great open space ... the barriers of personal limitations ... fallen ... at one with humanity, and ... humanity's mystical power'. For Eglantyne, still dealing with the grief of losing her brother, the idea of the spiritual oneness of the world and humanity was profoundly comforting. It was also deeply liberating. Class and gender distinctions had always frustrated her and the idea that such 'personal limitations' might be temporary constraints, nonexistent or irrelevant in a later, universal, spiritual life, struck a deep chord with her.

Against the advice of her tutors she now chose India as her special subject in her final year. 'International history ... is much more interesting than the history of one country by itself,' she argued. 'Besides, the story of each one separately is so very much elucidated when one knows the bearing of the whole.' Although she would never have the opportunity to visit India, in December 1897 she took a few weeks out to travel to Egypt with Dick as part of his grand tour, sponsored by Bun and Tye. After the constraints of college life, Eglantyne felt her spirits soar as she gazed across the expansive desert outside Cairo. 'Oh heavens, to walk out into it – there was nothing else between me and Algiers,' she wrote ecstatically. The pyramids, and the Sphinx 'with its half cynical, half gentle, wholly triumphant smile', also made a great impression on her. But while Eglantyne rather romantically admired one of her picturesque guides, 'a solitary Arab ... in trailing white garments and red shoes', the limits of her ability to see the 'oneness of humanity' were clearly demonstrated by her response to the attention she inevitably received as a wealthy tourist from what she called the 'natives ... those brown creatures [that] seethe around you, fighting for your custom and your bakshish ...' Of course Eglantyne, who had never travelled outside Britain before, was not likely to be prepared for the hassle and clamour of visiting the great sites of Cairo, and her language and attitudes were quite standard for the day, even if they seem unpalatable now. But not all late Victorian travellers were so distracted. Gertrude Bell also visited Egypt in 1897 where she was similarly fascinated by the scenery, ancient history and 'white robed, black cloaked Arabs', but her account does not appear so overtly racist. The history, heat and energy of Egypt all made a lasting impression on Eglantyne, but she found the trip exhausting and was relieved to get home to the silence and calm of Shropshire. Although she later made plans to visit India, Persia and China, she never had the chance to travel outside Europe again.

Eglantyne left Oxford with second-class honours in 1898. She was disappointed with her grade but philosophical about it, recognising she would probably have done better had she stuck to the courses laid down for her in the History Honours School, but unable to regret having repeatedly chosen her own lines of reading. She regarded her education as too important to be guided by the desire for good results alone, and had often scoffed that 'broken hearts seem to be the corollary of examinations since examinations first were'. Always seeing the best in her friend, Ruth Wordsworth later said that Eglantyne had an idealist's 'utilitarian attitude of contempt for anything but getting the power to live out of learning'.

Oxford would miss Eglantyne. Maud Holgate, the LMH Bursar, told Tye that her daughter 'will be a very great loss to us here, [and] to me personally ... There is no one whom interests one more or whom it is such a refreshment to be with, putting aside the deep affection one feels for her for what she is in herself ...' But looking back Eglantyne had mixed feelings about her college years. In some ways they had been a wonderful sabbatical, 'a blissful paradise of books, books, books', and yet when she left Eglantyne was not entirely sure what her Oxford education had equipped her to do. Eager to keep her promise to Gamul and start making a direct contribution to society, she was now frustrated not to have a specific qualification or immediate employment. For some time she felt despondent, at odds with both the world and herself, but Gamul's death had convinced her to have faith in God's plans however obscure they might at times appear, and she took comfort from her belief that 'Heaven will grant willing hearts the means and opportunities of serving one's fellow men.' As a result she let herself drift for a rare moment, wandering around the flower beds with Tye 'in an Arcadian way', learning to mow hay, helping Lill in the dairy, and taking solitary boat-trips on the mere; 'a very luxurious method of wasting time'. It would not be long before she would be up to her unqualified neck in hard work and until then, as her poem 'Answers', written in 1898, rather prettily records, she decided to enjoy waiting for inspiration:

Let all vexed questions lie;
I do not wish to know
The answers human thought may yet supply.
I wish to watch the glow
Which shimm'ring softly o'er the slaty sea
Brings wordless back its answer unto me.
A truce to questions, wrong or right.
This once for Truth's dear sake
Let's listen for the answers which tonight
God's world may make,
As we in silence list'ning sit and feel
The gathering dusk betwixt the hedge-rows steal.

Chapter 4

Testing the Maternal Impulse, 1898–1900

I don't care for children.

Eglantyne Jebb, 1900

Six months after my second daughter was born I officially became a bad mother. I absolutely, passionately, smugly even, loved my children, but at the same time instead of revelling in full-time motherhood I felt increasingly frustrated. Sometimes I thought I loved the girls best when they were finally upstairs asleep and I was downstairs looking at photographs of them awake. When they were downstairs I often found myself trying to get them to take a co-ordinated nap so that I could spend a few hours reading up on Eglantyne. When my new baby was two weeks and two days old we went on our first real outing, strapped together, across London to the Women's Library. To gaze at her in an archive library – it was all my romance and joy together – but it was clearly not going to help me get on with anything. I signed up for a readers' pass at the British Library. Why was it that when my own children were so young, and according to convention in need of endless motherly love and attention, I was choosing to spend time researching the life of another woman, and ironically one who championed children's welfare? And why was it that Eglantyne, who was to do so much for so many children, had no children of her own? Did Eglantyne love children, or not? Did she mean them to be the focus of her life, or just the focus of her intellect? What was this thing about loving children from a distance?

In 1899 Eglantyne embarked on a career that put her in daily contact with children: teaching in an under-funded school for working-class girls. It was an eccentric but reasonably socially acceptable choice of vocation for a woman of her class and background. Elementary education had been growing rapidly since the 1870 Education Act, which set the framework for the schooling of all children between the ages of five and thirteen in England and Wales. Increasingly women were being accepted as cheap teachers in the new schools being established, although feminists like Vera Brittain later caustically argued that this was 'merely a method of passing on limitations from one female generation to the next'. Eglantyne's father, Arthur, had been appointed a school inspector for the new Board Schools established by the Act, so Eglantyne was well versed in the merits of and difficulties with the system. After 1880 school attendance became compulsory for children up to twelve, providing new job opportunities for single women to teach girls of their own class. For women from the higher classes, teaching was still seen as a kind of maternal outreach work, a hang-over from earlier 'social mothering' which involved extending upper- and middle-class women's supposedly innate nurturing skills and moral sensibilities to the less fortunate classes. Championing wider maternal responsibilities had traditionally given single women a route to independence and authority in the civic sphere. Was Eglantyne experimenting with her maternal, as well as her social, impulse with some prototype 'child-saving' when she chose to become a schoolteacher?

'Since I saw you last', Eglantyne wrote tentatively to Tye in 1895, 'I have thought of a plan … The thing is I want to become a national school-mistress. It is a work which both wants doing and which I think I am fitted for.' Perhaps her interest in education was fuelled in

part by having witnessed her mother's good works in bringing vocational training to poor families through the Home Arts, and her
father's role as a school inspector. In any case she first hatched the
schoolteaching plan soon after she went up to LMH, and although it
was not a consistent goal, she kept a lively interest in education theory throughout her college years. 'Aristotle on education is very
interesting,' she mused in 1897, 'I had not realised before, though I
suppose I ought to have, that the Athenians educated their children
as though they were cooking characters … In our system of education the formation of character is … only an indirect end.' Soon she
had developed admirably progressive ideas about National School
education, adopting the 'Athenian' principle about the importance
of character formation, and adding a few ideas of her own such as the
value of practical work as opposed to pure book-learning. 'My views
on the subject are apt to cause great merriment,' she wrote to
Dorothy Kempe in 1898. In fact many New Liberals were turning to
Aristotle, among other political philosophers, for inspiration regarding education and citizenship at this time, and Eglantyne had unconsciously caught the political zeitgeist.[1]

The education debate was in full swing in the 1890s, fuelled both
by extensions to the franchise and fears about Britain's declining status in world trade, crystallised by John Stuart Mill's talk of 'collective
mediocrity'. Mass education was surprisingly controversial however,
as the idea that citizens needed to be educated in order to vote wisely
and work intelligently was countered by the fear that an educated
working class would be less satisfied and more inclined to revolt.
Eglantyne's Uncle Richard, now a distinguished Cambridge Classics
scholar and Conservative MP for the university, had thrown himself
into this public debate, supporting the expansion of both primary
and secondary education and emphasising the need for teacher training. However while he conceded that 'a certain mechanical rigour'
was essential in the education given to 'the common people', above
all he championed the broad promotion of the humanities, which, he

argued, 'tend to good citizenship, by enlarging mental horizon'. Eglantyne sat on the fence over this. Citizenship was rapidly becoming one of her own watchwords but, like Tye, she believed that education should be above all 'practical and active', and that manual work should be just as respected as literature and the Classics.

Eglantyne was fully aware that her own literary and academic efforts had so far failed to justify her dedicating herself to the life of writing she secretly aspired to, and as the end of her studies loomed she realised that she too was in need of some 'practical and active' work. At Oxford her growing disgust at class distinctions and social inequality had fed her determination to live a life of social worth. She was therefore drawn to Charlotte Toynbee, who was described by Ruth Wordsworth as 'one of the most practically useful and wise social workers in Oxford'. Charlotte was the widow of Arnold Toynbee, an economics lecturer at Balliol whose belief in the value of integrating the social classes had inspired the settlement movement. After her husband's death at the age of just thirty-one, three years before Eglantyne arrived at Oxford, Charlotte had thrown herself into two projects: the care of LMH's finances, and the welfare of children in National Schools. 'Mrs T's trim little figure', Ruth remembered, 'was part of the morning view … rather stiffly upright and severely dressed for bad weather, nothing unnecessary spent on herself. But her shrewd eyes and primly set mouth had a whimsical smile that belied their severity, and … stiff as she was, it was not long before she had succumbed to Eglantyne's charm and admitted her to a rare intimacy.' Charlotte supported placing well-born women as teachers in National Schools following the settlement model of integrating the social classes, so she took Eglantyne to visit a local Poor Law school and generally encouraged her. Although middle-class uptake was still limited, teaching seemed an ideal way to combine Eglantyne's interests in education theory and social reform.

'There is a great need of Ladies as National Schoolmistresses', Eglantyne continued selling her teaching plans to Tye, 'because of the good of the children's close contact with them.' Tye needed little persuasion, having years before publicly committed herself to the idea that 'women of the upper-classes might advantageously be employed in such guiding roles on a larger scale'. The idea that this was a reciprocal relationship however, and that working with children might in itself be attractive, was not mentioned by either of them. If anything Eglantyne seemed to think that schoolteaching was rather a bitter pill, but one that she was well placed to swallow. 'I am far from saying that teaching would be altogether congenial and delightful', she concluded her case, 'but ... I think it suitable.' She later told her cousin Gem that she went into it simply 'on the belief that she was too stupid to do anything else'.

With Charlotte Toynbee's help Eglantyne secured a place at the distinctly unglamorous but progressive Stockwell Teacher Training College in the autumn of 1898. Hoping to blend in a little, she trained back her golden-red curls and shyly entered the college 'wearing the oldest and severest of her green coats and skirts'. Nonetheless she was shocked by conditions at the college, and the level of illness among her new colleagues who were mostly from the lower-middle classes, and she was glad not to be deprived of all trace of privilege. 'This is an extraordinary great barrack of a place,' she wrote to her sister Dorothy, back at The Lyth. 'The Gods be thanked I have a room to myself. The dormitories are like giant beehives. The look of them makes a cold shiver run over me.'

Given her concern with social inequality, the extent of Eglantyne's initial snobbery about her fellow trainees, who all 'wear aprons and have accents', now seems surprising. But this was a very different group of daughters from those she had socialised with at Oxford, and although Stockwell ran a student magazine and had a flourishing literary society, Eglantyne chose not to join in. For their part, 'the girls ... just regard me as a pleasant idiot', she recorded miserably, 'and my first shock of absolute astonishment that anyone could venture to snub Me, has already given way, by frequent repetition of the experience, to the resigned belief that it is a part of the universal order'. Forced to re-evaluate her prejudices she soon admitted, 'it is a matter of perpetual wonder to me, that these people whom I used to think of as much as lamp-posts – the people … who live in villas all the same, on the edges of towns – have really got character, histories and interests and are sometimes very capable beings too … They teach me more, more, more than I can say.' Nonetheless not surprisingly Eglantyne made few friends at Stockwell. Within a few weeks her letters were sardonically marked from 'prison', and bemoaned the over-efficient, almost dehumanising management of the college. 'Indeed there is so much organisation', she sighed, 'that one is driven to wonder whether the thing organised does not disappear.' Whenever possible she escaped to explore London with friends, to church on Sundays, and otherwise to the college library, which she was relieved to find was 'really nice – often deserted'.

Eglantyne had gratefully accepted the offer to take her teacher training course over one year, instead of the usual three, in deference to her Oxford education. The downside was that she was thrown in at the deep end, facing 'a seething mass of students as a sham 3rd year!' Determined not to be rattled she 'wore a placid smile' but it is unlikely that she was fooling anyone. Unlike her lower-class peers Eglantyne had no personal experience of going to school, and no knowledge of many of the subjects like household management, sewing and nutrition that she was expected to teach. Not surprisingly classes hung over her 'like a thunderstorm', and when her student numbers increased from twenty to sixty she likened taking lessons to 'being put on the rack'. Nerves dulled her appetite and she soon lost weight and started catching every bug doing the rounds. Worst of all she discovered that she had no natural talent for teaching and flatly described her own lessons as 'execrable'. 'Yesterday I gave a lesson and they told me it was a "very" bad one,' she wrote with some self-pity. 'The assistant mistress, an uncompromising person with the clearest of brains, criticised me till there was really nothing left of me but my bodily presence.' Once again she felt as though she was physically disappearing under the various assaults made on her by life at Stockwell.

An escape route appeared when Sir John Gorst of the government's education department invited her to dine with a pioneering lady sub-inspector called Katharine Bathhurst. Dinner was quickly followed by an invitation for Eglantyne to become one of three new junior school lady inspectors. Realising that her sole qualification for the job was her social position, Eglantyne declined. Instead she determined to pull herself together and 'do better' at the job in hand by finding creative ways to catch her students' imagination. She soon brought history to life with stories and visits to the Tower of London, and, told to give a lesson on a rabbit, she bought a dead one and taught herself how to skin and dissect it. Slowly she was also beginning to learn what made children tick inside, and they began to respond to her unconventional approach. At the end of the year she had won many hearts if fewer minds among both fellow teaching students and pupils, and she later confessed that she only passed her exams when these allies 'brightly gave the right answers in a way that concealed the wrong questions'.

Eglantyne was also learning that her preconceptions about teaching had been misjudged. 'My life here is one long surprise,' she wrote to Dorothy Kempe. 'Everything which people told me about things here appears untrue … Indeed it is absolutely ridiculous for people to think that I make any sacrifice in coming here: it is the people I come amongst, who make the sacrifice – most nobly and generously – by enduring the affliction!' Teaching had turned out not to be about moral example, but passion, empathy and hard work. Sick of receiving pamphlets entitled 'Elementary Teaching as a *Career*!' Eglantyne swore she would write one herself, called 'Elementary Teaching as *Toil*!' 'I'd like to point out how these ladies entering the profession … under the banner of superior enlightenment, may rejoice in large possibilities of harmfulness, when they pretend to reform what they fail to understand.'

Despite her misgivings about the value of placing ladies in working-class schools, Eglantyne remained convinced that her own future lay in the classroom. What drove her was not a 'desire to be charitable', nor even 'love of the work'; in fact she seemed to be fully convinced that she had no talent for the job. 'I regard it as absolutely inevitable that I should fail daily in carrying through my work – perhaps for many years,' she wrote pessimistically. It was, she wrote, 'a matter of compulsion rather than enthusiasm ... Something tells me to follow, follow through thick and thin.' To Dorothy she explained that she had always regarded her work as her destiny. 'I can never resign myself to taking and taking, like a beggar, instead of giving like a Christian,' she wrote, 'but it seems so *odd* that the first should be thrust upon one by compulsion and the latter made so impossibly difficult.' Eglantyne's highly developed sense of social responsibility combined with her deep faith gave her no option but to pursue the vocation she had chosen. Furthermore she feared that if she abandoned her plans she might never have the opportunity, or the courage, to take them up again. 'My wish is so simple', she wrote in frustration: 'to fulfil the minimum of my obligations to my fellow men by a little work.' Children themselves did not seem to come into it.

Training completed, Eglantyne applied to various schools in the London docks and worst city slums, but to her intense frustration she was repeatedly circumvented by headmistresses unwilling to invest in an Oxford-educated lady who was realistically unlikely to remain in the position long. 'Can't get people to take me seriously,' she noted glumly, 'Headmistresses laugh in my face.' Finally, in September 1899, her Uncle James helped to secure her a position at St Peter's Girls' School in the lower-working-class neighbourhood in Marlborough, an attractive Wiltshire market town close to the ancient Savernake Forest. James had been the maths master at the prestigious Marlborough College for boys and now retired and recently widowed, he lived just three miles away at Ogbourne.

Ostensibly Eglantyne was supposed to spend her Sundays enlivening her uncle's invalid days, but no doubt the plan was also that he would keep a watchful eye over his rather unconventional niece, who should be at home arranging flowers but chose instead to spend long days teaching in a working-class school. Although it was never mentioned in their letters, it must also have been very much on Tye and Eglantyne's minds that Marlborough was the college where Gamul had boarded just three years earlier.

Eglantyne's main excitement when she came to live at Marlborough was that finally, at the age of twenty-four, she had a home of her own: an inexpensive cottage where she could enjoy the solitude she now habitually craved. From here she could easily cycle over to Avebury in the evenings, or tramp out across the Wiltshire Downs with Dorothy, Ruth, Charlotte Toynbee and other visitors at weekends. Still inspired to the simple life, she scandalised her uncle by insisting on living on her wages, and refused to accept the pretty new clothes he bought her as better suited to her youth and charm. In any case she had no need for them; she was utterly self-contained working on a new historical novel, researching Wiltshire history and archaeology, and being generally rather carried away by the luxury of her new-found freedom. 'The moon and the solitary star appear to be my companions and I am glad to have none others,' she gushed, 'Oh the depths of the silence of it: so full of meaning without a voice.'

Children are not known for their silence, and perhaps the solitude that Eglantyne loved so dearly was intensified by the noise and mayhem of her long days in the schoolroom. Compared with her London students however, Eglantyne's young country pupils were at least, she noted in that first autumn term, 'fresh and pretty ... steady and simple-minded'. On good days the school closed early so that they could go blackberrying. But on bad days, especially as winter set in, things were worse than Eglantyne had imagined possible. Conditions were miserable. There were not enough books, chalks, needles or fuel. Even in the spring Eglantyne had to make the freezing children clap their hands and stamp their feet every few minutes to keep warm. 'The noise of the former breaks the roof off,' she moaned, 'the thumping of the latter breaks the floor in ...' Her experience was only slightly softened by her developing relationships with her young pupils.

Eglantyne considered her school-class with humane concern but little sentimentality. Early on she described them with rather cool detachment as having 'pathetic faces with expressions of dull stupidity or animal cuteness'. She cultivated their interests and talents, and often visited them at home, where she was outraged by their appalling living conditions. But if anything she was bemused by their affection. 'They often wait outside the door of my lodgings and when I come out they fall upon me with shrieks and howls and inarticulate sounds resembling those of pigs when they see their food coming,' she wrote. 'They beam up at me all the way to school just as though they didn't know that I was going to bully them all day.' Her reservation was quite deliberate. Worried about the poor quality of her lessons, she took comfort from reading somewhere that 'no real or lasting harm is done to children by any teacher, however clumsy, if they have integrity of character'. The 'real evil', she decided, 'comes from attempts to attach them to oneself'. Eglantyne treated her pupils with the same spirited but rather aloof good humour that pervaded many of her relationships. Unable or unwilling to cultivate sentimental ties with them, she perhaps respected them more as individuals. 'She never talked down to a child's intelligence,' her younger cousins later testified. Instead she tried to help the children to think for themselves, and Miss Pullen, the headmistress, reported that although her pupils were not particularly distinguished in their exams, they did develop 'more than ordinary initiative and resourcefulness'. Eglantyne was, perhaps, a better teacher than she realised.

Preserving some emotional distance also enabled Eglantyne to observe her pupils better. She was fascinated by a discussion in *The Spectator* about the callousness of children, which the paper attributed to 'the fact of all animal qualities being predominant in children, the more distinctively human ones emerging only later'. Watching her pupils in the playground re-enacting the violence of the Boer War then taking place in southern Africa, or talking calmly about the deaths of sisters and parents at home, Eglantyne recognised this apparent callousness but attributed it to a different cause. 'Children have only the pain of the moment to bear, no painful retrospection and no anticipation of pain,' she wrote, 'and this is partly what makes them so irrepressibly cheerful and prevents their being alive to the possibilities of suffering ... This is a form of callousness', she concluded with some feeling, 'that I cannot help admiring.' 'I almost think I am getting fond of my children' she added wistfully in the closest concession to affection she allowed herself at Marlborough.

Eglantyne's spirits rallied over the Easter break, but her depressions returned with the new term. 'The prospect of returning to my work tomorrow makes me physically ill, my body and heart ache in concert,' she confided to her diary. 'If only I were going to the dentist tomorrow – but to stand mutilating the scripture to the detriment of inattentive children, I could shed tears.' The Rector's wife signed her off sick and wrote to let Tye know of her concern, remarking that 'she is a most loveable girl with the sort of longing for self-abnegation that would make a martyr but which in ordinary life is apt to make one tremble for her health'. Eglantyne meanwhile was writing to Dorothy, 'I have hailed every illness I have had as a means of temporary escape!'

Later that spring she hit her lowest ebb. 'The value of my work? Nil, the children have learnt nothing ...' she recorded miserably. 'So it goes: day after day into vacuum, and though one thanks heaven that they are gone, it is not without regretting that they are lost.' The work that was 'infinitely worse than breaking stones', the separation from her family, the physical strain and the concern that there was more harm than profit in the work was bad enough: the thought that this might last her lifetime was too much. 'The desire is in me once more to escape from the burdens and responsibilities of living,' she confided to her journal.

On a short break with Bun exploring the Vale of White Horse, Salisbury and Stonehenge in a pony and trap, Eglantyne told her aunt that she understood why solitary shepherds, from Joan of Arc to David, saw visions. Later she wrote that for her too that spring, 'in my trouble there came to me the face of Christ'. Eglantyne's vision arrived quite modestly and literally in the form of a 'cheap print' on her classroom wall. For Eglantyne however, finding Christ in her midst was a spiritual epiphany of the profoundest significance; a direct message from God in her moment of greatest need. She was now confident that she had been chosen to do God's work: 'He has chosen us, and not we Him,' she scribbled excitedly in her diary, to her sister and to several friends. At the same time, and with some deep relief, she could finally start to accept that this great work might not be teaching, and she drafted a short verse of thanks:

I have no words to speak my gratitude,
But, silent, lay my heart before thy throne.

Her sense of release developed over the next few months. By the end of July she confessed freely to her diary, 'I have none of the natural qualities of a teacher: I don't care for children, I don't care for teaching.' By October she was questioning her whole assumption, so strongly held before, that teaching had ever been her calling. Looking back she remembered passing the time on an uneventful family holiday when she was fourteen by hiding behind sand dunes to look down on the children coming out of school. 'In retrospect it is utterly impossible to account for this form of amusement,' she now wrote. 'How could it have given us any pleasure to watch the little wretches, the Dreadful Idea of closer acquaintance never entered my head.' In December she finally allowed Tye to insist that she gave up her job on the basis of her failing health. She still felt that it was wrong to suddenly throw over the work she had committed to do, but she was willing to abdicate the responsibility, in part to her mother, and in part to her freshly awakened faith.

Eglantyne never lost her interest in education. Returning to visit her uncle in early 1901, she took the opportunity to have an unofficial nose round some of the other local schools to see how they were run. 'It smacks of the customary futility of my proceedings', she wrote to Dorothy Kempe, betraying the knock that her ego had taken, 'that though I have so constantly refused to inspect on His Majesty's behalf, I seem to have no objection to inspecting on my own.' That spring she supported the controversial new Education Bill, which proposed to extend free secondary education to all, although she claimed 'it does not go quite far enough to please Miss Eglantyne Jebb'.[2] Two years later she took over the private history and literature education of two of her Irish cousins, Gem and another Eglantyne, inspiring them by taking them on regional history tours and by throwing 'a glamour of romance over everything she touched, whether it was factory legislation or the scansion of Chaucer'.[3]

Eglantyne also later served on the committee of the Cambridge Bureau of Education, overseeing the development of schools in the city. Education 'should not just be for the clever few, but to raise the standard across the entire class', she argued in 1906, before adding ruefully that 'teachers are needed with special, and it must be confessed, somewhat rare, gifts'. Increasingly she began to see education as an important way to prepare the next generation for active citizenship, taking the position that 'every boy and girl should be brought up in the knowledge that they have a ... duty to the community'. Ultimately education would also become a crucial programme area for Save the Children, promoting the pioneering principles of Eglantyne's contemporary, the British educationalist Margaret McMillan. But although Eglantyne would always keep up a keen interest in the area, by the end of 1900 she was sure that her own future was not in the classroom.

'The experience of elementary school work was one of inevitable pain,' Dorothy Kempe later commented. 'She did not really understand or care for the children – if they had made the absorbing appeal to her ... she might have stayed.' Ruth agreed; Eglantyne was 'not really "fond of children" in the way of normal motherly women', she commented. 'She was gentle, patient, unselfish, charming with them, and kept them happy, but they tired her very much and she was really happier when they weren't about generally. If she had cared for them individually as much as normal women do (instinctively, though not necessarily unselfishly) she could never have fulfilled her mission.'

Dorothy Kempe was right that it was not individual children that made 'the absorbing appeal' to Eglantyne. She did not enjoy teaching or directly caring for children; she found them loud, tiring and stressful. When duty called she would reluctantly look after nieces and nephews, but apart from her two teenage cousins she showed little interest in her younger relatives or the children of her friends, rarely even mentioning them in her letters. 'I don't think children appealed to her individually,' another college friend recalled, 'one had the impression of weariness, and perhaps distaste,' and her closest niece, Dorothy's daughter, later similarly remembered that Eglantyne 'was not a "child lover" ... at no time in her life did she take pleasure in actually looking after small children herself'.

Eglantyne never would have children of her own, and not only did she not express regrets about this; she never even seemed to consider it. 'All children are mine,' the educationalist Margaret McMillan often said, rather suggesting that she was left emotionally unfulfilled by not having had a family of her own. Eglantyne never similarly projected herself on to the children she taught or worked with; she had no need for such an illusion. She had not sacrificed the chance of having her own children in order to save the lives of the many; she had never wanted her own family. 'I suppose it is a judgement on me for not caring about children that I'm made to talk all day long about the universal love of humanity towards them,' she would write with dry amusement to a close friend after establishing Save the Children in 1919. Eglantyne did recognise the power of maternal sentiment, and was quite happy to harness this to generate support for the charity, but her own interest and passion for her life's work was differently motivated.

Does this make Eglantyne an unlikely children's champion? Aren't women, mothers and others, working in the area of child welfare meant to be motivated by irrepressible motherly love? Or is maternal love a distraction that must be put aside by any woman really wishing to achieve great things in the public arena? Throughout the nineteenth century women used maternalism strategically as a justification for social action either unconsciously or quite deliberately, both in private and in public. 'Oh my poor men: I am a bad mother to come home and leave you in your Crimean graves,' Florence Nightingale exclaimed publicly as she returned from Scutari in 1857 to reform the War Office, en route adopting a mantle of spiritual motherly responsibility for the dead and dying British soldiers. 'I address these words to you, as a mother to mothers,' Josephine Butler campaigned for the welfare of child prostitutes in 1881 after her own daughter had died in a tragic domestic accident. 'Listen to me while I plead for the children.' It didn't really matter if such statements were driven by sincere affection or strategic affectation; convincing maternal emotion conveyed moral authority, and sanctioned women's public social action. But by the start of the twentieth century the understanding of poverty and the premise of women's rights both began to shift, and social work became increasingly professionalised. As women gained new career opportunities, motherhood and maternalism again came to be seen more as a barrier than a bridge to social action. 'A thousand children have always seemed actually more worthy of self-sacrificing devotion than the "child in a sick fever" preferred by Mrs Browning's Aurora Leigh,' the childless Beatrice Webb wrote, implying that a choice had to be made between focusing on the well-being of particular individuals and working for universal welfare.

When I stopped working at Save the Children in order to raise a family I chose to prioritise my particular family, and their and my particular needs. As it turned out I soon felt that I would be a better mother if I did not dedicate myself completely to raising my children. I wanted always to have that energy and enthusiasm with them that seemed so hard to sustain twenty-four/seven, and I wanted them to have the example of a mother who lives some of her life for herself in the wider world, however much she loves her own family. However the irony of choosing to escape from some of my childcare responsibilities to investigate the development of Eglantyne's child welfare focus was not lost on me. Nor was the fact that Eglantyne herself never had children, or even seemed to like them much, yet remained committed to Save the Children from its launch to the end of her, admittedly short, life. My sense of empathy with Eglantyne waxed and waned. Unlike me, Eglantyne chose the universal over the particular. Her focus was not a personal, embodied child, but an unknown, universal, symbolic child, that represented social potential. 'The future of the world rests with the child,' she wrote the year before she died. But Eglantyne's concern for children was not entirely detached from the real children she encountered during her life. 'Grown-ups can adjust themselves to a certain extent … but children just stop developing', she wrote having witnessed the impact of severe deprivation on young children, 'and it is doubtful whether lost ground can ever be recovered.' Maternal sympathy is not a prerequisite for this kind of humanitarian concern and understanding. Ruth believed that perversely it was Eglantyne's guilt about her lack of maternal impulse, rather than a maternal love of children, that inspired her to dedicate her life to them. 'I sometimes think that the knowledge that she "didn't feel like that" ', Ruth confided, 'made her feel that she owed [children] a debt.'

Arguably motherhood also involves plenty of guilt. This idea plays itself out in my mind as a question of our times, both as I push the swings and as I shut the study door. But I don't believe that the question bothered Eglantyne much: motherhood, or her lack of it, never featured among her many later anxieties, unlike the nature of her love for her friends or her duties as a daughter. Certainly there was considerable social pressure for women to become wives and mothers in the early twentieth century, but in this as in so many ways Eglantyne chose to be a woman out of her time and felt comfortable with the choice she took.

Soon after she left Marlborough, on Christmas Day in 1900, Eglantyne wrote a poignant record of her 'Standard Three' girls. These moving and yet still slightly cool portraits show that Eglantyne did make an emotional investment in her pupils. It was not exactly maternal concern; it was humane compassion. Mattie Wild – later touchingly reinvented as Jessie Wild in one of her unpublished novels – Eglantyne remembered as having a huge capacity for happiness; she was kind and generous and should have been born a Duchess, but as a washerwoman she would probably die 'a hideous soured old hag'. Jane Russell was 'neither original nor imaginative', but had grown up among the books in her father's shop, and 'seemed to have sucked in knowledge from their presence'. Annie Howell was one of her brightest students, but already ill and unlikely to live long. 'Annie, your present ambition in life is to read right through the Encyclopaedia Britannica ...' Eglantyne wrote, 'but whether much reading is in store for you, alas I doubt.' Bessie Gray's mother had died in childbirth leaving her to help raise five younger brothers and sisters. 'Just a little bit of a thing she was in her long black dress, with a white face, a sad expression, scrubby features and puny arms ...' Beatrice Luck 'could never stand straight, but was always lounging and looking as dolls look when the wire that keeps them together got slack'. Finally Helen Willis: 'I almost wish Helen were too good to live,' Eglantyne wrote, 'for the world will spoil her, and I had rather she died.' Having written her final school report, Eglantyne prefaced it with the most personal words she was ever to write about individual children, likening them to wayside flowers, 'not cut back or trimmed in garden pots, nor nurtured in abundant soil and tended with care, but struggling up as they could, here blossoming in wanton luxuriance, and there pinched and stunted, but everywhere turning their faces to the sun':

Mine were such plants –
Mine no more! Nay, I will take you, my flowers, and place you one by one between the pages of this book, that you will wither not, nor perish. Your colour will fade, your scent vanish and your freshness be lost to my skill, yet for me you will live in here, the garden of my imagination.

And with that, Eglantyne closed the book, tied it with plain curtain ribbon, and put it, carefully, away.

Chapter 5

Happy Days, 1901–1902

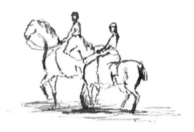

I never recollect being so happy before.

Eglantyne Jebb, 1901

Released from the misery of schoolteaching by a combination of doctor's orders and Tye's anxiety, Eglantyne returned to The Lyth in 1901. Here she and Tye tiptoed around each other as Eglantyne dutifully attempted to rest and recover. She was twenty-five but felt exhausted and bitterly defeated. Coming across her beautiful daughter reading in the garden, Tye described Eglantyne as 'the very pearl of the oyster – a tall white maiden as lovely as a dream princess, with golden hair, and the sweetest of dear human smiles'. But with little to distract her, and the atmosphere heavy with love and concern, The Lyth soon began to feel rather oppressive. Escaping on long walks through the open Shropshire countryside, the 'vastness of the earth and sky' finally lifted Eglantyne's spirits. That spring she took a series of short holidays with her sisters. In early May she and Lill went to the English

Eglantyne and Lill horse-riding around the margin of one of Eglantyne's letters to her aunt Nony, 1891

coast to paddle in the sea, and at the end of the month she travelled with Dorothy up the Rhine to the spa town of Bad Kissingen in Bavaria where they walked by the river, climbed the foothills of the Rhön Mountains where wild orchids grew, and went to church, a lot. At last Eglantyne began to enjoy the luxury of having no responsibilities. 'I am so delighted to think that I need do nothing at all,' she wrote to Dorothy Kempe, before adding less convincingly, 'Oh the horrid, dusty, noisy, pitiable world of human affairs – ugh! May I never get near it, touch it, go inside it again; how it jangles and creaks, and grinds one up! How glad I am no longer to be involved in the vain attempt to help on the machinery of society!'

When Dick left The Lyth to travel abroad, Tye decided that she had no reason to remain in Shropshire and that a change would do both her and Eglantyne good. Em, her eldest daughter, was already married and living in Ireland. For a while Lill, who had gained her Agricultural Diploma in 1897, the first woman to sit the exam, remained as the very able farm bailiff. Dorothy, the youngest, was finally away completing a year at boarding school in preparation for studying social economics at Newnham that autumn. So with Bun's ever-generous support Tye put the house up for rent, and took Eglantyne with her to live in Cambridge, close to her beloved brother Sir Richard Claverhouse Jebb. Bun was sad to leave The Lyth with all its ghosts and associations, but Eglantyne felt released. 'The moment of parting in a place where I have lived, is one of sudden and uncontrollable joy, and while I am saying goodbye with decent outward gravity, my feet are ready to dance in time with the marching of my heart,' she wrote secretly to Dorothy Kempe. 'Failures, follies, blunders, the heaviest part of my baggage, are all left behind in the detestable prison house, the beautiful world lies in front and the sun and air at once begin to heal the scars which the chains have left …' Strong language for someone who had enjoyed a fairly charmed childhood at The Lyth, but Eglantyne was raring to move forward again instead of dwelling in the past.

It was wonderfully refreshing to arrive in Cambridge as the new century stretched ahead. Cambridge, more than anywhere in England, combined a comforting, deep-seated traditionalism with a lively progressiveness rooted in the city's pre-eminence in the natural, and increasingly the social, sciences. Tye's brother Richard was among the many eminent academics drawn to the moral and social reform debate in the city. Shy, but sufficiently vain to be regularly 'amazed by his own tailor's bill', Richard was something of a figure of fun among the Cambridge dons. 'What time he can spare from the adornment of his person, he devotes to the neglect of his duties,' the Master of Trinity wrote caustically after he was elected a Fellow of the college in the 1860s. Although he and Tye were always close, affectionately teasing each other about birthdays and reading lists throughout their lives, Richard was gently mocked even within his own family. 'Poor Uncle Dick was the least considered in the Jebb household ...' one niece remembered. But academically he was brilliant. One of the elite Cambridge 'Apostles', he won the highest honours in Classics, was appointed Chair of Greek at the university, and earned international respect as the leading Greek scholar of his day. In 1891 he was elected Conservative MP for the University, a post he retained through three elections, and one that enabled him to promote his support for female higher education and suffrage. In 1900 he received a knighthood.

Soon after the Royal Commission had given dons the freedom to marry in the 1870s, Richard had married the cultivated and vivacious American émigré Caroline Slemmer. A Titianesque beauty, with dark eyes, auburn hair and a voice 'like red velvet', Carrie was 'a woman of whom any man might be proud' Arthur Jebb once rather tactlessly wrote to Tye, 'and her Americanism, so far from being a blemish, is as refreshing as a sea breeze'. Not surprisingly Carrie made quite an impact on Cambridge society. 'I understand that it was in this very house that you received three proposals of marriage in one evening?' she was once quizzed at a tea party, to which she replied,

'Nonsense, that would have been absurd; two of them were in the garden.'

Carrie and Richard entertained a great circle of friends at Springfield, their 'picturesque villa residence' in Cambridge, over the next forty years. Most were Fellows of Trinity, including George Darwin, son of the naturalist, whose wife Maud was Carrie's niece, and whose daughters, Gwen and Margaret, Eglantyne soon befriended. They also hosted Benjamin Disraeli and Thomas Carlyle among other politicians and social commentators, and many of the leading artistic and literary figures of the day, including William Morris, Robert Browning, Alfred Lord Tennyson and his son Hallam, Ellen Terry, William Thackeray, whose Becky Sharp Carrie liked so much better than Amelia, and George Eliot, who they counted as a friend. When they were visiting from America, Mark Twain and Bret Harte would drop by as well.

By the time that Tye and Eglantyne arrived in 1901, Richard and Carrie were well established in the highest echelons of Cambridge society. Carrie admired Dorothy when she went up to Newnham College, but she was enthralled by Eglantyne whose beauty, intelligence and quick wit made her sparklingly attractive and must have reminded Carrie of her own younger self. Soon she had taken her niece firmly under her elegant wing. 'My aunt does so much for me,' Eglantyne wrote happily, 'lending me her horse and half a hundred other kind things.' In return Eglantyne helped Carrie to raise funds for the Cambridge Women's Memorial for Queen Victoria, who had died in January 1901 in a sort of spirited admission that she did not belong to the new century. Carrie was a consummate lobbyist and Eglantyne learnt useful lessons in recruiting support from high places from her aunt, but overall she was not greatly impressed by her first experience of fundraising.[1] 'She said she felt like a Bishop and his Secretary as I followed her laden with papers into the houses,' Eglantyne described the scene to Dorothy Kempe. Nonetheless by strategically selecting what she called her 'victims', she could also proudly report that 'nobody has turned me away from their doors yet – indeed they cannot very well, as they … are all wives of Fellows or are otherwise connected with Trinity'.

Tye had had a house, which she called Inchmaholm, built at the edge of the city, although Cambridge was then small enough for this to be just a short walk or cycle ride from both colleges and town. 'Eleven fields face my bedroom window', Eglantyne recorded romantically, 'the house is a meeting place for the winds'. Soon it also became the meeting place of every kind of artist and author, once again fanning Eglantyne's own literary ambitions as the pleasures of wealth, connections and culture opened for mother and daughter. Eglantyne embraced her new life enthusiastically. By October she had happily settled into a round of dinner parties and college balls, picnics, poetry readings and general intellectual debate in the company of some of the most distinguished men and women of the time including the Darwins, Keynes and Trevelyans.[2] 'I never recollect being so happy before, which seems rather extraordinary after the collapse of my plans,' she now wrote breezily to Dorothy Kempe. 'I do not know whether to be ashamed of so much appreciating mere idleness and luxury. It is not perhaps that which I care for so much, however, as the feeling of being once more among friends.' Eglantyne dated her change of mood from an 'At Home' in Trinity she attended soon after arriving in the city. 'You know the feeling when you have been long cold and somebody rubs you warm …' she told Dorothy: 'Suddenly, in those bare rooms crowded with people, the world seemed to sweep back upon my gaze. I felt once more the steady, strong pulsation of life – I never thought it would come back. It seems odd that when you have failed yourself you should yet take such delight in the companionship of people who have done things and succeeded, but so it is.'

Left untold was another, very specific reason for Eglantyne's new-found happiness. Three years earlier her brother Dick had introduced her to one of his Cambridge friends, the charismatic Marcus

Southwell Dimsdale. Marcus made enough of an impression for Eglantyne to write home about cycling out with him that May, chaperoned by Gwen Darwin at Aunt Carrie's request, to collect cowslips in a field outside Cambridge. But Eglantyne was then just twenty-two, the end of her studies was looming, and her attention was closely focused on pursuing a socially valuable vocation. Romance was not on her agenda. In any case she had rather enjoyed being devastated, just a few years before, when her first university mentor, Mary Talbot, married and was consequently removed from college life. 'The mournful news about Miss Talbot is but true ...' she had written to Dorothy with self-mocking melodrama: 'O ye heavens! Ye earth! Ye sea! Ye sky! Ye fowls of the air and green herbs! Hear me vow an undying and perpetual grudge against Miss Talbot! Why can't she leave marrying and being given in marriage to the world's great motly crew of ninnies?' Lamenting that there were too few reasonable people to be able to 'offer one on the altar of matrimony', Eglantyne mischievously stuck pins into a wax effigy of the groom-to-be with her Crick Road housemates. Tragically Mary Talbot died in childbirth just two years later. Eglantyne was clearly not planning on risking that sacrifice herself in the near future. But by 1901 things were very different. Eglantyne had fluffed her teaching career and was back living with her mother. Perhaps it was not surprising then that Marcus, still conveniently unmarried, now held rather greater appeal.

Now a respected Cambridge don, Marcus was clever, witty, kind and charming, and adored by everyone who knew him. Essentially he was a college man, focused on his brilliant academic career, although he was not yet in the elite circle of scholars that included Eglantyne's impressive uncle Richard. An Eton scholarship had taken him to King's, where following a double first in Classics he taught Latin, then regarded as rather a lesser subject than Greek. Until 1861 King's had only admitted Etonians, and the connection with Eton still distinguished King's from other Cambridge colleges.

Incredibly Eton scholars at the college were awarded automatic degrees, creating huge tensions between old Etonians and other undergraduates. Marcus seems to have navigated these waters rather skilfully, forming close friendships with men on both banks. Many of these friends – like the popular writer Arthur Benson, the privileged and repressed son of the Archbishop of Canterbury, and college rivals like the Provost Shepherd, who taught Greek – were romantically attracted to young men, though not always active in their pursuit. Marcus was not. 'Whatever may be said of Latin literature', he once made a passing dig at Shepherd, 'I for one prefer the Roman virtues to the Greek vices.' Remaining single at forty in no way belied this; Cambridge dons still traditionally lived in their colleges and Marcus was simply happier devoting himself to academia than to the search for a wife and responsibilities of a family. Arthur Benson's warm description of a college friend in an essay based on his vast and detailed diaries might well have been inspired by Marcus. 'His table is covered deep with books and papers', Benson wrote, 'but he will work at a corner if he is fortunate enough to find one; and if not, he will make a kind of cutting in the mass, and work in the shade, with steep banks of stratified papers on either hand.'

In Marcus Eglantyne saw an intellectual partner who shared her love for books and study, but also someone with a sense of humour and a deeply romantic soul that seemed to echo her own. Like both her and her father, Marcus was passionate about literature, history, the British countryside and the beauty of nature. These interests merged when his imagination was stirred on solitary rambles through the Gog Magog hills outside Cambridge, while exploring the sites of historical events, or even just considering the pages of a map. Eglantyne recognised and was entranced by this passion for rural England, the 'smooth downs' and 'breezy wolds', and the traces of history left on the land whose secrets were so willingly revealed to the enquiring and imaginative mind. Marcus and Eglantyne would both later become enthusiastic organisers and guides on rambling and riding holidays, and in 1903 Eglantyne took two of her young Irish cousins on a series of history tours where they were encouraged to 'wander about in overhanging ruins' as Eglantyne began to instil this love of British history and geography in another generation.[3]

Marcus meanwhile would later write and publish rather rambling and charming essays on the places he had found of interest. Language, from 'polysyllabic Latinity' to the Welsh 'jungle of consonants', delighted him. He relished place names, enjoying their variety, suggestiveness and charm as much as their etymology. 'How absurd to take a ticket to Stoat's Nest! How absurd for Stoat's Nest to be provided with a platform, and a waiting room, and a parcels office!' he wrote. 'And Mumby Road; how depressing!' Yet other place names sent his spirits soaring. 'Lydiard Millicent', he wrote of a Wiltshire village, 'is an idyll in itself, and Compton Winyates a romance.' Did Eglantyne wonder what he made of the poetry within her name? Perhaps it was something he once commented on, firing her all too fertile imagination, as not long later she made her fictional Hugh Overford wax lyrical about the name Frieda Jones. 'Even writing it I linger over it, loving the very curve of the letters ...' Hugh gushes in Eglantyne's manuscript. 'And when I have written it, I look at it, and it wears the air of a magic spell.'

Eglantyne and Marcus had much else in common besides language and literature. Like her, Marcus had imbibed his romantic love of time and place from childhood, having been born and brought up at the family estate, Essendon in Hertfordshire. The first Baron Dimsdale, a pioneering doctor before Jenner's vaccination breakthrough, had made title and fortune by successfully testing smallpox inoculations by invitation, but nonetheless courageously, on Russia's Empress Catherine. A hundred years later, as a boy playing cricket on the lawns, or casting lines across the ponds for perch and roach, Marcus would regularly get a thrill from imagining 'that somewhere in the dark wood behind, the coach in which an ancestor of ours had travelled to Russia was rotting unheeded to decay'. It was not unfounded fantasy: the first Baron's (third) wife was a very good tourist and together they had brought back from Russia not only her wonderful journal, but also numerous portraits of Catherine the Great and even collections of the young prince and princesses' court clothing. Like Eglantyne Marcus had grown up surrounded by the romance and relics of a noble and adventurous family.

The Dimsdales were also an intellectually demanding family with high expectations of their sons, and more than his elder brother Charles, Marcus was the Dimsdale golden boy. Blessed with blue eyes, fair hair and sunny temperament, Marcus also had an easy intelligence, and every prospect of greatness. His father, the sixth Baron, was a busy and well-connected politician who supported suffrage amongst other progressive causes. His sisters collected letters from some of the great and good corresponding with the family in a leather-bound album: Robert Peel among many other politicians features, as do Tennyson, Dickens, Trollope, Wilkie Collins and Laurence Alma Tadema. The terrifying Essendon visitors' book meanwhile required contributions in verse. 'He loves to lie on the river's brink, it is there that he has quiet to think,' one childhood friend teased Marcus on these pages, while an entry by one of his sisters paints an endearing portrait of him as a conscientious undergraduate, trying to distract himself from impending finals results:

> Warm and weary, asleep he falls,
> tired by concerts, sisters and balls
> to dream weary dreams –
> of lists, without the name of Dimsdale
> and feeling sure that he must fail.

It is easy to see what attracted Eglantyne to Marcus. She would have recognised much in his childhood home and gently demanding upbringing: the cabinets full of eccentric family souvenirs and the walls heavy with obligatory portraits, ancient weapons and cases of stuffed owls and hawks, as much as the expectations invested in the children. Certainly her and Marcus's outlook was framed by similar experiences of growing up insulated by family history, social connections and well-stocked libraries, and aerated by a love of the great outdoors.

Above all, Eglantyne and Marcus shared a passion for riding. Eglantyne was a natural horsewoman; she had always loved long rides across open country and had joined her first hunt when she was just fifteen. Some of the most touching and personal lines she ever wrote were to horses, among them a 'Farewell to Jack', a cob who had been sold to pay death duties when Eglantyne was fifteen:

Short times were we together, Jack,
My horse without compare,
Two summers saw us race the breeze
Across the country fair.
Two winters saw us beat the turf
Along with pastures bare –
All that was left to me then, Jack,
Was a lock of chestnut hair.

Eglantyne had kept up her riding during college holidays, often alone on whichever working horses could be spared from the farm at The Lyth. 'To mount a very tall horse, which does not always stand still, is by no means devoid of interest,' she once wrote cheerfully to Dorothy Kempe. 'One has to bring him as near as one can get to a gate, climb up it, gather one's skirts, and give a flying leap through the air into the saddle: the question being, will he, or will he not submit to the process.' Soon she and her brother Dick would arrange to go out riding together for forty or fifty miles in a day, deliberately peeling off from each other once out of sight of the house so as to ride at their own pace. 'Make a point of saying nothing on the subject,' Eglantyne cautioned, before riding as hard as she liked, and over as many hedges as she chose. She would have cut a striking figure riding out alone, whatever the weather, especially on the day that a bough knocked off her hat, pulling down her auburn hair in the middle of a run. 'I was not going to stop for fifty hats,' she later swore, despite admitting being 'rather distressed at finding myself riding like the young lady in the advertisement of "Koko for the hair".'

Riding was considered good for Eglantyne's health, and it was not long before she was again racing through the countryside, no doubt scattering hairpins throughout Cambridgeshire. Carrie had kindly given her the use of her own fine horse, but this well-trained mare was more used to pulling an elegant and lightly built Victoria than racing the winds unharnessed. Soon Eglantyne splashed out on her greatest personal indulgence, her 'wonder horse', Estelle, whose temperament better suited Eglantyne's own fearless enthusiasm. 'Like the horse in Northanger Abbey it can't go less than ten miles an hour if it tries,' she boasted to Dorothy. 'It is perfectly quiet all the same, if you are content to go at its own pace, and race the motor cars!'

Riding out with Estelle across open fields, through woods and fells, was one of Eglantyne's greatest pleasures, both for the joy of the ride, and for the discovery of 'all sorts of strange, delightful nooks – haunts of ancient peace' out of reach by foot or bicycle. On such rides, as Estelle 'plunged knee deep through tangles of daisies and trailing vetch, and sorrel and clumps of flaming poppies', Eglantyne was again inspired to poetry:

Morning breaks, Estelle, Estelle,
O'er wood and wold, o'er field and fell
Morning breaks in glimmering gold
My wonder horse, my horse Estelle.
Beckoning to me is the long road,
And the hills are calling come,
And the wind is sounding
Marches, like a drum ...
We will rest beside the track-way,
When there falls the noon day hush,

Plunged in clover scented tangles
Where the grass grows long and lush.
There I'll lie and idly trace
The wanderings of tiny wings,
Through the leafy mazes
Where the goose grass clings ...

This was the daring and yet day-dreamy and romantic horsewoman
that Marcus now again encountered. Eglantyne for her part met her
match in Marcus who, after many years of solitary hacks and hunting
at Madingley Hall just west of Cambridge, was also a skilled rider.
Soon they regularly rode out together. 'I generally enjoy those rides,
when, as occasionally happens, the womenkind don't turn up,'
Eglantyne scrawled conspiratorially to Dorothy Kempe. 'Yesterday,
no women, but two men. Mr Dimsdale came, he is always a trump
card, from his knowledge of hedges, gaps in hedges, distances, nature
of soil, ditches, flowers, views, histories and last but not least, horses,
his own being matchless and a joy to look upon.'

The prowess of Marcus's horse is not actually certain. He himself
described it as 'mighty dull'. 'Perhaps like that horse in Tennyson',
he later looked back modestly, ' "he would have flown but that his
heavy rider kept him down". But I don't think so, for it seemed a
fixed principle with him never to leave the ground.' However there
is little uncertainty about Eglantyne's growing feelings for Marcus.
Even when 'the womenkind' did make a show, Eglantyne would
enthusiastically leave them far behind, making the most of the
opportunity to enjoy some unchaperoned time with Marcus. 'A
sense of oneness with things about her came over her,' Eglantyne
would later fictionalise these rides in her novel about Frieda and
Hugh:

She and her horse were one, as she felt his strong limbs fly beneath
her with delight, his excitement came throbbing through to her
and hers to him. His life and her life indistinguishably pulsed ... And

looking straight in front, always she fixed her eyes on the same figure, the man that galloped recklessly up hill and down dale. There in the midst of it all he was. He was framed in a tempest of joy.[4]

Although clearly attracted to Marcus, Eglantyne was also left uncomfortably conscious of a new-found vulnerability which grew as he failed to make any formal commitment to her. She reflected this in her fictional narrative by making Frieda wake in a panic from dreams about Hugh: 'It vexed her that since they had gone out hunting together he seemed slowly to be taking possession of both her sleeping and waking thoughts.'

Eglantyne's sister Dorothy had also met someone. In the summer of 1897 Lill's Newnham friend Victoria Buxton had invited Dorothy to join a Newnham–Trinity reading party in the Lake District. Victoria's brother Charles Roden Buxton, known as Charlie to his friends, was also invited. Like Dorothy, Charlie was passionate about poetry, and the two soon hit it off. 'We walk all the afternoon …' Dorothy wrote home dreamily, 'I am every step reminded of some part of Wordsworth – especially when the glory and the wilderness of the mountains raises a fever in the blood.' It was, she felt, 'an ideal kind of life'.

Brilliant as well as handsome, Charlie had taken a first in Classics and was President of the Union at Trinity College where he had studied under Richard Jebb. According to his proud sister, he performed his presidential functions 'wearing evening dress which showed off his good looks'. But like Dorothy and Eglantyne, Charlie had also inherited a strong social conscience from an impressive family. One of ten children brought up at Warlies, the somewhat ostentatious Buxton family home in Essex, he was the great grandson of Sir Thomas Fowell Buxton who brought the 1833 bill to abolish slavery in the British colonies, and whose wife Hannah Gurney was Elizabeth Fry's sister. Sir Thomas had believed that 'the great difference between men, between the feeble and the powerful, the great

and the insignificant, is *energy – invincible determination'*. It was a philosophy that Charlie took to heart, resolving never to be distracted
from a life of worth and purpose. Correspondingly although as a
child he had had every advantage, and was remembered for hunting
cats while dressed in a green velveteen suit, by the time he was an
undergraduate inspired by the settlement movement, he and his
close brother Noel were more likely to be found dressed in old
clothes and spending nights in 'common lodging-houses' to get
closer to the poor.

But Charlie was not looking for love any more obviously than
Marcus appeared to be. Eglantyne and Dorothy compared notes on
their slow-burning romances, the hopeful anxiety of each reassuring
the other, but in 1902 it all went disastrously wrong for Eglantyne.
On a clear bright day at the end of August Marcus took Elsbeth
Philipps, the well-connected daughter of the Prebendary of Salisbury
Cathedral, down the aisle. It was, friends agreed, a 'quite peculiarly
happy marriage'. Only Dorothy knew the strength of Eglantyne's
feelings and understood the agony of her distress. In March the following year the newlywed Dimsdales moved, with their servants and
furniture, into the Old Granary, part of the Darwins' converted mill
house Newnham Grange, just across the road from Richard and
Carrie. Accepting the unavoidable Eglantyne forced herself to pay a
courtesy call, but confronted with the reality of their happiness she
was overcome with despair. After the minimum polite stay she fled
the house in the direction of Madingley where Marcus used to hunt,
her mind 'obsessed' with reaching the local medieval ditch, although
'an inner voice' told her that 'if she went that way she would never
come back'. For some hours she dithered about in these lowlands,
romantically considering drowning her grief in the 'darkening
marshes', before eventually returning home.

Eglantyne's letters present an intriguing love story, but one that
seems rather one sided. How could this marriage disaster have happened, and why was it such a shock for her? Was Marcus, contrary to

all the evidence, a ladies' man, toying with her emotions while he courted several women on different bridle-paths? Eglantyne's feelings and expectations, and the force of her disappointment, were all too clearly sincere. Afterwards the affair was quietly put aside and Marcus was not directly mentioned in any later letters that survive, or in any biography. Letters are the biographer's fossils; the residual evidence of emotion in history. Without any surviving letters between them, or any at all from Marcus mentioning Eglantyne, it is hard to know how much this was a flourishing romance and how much a rose-tinted fantasy of Eglantyne's.

A call to the Public Records Office provided a rather shocking conclusion to Marcus's story. On 28 July 1919, an appropriately miserable and overcast day, Marcus, then fifty-nine and 'not being of sound mind, memory and understanding, did shoot himself with a shot-gun causing injuries from which he then and there died'. *The Times* records his funeral as taking place at Essendon three days later. A memorial service was held at King's College Chapel in Cambridge. Then, rather appropriately, the trail went cold.

I was also moving house, ending up twenty miles south of Cambridge, just as I was pondering the Marcus mystery. Out for dinner in the local Thai restaurant one evening, an ex-Save the Children friend who lived nearby mentioned, out of the blue, a friend of hers called Katherine Dimsdale … Sometimes I have felt I am sort of psycho-stalking Eglantyne, hanging around her houses, touching her possessions, riffling through her letters and emotions. It is an uncomfortable feeling. But it is wonderful when you are given the illusion by some unlikely coincidence that 'they' just might be stalking you instead.

Three weeks later I was invited to dinner with Marcus's grandson, Nicholas Dimsdale, and his wife, at his cousin Robert's romantically eccentric Hertfordshire country house. Dinner with the Dimsdales was a wonderful experience. Everyone except the dog, a deerhound, had a good thirty years on me, and all were much better turned out.

Elegantly efficient, Robert's wife Françoise ushered me through the fabulous entrance hall, any light in which had long since been soaked up by the mahogany staircase, clocks, cabinets, huge Victorian dolls-house and at least three stags' heads labelled from 1911. Carefully passing the dining-room so as not to disturb the table piled high with letters, chronologies and maps for Robert's biography of the first Baron Dimsdale, we had drinks in the drawing-room surrounded by portraits of various handsome Dimsdale eminents and several Catherine the Greats. The house was vast but so full of the concentrated souvenirs of ancestral country homes that it felt as though social history was the essential mortar holding it together, and if the pictures were unhung the whole place would collapse.

That evening, as we politely discussed manic depression and suicide in turn-of-the-century Cambridge over dressed avocado, it struck me how inconceivable this gathering would have been to Eglantyne. One hundred years ago a fragile Eglantyne, her ego just recovering from her miserable failure at teaching, was left heartbroken amid thoughts of suicide in the soggy landscape outside Cambridge. Some years later Marcus went into his library, where his wife would find him the following morning, and blew off the top of his head with a 'double-barrelled ejector sporting gun' in his own private moment of despair. And here we were, two generations later, companionably piecing together the strands of these lives that had unravelled so dramatically. Time was all that was needed to remove such once-insurmountable barriers, but more time than was allowed to either Eglantyne or Marcus.

Marcus had died in 1919 when Nicholas's father, Wilfrid, was just thirteen, and perhaps understandably Wilfrid had hardly ever spoken about him. Photos in the family album, however, show that Marcus had been a proud father; sharing a joke with his eldest daughter on the beach at Bamburgh where the family holidayed every year, looking stylish with children, toy boats and trilby at Overcourt Ferry, and sitting surrounded by all four kids on a windblown Royston

Heath. There had been five children, but the youngest, born in 1912, died three months later after drinking cows' milk infected with TB. Nicholas remembered his grandmother Elsbeth 'Elsie' Dimsdale very well. She was 'a remarkable woman', he told me, 'fearless, highly intelligent, and a pushy outgoing networker'. Elsie came from the well-connected Philipps family. Her father, the Reverend Canon Sir James Erasmus Philipps, was the twelfth Baronet, Prebendary of Salisbury Cathedral and a typical Oxford Movement man. Three of her five brothers, all MPs, once caused a sensation walking through the doorway of the House of Commons together – three giants each well over six feet high. They were all colourful characters and had meteoric careers, becoming rich and famous recovering lost family estates and fortunes.[5] Elsie was made from the same impressive mould. Known by her fellow students as 'the Phoenix', she was brilliant, dominating and rather arrogant at college where she read History at Somerville, leaving Oxford with first-class honours the year that Eglantyne went up. She went on to become the first woman to hold a research fellowship at Cambridge, where she founded the Women's University Club while Eglantyne was wrestling with teaching. Later she worked for the Ministry of Health, as well as undertaking considerable voluntary work. In 1912 she responded to her baby's death by co-founding the Papworth Tuberculosis Colony, the Cambridge Midwifery and Nursing Association, and throwing herself into a campaign to eliminate TB from the milk supply, work for which she was later awarded the CBE.

It seems that Marcus was attracted to forceful women with strong social consciences. Although in some ways the 'pushy', outgoing Elsie, more matador than doormat, did not appear a good match for the introverted scholar, perhaps her strength of character was what attracted Marcus most.

When Marcus met Eglantyne he had been suffering from depression for some years, and was probably in the down phase of a manic-depressive cycle. Soon after his early brilliance at Eton and King's, he became both academically and socially crippled by this condition, which sapped his energy as well as his confidence. His great published works, wonderful editions of *Livy* and his *History of Latin Literature*, which leaps off the page and once leapt off the shelves, would not appear until 1912 and 1915 respectively. Arthur Benson, Marcus's college friend who also suffered from manic-depression, recognised Marcus's 'weary fluctuations of energy, causeless dejection, [and] dark overshadowings of the inner spirit', and concluded that his friend was naturally susceptible to failure. Marcus must have been aware of this tendency within himself, and perhaps Eglantyne, with her bitter self-reproach over her own failure at teaching, her weak health and emotional vulnerability, seemed too much like himself for Marcus to take her on.

Elsie's cool confidence and consistent, unstoppable energy would certainly have presented an attractive alternative. Soon they moved to the Cambridge countryside, breathing in the wide views from their hilltop garden, and for some years the joys and distractions of family life did seem to help Marcus. But then his illness started to return more frequently; the depths of his recurring depressive cycle ultimately proving unbearable. A year after Marcus's final act Elsie collected his private papers and published a selection in an anthology called *Happy Days and Other Essays.*[6] Perhaps ironically the happy days that Marcus had recounted focused mainly on his childhood, the pleasure of solitary country walks, and not a little on his horse-riding.[7]

Margaret Keynes, the sister of the economist John Maynard Keynes, who soon became a close Cambridge friend of Eglantyne's, later reported that Eglantyne received several other marriage proposals but was so unselfconscious that they came as a surprise; a rather disturbing surprise, as she hated to cause distress. Eglantyne never married, and I could find no further record of these proposals. The romantic idea that everyone had someone destined for them, and that it was not morally right to give your love to anyone else, was fairly fashionable at this time. Possibly Eglantyne, romantic as she was, believed that Marcus was her one and only, and for a while refused to consider anyone else. If so she later managed to put him to the back of her mind very effectively. Perhaps she just never found another man she liked so much. In any case there were other, more positive reasons for staying single.

In the early 1900s there were still obvious advantages to be had in marriage. Financial security and the chance for a family were not the least of these, but neither particularly concerned Eglantyne, who had sufficient family income for her modest needs and tastes, and no desire for children of her own. Meanwhile Queen Victoria's advice to her eldest daughter that 'being married gives one one's position, which nothing else can' had long been challenged. Upper-class women now had access to higher education and respectable voluntary and paid work, particularly in the civic sphere of schools, hospitals and general social welfare. 'There is a marked difference in the education of women in the last ten years,' Eglantyne's Aunt Carrie had noted even in 1879. 'Every kind of advantage is thrown open to them and arranged for them, and as a reaction from husband-hunting they are throwing themselves into all sorts of things that promise an interest or a career.' Women like Elizabeth Garret Anderson, whose family Eglantyne's uncle Richard knew, Beatrice Webb and Jane Harrison, who taught Dorothy at Newnham, were even taking on the previously male-dominated worlds of practising medicine, public social policy and classical scholarship. The spirited and academically brilliant Harrison, who also never married, might have presented a particularly appealing example to Eglantyne, and it is quite possible that after her 'disappointment' Eglantyne began to believe that she too was reserved for greater things.[8]

Although many other women, including Garrett Anderson, Webb, and of course Elsie Dimsdale, did manage to combine marriage and vocation successfully in different ways, the fear that the two were incompatible was a common concern. 'In my days of deep depression I brood over matrimony', Beatrice Potter had written in her 1890 diary before accepting Sidney Webb, 'but it is as an alternative to suicide … That is *exactly* it: marriage is to me another word for suicide.' Even women not so vehemently set against marriage often had principled objections to making it the be all and end all of their existence. This was Gwen Darwin's position in 1905, when she offered her support to Eglantyne's current social project on the basis that 'I can't bear to just be a young lady living at home and waiting for someone to come and marry me as most girls are.' And some of Eglantyne's married friends, like Dorothy Kempe, now Mrs Thory Gage Gardiner, soon found their lives seriously constrained as a result of their marriage. 'Gardiner was such an old bachelor,' Eglantyne's college friend Maud Holgate wrote euphemistically, 'he never seemed to care for any of her friends to go there.' As a result Dorothy, who had been close to Eglantyne for years, lost touch with her almost altogether after her marriage.

Eglantyne soon also had examples of marriage within her own family to consider. Her eldest sister, Em, was living in Ireland happily caring for her schools inspector husband and their two young children.[9] Dick had also married in 1900, and was supported in his career as an authority on Empire by his wife Ethel. Lill was more adventurous. In 1902 she travelled across Asia Minor with her college friend Victoria Buxton, two rusty revolvers and a geological hammer to test the soil, rocks and agricultural operations. Their route deliberately crossed countries that, Lill wrote, had 'not yet been ticketed and docketed for the tourist', and highlights included being held up by armed men while floating down the Tigris on a raft made of inflated goatskins:

'Why, Victoria,' I exclaimed ecstatically, 'we're held up!' Victoria looked at me with a rather pitying expression. 'You've been rather a long time taking that in …'

'These [revolvers] are loaded', I said, 'but they seem rather sticky and rusty; I wonder if they will go off.'

'I do not think I shall fire', said Victoria, 'because I cannot do it
without shutting my eyes. I will just point …'

My heart suddenly warmed within me, 'Victoria,' I said, 'isn't this
a splendid piece of luck?' 'Glorious!' said Victoria; and we gave
ourselves up to the full enjoyment of the situation.[10]

When Lill's account of her adventures, unofficially edited by
Eglantyne, came out in 1908 it caused a sensation. But by then she
had already built up an impressive career promoting agricultural
reform, and married a rather uninspiring Treasury official. The wedding was romantic: Lill was dressed in white satin with a crown of
orange blossom. The marriage was not. The relationship fall-out
from Lill's hugely successful career, even after she had had two
daughters, presented Eglantyne with some salutary marital lessons.

Edwardian marriages were not all either domestic bliss or vocational blight however. Charlie Buxton was pretty much the inde-
pendent and politically minded woman's ideal marriage prospect. In
March 1904 he wrote to Dorothy, addressing his letter 'Dear
Comrade', to reassure her of his resolve 'never to sweep a woman
from her own unfettered judgements'. They were married that
August. Although Charlie's shares in the family brewery in London's
Brick Lane made him relatively wealthy, the couple quickly adopted
the simple, frugal dress and lifestyle that reflected their rather austere
Christian principles. Soon after their wedding they moved to a
working-class Kennington terrace, and on walking holidays in the
south of England they were sometimes mistaken for tramps. 'It is a
dream marriage,' their college friend Jane Harrison commented, 'I
have sometimes felt that marriage would be a desecration, she is so
original; but with this marriage I am content.'

As the only unmarried daughter, it was left to Eglantyne to dutifully care for their increasingly sick mother. At first she did this at
home in Cambridge, and later by escorting Tye around the tedious
health spas of Europe. Meanwhile Dorothy and Charlie dedicated

themselves to social and political reform, Lill doggedly pursued her remarkable agricultural career, and Em and Dick enjoyed the luxury of domestic happiness. Far from a tie that binds, to Eglantyne marriage might well sometimes have seemed to provide an enviable escape from family duties.

Had Eglantyne married Marcus, with their shared love of the countryside, history and writing, his ongoing depressions, and the likelihood of a large family of children to bring up, it is unlikely that we would now have the international development agency Save the Children. But for just one moment, in the spring of 1902, Eglantyne might quite cheerfully have exchanged her vocation for the prospect of marriage to Marcus Dimsdale. Instead, her broken heart strengthened her determination to live a life of social service, thus finding a rewarding escape from the tedious duties of an unmarried daughter and maiden aunt, without taking on the responsibilities of motherhood.

Chapter 6

Brief Studies in Social Questions, 1902–1910

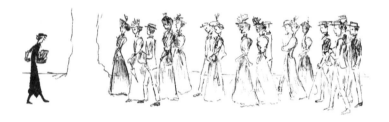

Large economic and political questions lie at the root of our relief problem.

Eglantyne Jebb

D espite developing quite different social and political perspectives the four Jebb sisters, Em, Lill, Eglantyne and Dorothy, remained fiercely loyal to one another throughout their lives. Occasionally they would collaborate bilaterally on research or writing projects, and they were always quick to support each other through letters, visits or introductions. But it was Eglantyne and Dorothy who were the closest, and whose lives were to become the most deeply entwined.

While Eglantyne was letting herself enjoy a social life in Cambridge, Dorothy was growing up into an increasingly serious young woman. Always the quiet voice of reason and restraint in childhood games, Dorothy was naturally both sensible and sensitive

Eglantyne, relishing the 'austere domination' of her ideals, draws herself in black and laden down with papers, while walking against the tide of fashionable Cambridge society, c.1906

as a child. Unlike Eglantyne she was handsome rather than beautiful, with dark chestnut hair and large, rather doleful brown eyes – although these were quick to light up with concern and determination whenever any injustice attracted her attention. Dorothy was just fifteen when Gamul died, and his death affected her perhaps more than any other member of the family. The two of them had been kindred spirits; fellow worshippers of Eglantyne's vivid imagination in the long afternoons at The Lyth, but when Eglantyne was elsewhere, equally happy to pass gentle hours together lying on their stomachs, investigating the wonders of the Shropshire fields. When Gamul died Dorothy developed an overwhelming desire to apply herself to the problems of human society in tribute to her brother's ambition to become a doctor. 'Dorothy' means a gift of God, and Dorothy's name suited her conscientious sense of Christian duty as much as Eglantyne's prickly wild-rose tag captured her own less disciplined approach to creating some meaning in life. But although Dorothy shared little of Eglantyne's wayward nature, from her unruly curls to her mischievous sense of humour, the sisters were intimately bound together not just by their shared love of books and nature, but by their unshakeable sense of social responsibility.

Dorothy's social conscience at first found greater direction at Cambridge than Eglantyne's. Eglantyne had chosen to study history at college, a subject close to her romantic heart and one that she hoped might help her to write the social novels whose plots and characters, particularly romantic intrigues, would sugar-coat the contemporary social ills she intended to expose. Dorothy took a more direct route to taking on social injustice, choosing to study political economy and social economics at Cambridge. She was therefore rather aggrieved when at first Eglantyne seemed to be spending more time on her horse and in her party dress than she was at her desk writing, let alone taking on Cambridge social work. Later Dorothy rather disdainfully referred to Eglantyne's first few years in Cambridge as her 'worldly period', but she nonetheless claimed that 'an intense desire to be of service left [Eglantyne] no peace', and this was also true.

Eglantyne had never entirely ignored her social conscience, even when daydreaming about Marcus, or plunging Estelle through vetch and poppies on her solitary hacks through the countryside. For a long time she felt torn between what she aspired to as her 'ideal life', i.e. a life of social service, and what she could not help but refer to as her 'natural life', by which she meant her surprisingly enjoyable new social life. 'I keep wavering,' she confessed to her college confidante, Dorothy Kempe, 'I am never quite sure which [life] it is I am living or trying to live, or which is the real life. Impossible to reconcile them – different sets of principles rule the two and almost every practical question settles itself in different ways according to the life one is in at the moment.'

Having struggled to live among working people for the last couple of years, Eglantyne was enjoying some time relaxing with like-minded people of her own social class. Meanwhile she salved her conscience by dipping in and out of social debates and contributing to charitable appeals as the mood and moment took her. She kept up her interest in education, occasionally visiting local schools, and becoming a rather inactive member of the Cambridge Education Committee. She also joined the executive of Lady Darwin's 'Cambridge Ladies' Discussion Society', a more genteel version of the Oxford inter-collegiate debating society, which discoursed 'on any problem they wanted to understand a little better'. Ebenezer Howard's 'Garden City Project', which advocated town-planning to benefit the community above corporate profits, also caught her attention. And in the summer of 1902 Eglantyne suddenly took up a new interest, joining Maud Holgate on a trip to Copenhagen to visit farming co-operatives, and only returning after Marcus's August wedding to Elsbeth. But none of these projects inspired Eglantyne enough to attract her full attention, and she moved between them as gracefully as she had once negotiated groups of friends at Lady

Margaret Hall, managing to show interest all round while avoiding any serious commitments. Still the desire to be of service persisted, it was too ingrained to fade from her agenda altogether, and once Marcus was a painful memory she began to search for a new way in which to make her contribution. There were plenty of options.

By the 1900s philanthropy and civic good works were well-established avenues for upper-class women to network outside the home and gain some public authority.[1] Meaningful social work had been at the centre of single women's lives for at least a century. Rapid population growth, industrial development and urbanisation all combined to make poverty increasingly visible during the nineteenth century, and as concern about social unrest developed, women's voluntary work seemed to offer a potential source of social cohesion. The idea that destitution was caused by individual moral failure rather than structural or economic causes had led to a harsh New Poor Law in the 1830s. Middle- and upper-class women, respected for having innate nurturing skills and drenched in moral authority, were seen as perfectly placed to promote the required moral standards among poor families at an individual level. Thirty years later this moral diagnosis of poverty became the founding principle of the Charities Organisation Society, popularly known as the COS, which championed the personal approach while working to improve the efficiency of the charitable sector as a whole. This was the climate that had inspired Tye to found the 'Home Arts and Industries Association' when Eglantyne was a girl, giving her daughters a powerful example of what women could achieve even within the constraints of social decorum.

Ten years on, enormous numbers of women were regularly volunteering, forming the largely unpaid backbone of the developing social services system.[2] In the late 1880s research by Charles Booth and others precipitated a re-evaluation of both the extent and the causes of poverty. As the premise of organisations like the COS started to be questioned, the idea that poverty could be eradicated by social reform began to gain currency. Women like Elizabeth Wordsworth, Charlotte Toynbee and Florence Keynes in Cambridge inspired Eglantyne not only with their service in social welfare but also their reform work in the civic sphere, in education and local government. By the start of the twentieth century the new generation of college-educated women like Eglantyne and Dorothy were less likely to be satisfied by the amateur philanthropy of their mothers and were demanding more professional roles. The Fabian Society, established in the early 1880s, had become the pre-eminent think tank addressing these questions. Instead of the diverse charitable initiatives proposed by various philanthropists, the Fabians called for a state solution through the overhaul of social services and promotion of a national minimum wage. This shift in perspective ultimately led to the pioneering liberal welfare legislation between 1905 and 1911.

Eglantyne and Dorothy had moved to Cambridge right in the middle of this dramatic shift in thinking. Dorothy could not have picked a better moment to study political economy under, among others, Alfred Marshall, a leading advocate of the New Liberal notion of citizenship that had been promoted by the revolutionary academic Thomas Green and his friend and disciple Arnold Toynbee. Knowing of Eglantyne's friendship with Toynbee's widow, Charlotte, Dorothy regularly updated her sister as she applied herself to the mysterious problem of what she called 'the motive forces' that kept the working classes in their 'horrid state'. Dorothy's own motivation in this work, part traditional Christian duty and personal moral conscience, part guilt and distaste, were perhaps more complex than the reasons she initially attributed to the working classes for their own distress. 'The more I have to do with them the more depressing do I find the condition of their morals,' she bluntly informed Eglantyne: 'liars, thieves – indifferent lazy beasts. I would do anything not to be surrounded by them.' Although this was still an accepted view, it was not Eglantyne's experience of the Marlborough poor.

Eglantyne's interest was piqued and chastened by her more dili-
gent sister, and from the spring of 1902 she occasionally joined
Dorothy at her lectures. But it was only after her return from
Denmark that she realised how much she was in need of a new occupation to fill the space left in her heart and her diary by Marcus's marriage. It was with some strength of mind that, after her depressing
social call on the newlywed Dimsdales, Eglantyne saw she was at risk
of slipping back into the despair that had followed her failure at
teaching. That afternoon she remembered it was Mrs Alfred
Marshall's 'at home' day. Pulling herself together she grabbed her
hat, pen and papers, and took the brisk walk round to the Marshalls'
house, Balliol Croft, arriving just in time for the weekly lecture on
political economy.

As Mary Paley, Mrs Marshall had been among the pioneering
Newnham students of the 1870s. After marrying her lecturer, Alfred
Marshall, she went on to become the first female lecturer in political
economy, sometimes teaching alongside her husband and co-
authoring his publications.[3] She was now, in Eglantyne's estimation,
a 'very undoubtedly sane and sage and middle-aged woman', which
was just what Eglantyne was looking for. After the others had left
Eglantyne asked for some advice on a suitable occupation. Mary saw
that Eglantyne was intellectually gifted as well as charming, but dis-
trusted her restlessness. Without any high expectations, she suggested that Eglantyne consider the well-worn path of philanthropic
good works while continuing to attend weekly lectures.

For some months it seemed that Mary's cautious assessment of
Eglantyne had been right; attending lectures and writing papers for
her new mentor remained the sum total of Eglantyne's engagement
in social issues. But in November Eglantyne started quietly going to
local COS committee meetings, as a visitor rather than a member, to
see for herself how cases of the 'deserving' poor were assessed, and
what impact the work had. Although she approved of the principles
of research and analysis promoted by the COS, Eglantyne was not

entirely convinced by the organisation's methods or motives. There was no suggestion at the meetings that there was a fundamental problem with the existing social set up, or anything inherently wrong with a system whereby the wealthy regularly distributed charity based on their assessment of the moral character of the less fortunate. In a typically tongue-in-cheek review produced for Dorothy Kempe, Eglantyne wrote that the people on the committee amused her, before sharply observing the 'diamond rings on very white fingers turning the pages ... case after case read, case after case ticked off, a jotting in the account book, an entry in the journal, then the flare of the gas lamp in the ugly dark room, and earnest faces coming out of the shadows, stories of drunkenness, debt, disease: one goes on then to the next tea party'. Eglantyne was not advocating government intervention, but something about the COS approach of charity as a benevolent gift, rather than social justice as a civil right, already made her uncomfortable. Unsure of her ground, she hoped that if she attended enough meetings 'the missing links ... might become apparent, [and] one will catch the connection as one turns the page, but at present I feel bewildered, like a person who in reading a book has forgotten to cut it – Greek one side, Chinese the other!'

In February 1903 Mary Marshall confronted her young student as to why, given her evident earnestness, she had not done more. Eglantyne had a fair idea of her mentor's opinion of her and nervously 'felt sure she would think it was owing to my love of dancing', but being suddenly asked point blank she gave the real reason without expecting to be believed. 'I told her I felt convinced I wasn't able to do it, always having failed in what I attempted, I had come to the conclusion that I would do nothing.' Already shaken by her failure at teaching, and depressed by her mediocre degree result and her inability to produce the social novel that she still felt sure was inside her, the last of Eglantyne's self-confidence had been crushed by Marcus's apparent rejection. But she had underestimated both herself and her tutor. Striking a judicious balance between sympathy and practical advice Mary pointed to Eglantyne's excellent ability to express herself in her political economy papers and suggested that this strength might be put to good use by writing on social and economic subjects. Eglantyne knew her well enough to appreciate that she did not hand out praise lightly, and soon she was writing excitedly to Dorothy Kempe that 'the suggestion of the possibility, and her apparent conviction about it has – well, it has kindled hope ... LIFE HAS CHANGED!' Life did not change immediately of course. A month later Eglantyne was still attending lectures and moaning that 'the economics has been as dull as last week's bread'. What had undergone a transformation though was her self-confidence; she now began to get almost nervous about the exciting height of her new aspirations. 'Like a man never confesses to the full extent of his debts', she at once worried and bragged to Dorothy Kempe, 'I am always much too ashamed to confess quite how impracticable and how visionary are the ideals from whose austere domination I am always attempting to escape.'

Mary followed up her conversation with Eglantyne by recommending her as an assistant to Florence Keynes, a leading figure in local charitable circles. Florence was an intelligent and handsome woman, with a permanent crease between her eyebrows, furrowed, no doubt, from thinking so hard and so publicly. She had inherited the dark eyes and hair of her exquisitely beautiful mother Ada, along with her passion for the COS and Liberal politics. Her father, John Brown, was the Congregationalist Minister of the Bunyan Meeting House, and not surprisingly Florence, their eldest child, had developed a sense of social obligation from knee high. Like Mary Marshall, Florence had been an early Newnham student studying alongside Jane Harrison and Helen Gladstone, daughter of the then Prime Minister. In 1895 she became the Secretary of the Cambridge COS, and started encouraging female students to take up social work. As a result numerous projects were set up including open-air schools, classes for children with special needs, and following the lobbying of Lady Darwin, the radical introduction of two women police officers. In between all this good work, Florence married John Neville Keynes, a respected Cambridge don, 'whiskered, modest and industrious … with firm habits and buttoned shoes'. Together they produced three handsome children, each destined for brilliant careers. John Maynard Keynes, the revolutionary future economist, arrived first, soon followed by Margaret, who was strikingly beautiful with thick curls of dark hair and piercing eyes, and just as independent-minded as her brother. Margaret and Eglantyne would later form a close friendship. Fair-haired Geoffrey was Florence Keynes' younger son, later a highly respected surgeon and bibliophile who married Margaret Darwin. As soon as her three children were out of the nursery, Florence picked up her community work again, becoming 'a familiar if unsafe figure on her bicycle' as she rushed between local good causes. This was the energetic but well-dressed woman in her early forties, a robust Liberal intuitively concerned with the welfare and rights of the poor and disenfranchised, to whom Eglantyne was introduced in 1903.

Florence's first impression of Eglantyne was that she was 'extraordinarily beautiful', with her red–gold hair in 'full bloom' and her white skin always quick to betray any emotion, which was apparently quite often. Eglantyne was well aware of this tendency, an irritating trait that she naturally passed on to one of her less-loved fictional characters who 'blushed easily, even when alone', and it cannot have made her first interview with the redoubtable Mrs Keynes any the easier. Nonetheless Florence was greatly impressed with Eglantyne's sincere social conscience, and rather amused that this attractive and seemingly nervous young volunteer was so grateful to be made use of, when many might think that the boot was on the other foot. Eglantyne, for her part, was delighted when Florence commissioned her to research and compile a digest of the existing charitable work being carried out in Cambridge. Despite its obvious merits such a project had never before been undertaken, and Eglantyne threw herself into the work enthusiastically. 'A hope has been dawning on me that perhaps I have after all been rescued from the ranks of the unemployed,' she wrote gratefully to Florence, continuing with typical good-humoured cheek, 'The COS must often receive letters of gratitude from persons it has set upon its feet.' By 1904, as well as working on her charity digest, Eglantyne was on the committee of the Cambridge COS, producing a series of short reports, and coming up with the innovative idea of a Social Training Bureau for young people, with herself acting as Honorary Secretary.

Later that year Dorothy, who had not after all been entirely focused on work, married Charlie Buxton. After their wedding the couple moved to London where Charlie was the Principal of Morley College. He was also a serving barrister, but soon gave up this career for politics. He and his brother Noel were among the leading New Liberals pushing for social reform in the 1900s, and they counted Leonard and Virginia Woolf, Leonard Hobhouse and his sister Emily, Bertrand Russell, and Sidney and Beatrice Webb among their many progressive friends. Although in principle Charlie respected Eglantyne and Dorothy's views, inevitably he was soon exerting a liberalising influence over the sisters.

Eglantyne had never been much interested in politics, unless debate touched on the social causes she was involved with. At Oxford she had come down theoretically in favour of universal suffrage, but watching the local elections played out in Marlborough in 1900 she quickly revised her position, coming to the conclusion that 'one man one vote is a horrible idea. It is bad enough that the fate of the county should be determined by such people as the high street shop-keepers, and that our representatives should have to go round calling attention to the price of coal and promising cheap candles,' but 'the ignorance of the voters is something incredible ...' Reflecting again in the quiet of The Lyth the following autumn she came back round to the extension of the franchise, blaming 'the smoothness, artificiality and material character of modern life' for making her focus on the petty and trivial. 'If one could live as a citizen, live as a Christian!' she exclaimed, 'try to live out one's ideals: instead of saying that they are impossible and then sitting down to sleep'. But for Eglantyne living out ideals did not necessarily mean through political engagement.

She was still describing herself a 'staunch Conservative' at a 1905 Christian Social Union conference attended by Henry Scott Holland, the organisation's founder, the Liberal MP Charles Masterman and the writer G.K. Chesterton. Still politically naive, she was rather surprised to find herself mixing in such progressive company. But this was a moment of great political upheaval, causing many people to re-evaluate their political and social beliefs. That year the Conservatives were thoroughly defeated in the 'Great Landslide' led by the Liberal MP Sir Henry Campbell-Bannerman, who was decisively returned as Prime Minister on 5 December. Campbell-Bannerman's premiership saw the introduction of many of the great Liberal reforms, including sick pay and old age pensions, designed to square concepts of individual human rights with the notions of citizenship, social reciprocity and responsibility that were at the heart of New Liberal thought. Charlie contributed enthusiastically to this public debate.[4] He was convinced that private philanthropy was not sufficient, not even appropriate, to tackle the root causes of poverty and social distress. Social progress would only be achieved through an extension of state activity, he argued: 'the power behind this machinery is enormous. Here at least is an organisation which can grip and grapple with social evils.' Nonetheless he respected and encouraged Eglantyne's social investigation in Cambridge, believing such work laid the foundations for state-sponsored reconstruction. Eglantyne now began to question her political perspective and enthusiastically support a range of Charlie and Dorothy's public campaigns for reform and social justice.

The end of 1905 was Eglantyne's political turning point. Her uncle Richard had become increasingly frail, described two years earlier by Arthur Benson as looking 'like a dissipated hairdresser … very much bowed, with tremulous leg on a bicycle'. He died in December 1905, aged sixty-four, prompting a by-election. Far from supporting the new Conservative candidate Eglantyne 'flew herself into the thick of the battle', even making street corner orations for the Liberal who stood for Cambridge in the 1906 elections.

Although she now permanently abandoned her romantic Toryism, Eglantyne never went as far left politically as Charlie and Dorothy, who would end up as active members of the Independent Labour Party. But in many ways Eglantyne was more liberal in social policy than her reverence for the past and her upbringing would allow her to be politically. Maynard Keynes once defined Liberalism in the following terms: 'Let there be a village whose inhabitants were living in conditions of penury and distress; the typical Conservative, when shown this village, said: 'It is very distressing but it cannot be helped;' the Liberal said, 'Something must be done about this.' Charlie had a more idealistic perspective. 'If I did not believe that the world is advancing ever nearer to the ideals of the best men … I should be a Conservative,' he wrote as a student. 'The real foundation of liberalism is the belief in the higher world than the world around us of palpable facts.' By either definition Eglantyne was a Liberal long before she admitted it to herself, but in 1906 she became an enthusiastic convert to the Liberal Party. Profiled for the 'Liberal Portrait Gallery' in *The Cambridge Independent Press* she explained, 'I was a long time realising that social reform on the part of the Conservatives … is like charity in the hands of Lady Bountiful – everything to be made nice and pleasant, but the "upper class" to be respected and obeyed. The corruption around elections opened my eyes, and I came to believe that no social reform could be of use which did not promote the independence of the people.'

Despite many distractions, Eglantyne's COS register of Cambridge charities was slowly progressing. It had evolved into a much larger project than Florence Keynes had originally envisaged in 1903 when Eglantyne grumbled to Dorothy Kempe that 'they want it done immediately, which is rather inconvenient for me'. In September Eglantyne admitted there was no way she was going to make her October deadline. She blamed the 'yards and yards of these hard mechanical letters' in response to her enquiries, along with the inability of charity secretaries to state the correct income of their organisations. 'It was really a relief', she wrote, 'when the Colchester Asylum for the Feeble-minded broke the monotony by thanking me effusively for my "kindness".' But in November she found a renewed enthusiasm for the project: 'I have refused all invitations to comfortable lunches and teas in the rooms of dear fellows of colleges etc., – and work all day,' she now boasted. 'I have just written to seventeen parochial clergymen …' Bun noted approvingly that Eglantyne's schemes were colossal, and Dorothy proudly wrote that 'only my Achilles of an Eglantyne' could take on such a project. But Eglantyne's research was so meticulous that Florence later commented with some palpable polite frustration that for Eglantyne, 'enthusiasm was … no cover for hasty or ill-informed action. She spared no trouble to acquaint herself with the causes of unsatisfactory conditions, and the best methods of dealing with them.'

Eglantyne was aware that her subject matter might not be the most riveting to the casual reader, and also that many Cambridge charities were in fact far from effective combatants of urban poverty. At one point she even sent a wry letter to Florence suggesting that the whole thing might be better written in verse, and enclosing the following sample:

This is the BRIGHT YOUNG WOMEN'S CHEERY DAYS ASSOCIATION.

ITS OBJECT IS: To practise standing without turning giddy on a high moral elevation.

THE METHOD IS: To start branches everywhere. They pay affil-
iation fees – and then they've all the privileges of the B.Y.W.C.D.A.

We've meetings too, in every three years at least one, and before we
have our tea the Secretary reads our report and tells us what we've
done ...

But rhymes aside Eglantyne was inspired by the project, seeing herself as continuing the important tradition of social reporting established the previous century. Increasingly instead of concealing their
slum explorations as shameful voyeurism, well-to-do philanthropists
had done their best to publicise them, using the information gathered
to promote a better understanding of poverty. Eglantyne now developed her charity digest into a comprehensive social survey, which
was only finally published in 1906 as *Cambridge: A Brief Study in Social
Questions*. It was not that brief, at over two hundred and seventy
pages, but was at least much shorter than Charles Booth's *Inquiry into
the Life and Labour of the People of London*, published in sections
between 1886 and 1903, on which it was modelled.[5]

'We make our occasional descent into the slums as from another
world, and are like men from Mars to the inhabitants,' Eglantyne
wrote engagingly at the start of her report, inadvertently perpetuat-
ing the middle-class idea of the 'strangeness' of working-class people.
And her use of loaded description, in the style that came naturally
after years of rather tortured poetic constructions, also reeled her
readers in. 'What has become of the orchards and the flowers?' she
lamented early on. 'Here is the blackened stump of an old fruit tree,
forlorn against the litter and rubbish heaps, here is a bit of bare
ground with more paper than grass ... The names alone recall the past
– Orchard Street, Flower Street, Blossom Street!'

Such passages also served to emphasise that a large part of
Cambridge's problems resulted from its transition from a small agricultural and academic centre into a modern city whose population had
quadrupled since 1830 without the requisite investment in housing,

sanitation, education or employment. Eglantyne had adopted Booth's distinction between the 'true working-classes' and the 'casual residuum', by which he meant the idle poor who should not be encouraged by charity. Though 'the residuum of society may need help most, it does not therefore follow that they will profit by it most' she wrote, proposing that 'private charity should ... leave to the state the hopeless and incurable cases'. The working poor were of far greater significance, and most of Eglantyne's report is given over to exploring the causes of their distress, including industrialisation and urbanisation with what she termed their 'evils attendant': unemployment, ill health, lack of savings, bad housing, limited education, misdirected charity and declining faith. Eglantyne was not opposed to the capitalist system per se, but critical of the uneven distribution of its rewards. It was a position she would never deviate from, arguing seven years later that 'instead of condemning wholesale our industrial system, what we should try to do was obtain a fairer division of the advantages'.

Meanwhile, borrowing the increasingly influential New Liberal concept of citizenship, Eglantyne saw the crux of the problem as being one of injustice rather than misfortune. 'The wretchedness of the urban poor can no longer be taken for granted, or their circumstances be regarded as unalterable ...' she asserted: 'we have created them ourselves and are responsible for combating them.' She was therefore dismayed at the lack of citizenship evident in Cambridge, the scant amount of voluntary work undertaken, and the limited use made of the franchise. 'Not half the voters concerned trouble to record their votes', she noted, 'we are all citizens bound to make the best of our town, our duties of citizenship ... the task of dealing with social problems, involves us all'. Inspired by settlement ideals of breaking down class barriers, she emphasised the importance of finding inter-class solutions, and argued that 'working men are the best people to solve working-class problems'.

Eglantyne's understanding of citizenship had an innovative angle however. Ultimately as she believed that 'everyone is born to work for others', she was struck by the importance of children as the next generation of citizens. ' "Boys will be boys" is a common saying,' she noted, 'but "boys will be men" is perhaps a fact which demands more consideration.' Attitudes towards children had changed dramatically through the Victorian era. According to George Trevelyan, whom Eglantyne knew as a 'fiery youth' fascinated with social problems, and who would later become famous as the Liberal social historian G.M. Trevelyan, 'enlarged sympathy with children was one of the chief contributions made by the Victorian English to real civilisation'. Certainly a raft of much-needed child protection legislation came into place in this period, and Ragged Schools, Barnardo's Homes, National Children's Homes, the Children's Society and the Society for the Prevention of Cruelty to Children were all founded between the 1840s and the 1890s.[6] Increasingly children were being seen and valued as national assets, upon which the future health and strength of the nation depended. Eglantyne's thinking was clearly influenced by this changing perspective as much as by the New Liberal ideas endorsed so enthusiastically by Charlie. Although still focused on the domestic agenda, her association of citizenship with children was a crucial step in the development of her social thought.

'To avoid the worst errors and mitigate the worst evils, if not to help in building up new and better organisations of society,' Eglantyne concluded her report, 'it is essential to act upon intelligible principles, and, if we reject one theory, to reject it only because another seems … to offer a better basis for increased justice in social dealings.' Her survey had endorsed many existing initiatives to alleviate poverty and foster better social relations, including donations of time and money through COS-endorsed routes such as education, savings and, rather more innovatively, a juvenile labour exchange, but she felt that none proposed a comprehensive solution. Eglantyne had begun to realise the question she wanted to address, but she was not yet ready to propose any strategic answers. 'Let us at any rate know what it is we do think on these subjects,' she urged pragmatically:

'it is for this, rather than for any particular set of opinions, that I contend.'

This seems quite a tame conclusion after a report which was in many ways innovative and challenging. Probably Eglantyne had modified much of her manuscript on the advice of Mary Paley Marshall, Florence Keynes and Florence's daughter Margaret, who was now Eglantyne's friend and ally at the Cambridge COS. As late as October 1906 Margaret was still sending criticisms and suggestions to Eglantyne, most of which were gratefully accepted, and some spiritedly rebuffed. 'If I have exaggerated (– either in the description of fact or the expression of principles)', Eglantyne told Margaret:

> I have at any rate weighted and modified my words until I know that they convey far less than what I myself believe to be true. Of course the condition of large towns is incomparably worse again – but then my vocabulary is by no means exhausted!! I only mean to say – what I have written may go beyond the truth, but of my idea of the truth it falls very much short. This has all along made it difficult to write – and the more I write the worse in this respect it seemed to get: my own ideas which, after all may be one-sided, kept coming out. But I will see if I can't tone down a few phrases.

A week later Eglantyne was sending off more chapters to Margaret, worrying particularly about her 'pious ending to the chapter about girls'. Incidentally anticipating the invention of the Post-it note, she continued, 'I must say when I think how revolting piety is to most of my friends, I turn a little green at the thought of their reading the book: I console myself however by the assurance that they won't read it. Wouldn't it be a good plan to have little red flags, stuck in the margin, so:- Flag pic The Christian Church etc. etc., as a warning to them where to skip?' There is no record of what Eglantyne's friends made of her report, but it was generally well received by the press, being reviewed in the *Daily Telegraph*, *Westminster Gazette*, *The Spectator*, various locals papers, and even some of the German and Italian press.

Almost exactly a hundred years after Eglantyne's report was published I found myself researching an essay on the development of her social agenda. Eglantyne loved libraries, often seeking refuge in them at The Lyth, in Oxford, and at her Stockwell teacher training college. It therefore felt appropriate to find a quiet desk at the British Library and search for Eglantyne by calling up some of the primary sources not requested for perhaps fifty years or more, in the vaults below 'Humanities One'. At the end of one long day looking at COS reports from the 1900s I was ready to pack up. I had achieved very little, having been rather distracted by the man opposite, who had sellotaped a pair of flexible plastic magnifying glasses in place below his bifocals. The whole lot kept slipping below his nose as he made his copious notes in felt-tipped pen. Feeling insufficiently committed I turned back to my own pile of books and opened a rather heavy anthology entitled *Tracts on Social and Industrial Questions, 1860–1911*. I was rewarded by finding a copy of Margaret Keynes' 1911 publication on *The Problem of Boy Labour in Cambridge*, still carrying an advertisement for Eglantyne's 1906 report on its back cover.[7] The advert quoted the review from *The Spectator* congratulating 'Miss Jebb and her friends' on 'an admirable little book …' How pleased Eglantyne would have been by this patronising praise is debatable.

Eglantyne had gone much further than her original brief for a digest of existing charities; her report was the first thorough social survey of Cambridge, and it later served as a model for social reports of Norwich, Portsmouth, Worcester, Liverpool, Edinburgh, Leeds and Oxford. Just how widely she had interpreted her commission was illustrated by another article in the *Tracts* anthology: 'The Cambridge Register of Social and Philanthropic Agencies', published in 1911, just five years after Eglantyne's report came out, and from the same Cambridge COS office.[8] A terse introduction to this alphabetical directory states, 'it is the design of this Register to furnish a kind of information always in demand but seldom easy of access'. Wasn't this what Florence Keynes had first commissioned Eglantyne to produce? It is tempting to imagine Florence sighing over Eglantyne's much more ambitious social report, and then quietly setting to work on the more basic register once Eglantyne had left Cambridge.

After she had finished her social survey in 1906 Eglantyne's health took another turn for the worse, and she took some months off, visiting Dorothy and Charlie, and spending time with her college friend Ruth Wordsworth who was ill with typhoid in Salisbury. No one, including the doctors, knew what the matter was with Eglantyne however, and Tye simply assumed that her daughter had inherited her delicate constitution and did not cope well with much physical or mental exertion. Eglantyne and Ruth spent March 1907 convalescing together at a 'delectable' isolated Dartmoor farm where Eglantyne threw herself into a new novel about a girl who escapes from a nunnery, reading passages aloud in the evenings to entertain Ruth. When they both felt stronger Eglantyne taught Ruth to ride. It was, Ruth said, 'a glorious experience of a month's solitude in company'. More trips followed. That July Margaret joined Eglantyne and Bun on a short walking holiday: 'The general objective of our expeditions is a wild and savage life with the possibilities of sudden death,' Eglantyne wrote to Margaret enticingly. 'I need hardly say we should much enjoy your company.' And not long later Eglantyne led Ruth and Charlotte Toynbee on a rainy riding expedition, Charlotte in a pony-cart but the others in the saddle, across the Berkshire Downs to the White Horse via the Silchester ruins. Eglantyne had evidently recovered much of her strength and energy.

1906 had also been a busy and sometimes trying year for Dorothy and Charlie. Their first child, Eglantyne Roden Buxton, had been born in July, and proved to be one of the few babies to inspire her aunt's affection.[9] Eglantyne joined them to help before the birth and stayed on afterwards, happily writing up her Cambridge research and later working on her current novel in between taking her turn at rocking the cradle.

Charlie welcomed Eglantyne's help as much as Dorothy, as he was busy fighting his first election. In the event he was not returned. 'Better that he should fail than sacrifice his standards,' Eglantyne consoled Dorothy. 'Charlie's mission, as everyone knows, is to hasten the day of juster social relations, greater equality of opportunity, a wider diffusion of happiness and well-being.' Soon Asquith's Liberal government began to deliver the progressive welfare policies initiated by Campbell-Bannerman, and Eglantyne witnessed the introduction of government pensions and health insurance, confirming her faith in political solutions and Liberal policies in particular. 'A great cause is entrusted to this generation: as great as to the generation of Cromwell and Wesley – the emancipation of the working classes,' she now enthused to Dorothy, adding with some foresight, 'We may have embarked on a longer struggle than we know.'

In 1909 Eglantyne's brother Dick, now well known as an authority on Empire and correspondent for the *Morning Post*, stood as an Independent Conservative MP. This time Eglantyne felt duty bound to accept the unmarried-aunt role of looking after Dick's two boys while he and his wife Ethel ran their campaign, but not without teasingly vowing to 'take my revenge by turning his sons into Radicals'. Dick lost his deposit. No comment made by Eglantyne.

That autumn Charlie and his brother Noel joined Bertrand Russell and the Webbs among others to support the newly formed 'People's Suffrage Federation' chaired by Emily Hobhouse. Advocating including all women in the proposed electorate, the position taken by the group was even more radical than that taken by the 'Women's Social and Political Union'. Soon Dorothy, Eglantyne and Margaret Keynes had all joined suffrage demonstrations, Margaret reporting from a march through Guildford in 1911 that 'a few men booed, a good many laughed' and that there were 'some motors … of ladies who were shocked, hurt, saddened!' But the cause failed to inspire much more active support from any of them. 'I wonder', Margaret wrote to Eglantyne, 'if suffrage speeches now can ever be anything but dull …' and later her plans to paint suffrage posters proved rather half-hearted when 'the ink could not be found so we played backgammon and drafts with the greatest of energy'. 'I hope that you and Eglantyne appreciate your position in a country where you are allowed to have … some rights, even if your voting powers are sadly restricted,' Florence chastised them. Margaret was gripped, however, by a visit to the Ladies' Gallery of the House of Commons to hear Lloyd George bring forward his great insurance bill. 'It was very interesting indeed – thrilling' she told Eglantyne; 'a plan which will affect closely the welfare of millions of the community being calmly laid out, one Utopian idea after another. And the low applause at intervals … the kind of noise the sea makes when each wave falls back into place over the loose shingle.'

Charlie was finally successfully returned as a Liberal MP in the first General Election of 1910. Although the overall result was a hung parliament without an effective Liberal majority, Eglantyne celebrated Charlie's seat with him and Dorothy, praising his persistence while commenting with new insight that 'this election has represented a much greater crisis in political history than any I have ever known and I have felt more deeply than about any question previously'. It was an amazing turn around for a woman who until five years earlier had always accepted the Conservative family line.

Charlie was voted out again before the end of the year. Part of his electoral difficulties was that although he was passionate about human and civil rights, he would rather hide from his potential constituency in the company of a good book than go out to solicit for their votes. Even as an MP he preferred to lecture on cultural subjects than campaign for his own policies, once producing a collection of literary essays under the title 'A Politician Plays Truant'. Lady speakers were still a relative novelty, but Dorothy's support for Charlie's election campaigns was more proactive. 'If one is not too anxious an election is great fun,' she wrote cheerfully to Eglantyne. A natural and confident orator, Dorothy was delighted to have found such a congenial way to serve both husband and society: 'How well I know that to try to live out your ideals is to plunge into fire storm and whirlwind. But so long as the stars of love shine brightly over head, all is well,' she continued rather tactlessly.

Back at home with Tye, Eglantyne was beginning to suffer another minor crisis of confidence. Increasingly aware that her own party political campaigning put a strain on her mother, she restricted her activity in the 1910 elections to publishing a non-partisan *Manual of Prayers for Private Use during the General Election*. Although not a campaigning document it was a sincere gesture that reflected her belief in the power of prayer, and her religious motive in much of her civil activities. 'Prayer and action should be as the weft and warp in life,' she wrote in the preface, 'for even he who seems to stand entirely aside from the struggles of his generation, will yet find that the closer he interweaves his prayer with what he actually sees and knows in the world about him, the nearer is his spirit drawn to the Visible and Invisible Realities.' The possible occasions Eglantyne listed for the prayers make rather more amusing reading, including a 'prayer for deliverance from the temptation to make false statements in political speeches'. Nonetheless Tye now gave up her Cambridge house partly because of Eglantyne's support for the local Liberal MP, leaving for the continent with Eglantyne in tow as her frustrated travelling companion.

Eglantyne's work would be closely tied to Dorothy and Charlie's political agenda for many years. Charlie was adopted as a Liberal Party candidate again in 1912 but, never a successful career politician, he would be expelled by his local Liberal Association within three years because of his opposition to the government's war policy. Eglantyne meanwhile had found her forte in social economics, working alongside Florence and Margaret Keynes, and the combination of these disciplines would inform all her later ideas. For

Eglantyne, poverty was neither a result of natural law or providence, nor purely a government policy issue, but a collective social responsibility that could only be addressed through the promotion of active citizenship across all social classes and generations. These were the 'large economic and political questions' that she now believed 'lie at the root of our relief problem'.

Chapter 7

Love Letters, 1907–1913

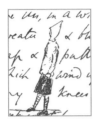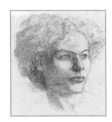

Margaret's friendship, the greatest blessing of my life.

Eglantyne Jebb, 1913

After dinner one evening on my second visit to The Lyth,
Lionel Jebb produced a mock-croc-print box-file neatly
packed with several hundred letters. Nearly all were closely
written in Margaret Keynes' neatly looping ink, much easier to read
than Eglantyne's scratchy writing. Many were carefully refolded and
tucked back into their envelopes; others had been stapled or paper-
clipped together, the rust drying out the corners of the pages so that
they had splintered apart again like peeling paint. Together they
formed half of a correspondence that ran for over twenty years from
1907 to 1928. Even for a time when letters were the main form of
communication it was an impressive cache, particularly between
1908 and 1912 when Eglantyne and Margaret were both writing
several times a week. When the intensity of their correspondence
raised eyebrows, Eglantyne demurred that writing regular letters was

*Eglantyne in her tobogganing clothes, drawn to amuse Margaret in a letter from Switzerland,
1910, and pencil portrait of Margaret Keynes by Gwen Darwin, later famous as the artist
Gwen Raverat, August 1910*

less artificial than keeping a diary, and Margaret told her mother that it was easier to write every day than once a month. Between themselves they took a different line. 'If you were here you would not think me importunate if I bid you morrow every day; and such patience will excuse my often letters,' Margaret quoted John Donne, whose poems she was binding, to Eglantyne in October 1908; 'No other kind of conveyance is better for knowledge or love.' Then, in case they had been slacking, in 1910 their Christmas present to each other was the promise of *daily* letters. 'My sweetheart, I have had no letter from you today,' Margaret complained teasingly on 26 December. 'Do you think suffragettes have been at the Congresbury postbox!' Taken together what emerged from the collection was a moving story of shared dreams, lonely mountains, love tokens, Hungarian frogs, and perhaps too much time spent thinking and writing.

'Miss Keynes is very good, but too nervous for me to deal otherwise than gently with her,' Eglantyne wrote rather patronisingly when Margaret started as her trainee assistant in the COS office in 1908. 'Exceedingly pretty and winsome', Margaret was just twenty-two, nine years younger than Eglantyne. But she already shared Eglantyne's uncommon passion for social service and over the next few years the two women formed a close friendship that would grow into the most complete emotional relationship of Eglantyne's life.

Margaret had grown up at 6 Harvey Road, then on the outskirts of Cambridge overlooking the grazing fields that stretched out towards the Gog Magog Hills. The house was double-fronted with large bay windows, but was still a slightly depressing-looking building, made from the dark yellow bricks once called 'corpse-bricks' by the Keynes children. Florence Keynes had decorated the place sombrely inside, as was then the fashion, with expensive dark blue Morris wallpaper, Raphael prints and heavy inherited Victorian furniture. Now a student residence, these have long been replaced by magnolia paint, cork-boards and fire exit signs, but two solid wooden fireplace surrounds still boast their carved 'K' for Keynes motifs, betraying the property's richer and prouder past. This had once been an ostentatiously intellectual household, where a rather precocious Maynard, not quite two years older than his sister, enjoyed testing his wit at Margaret's expense, once reducing her to tears by logically proving that she was just a 'thing'. Margaret clearly had a bit of a time of it – one rather recriminatory article in the Keynes' family journal ends 'moral deduction: it is better to be a naughty boy than a teased sister'. But overall, all three children, Maynard, Margaret and Geoffrey, got on well, and the elder two, closest in temperament as well as age, held each other in great esteem throughout their lives.

Unlike her brothers Margaret was not obviously academic. Having driven several German governesses to distraction, when Maynard and Geoffrey went to Eton Margaret focused on gardening and art while boarding at Wycombe Abbey in Buckinghamshire, the same school coincidentally that Tye had chosen against sending Dorothy to some years before. Although clever and creative, Margaret later forcefully eschewed all intellectual pretentiousness. Gardening, bookbinding and social work would be her lifelong passions; she would later set up a book-binders guild, and bind books for Eglantyne, and Maynard's friend Lytton Strachey among many others.[1] When Geoffrey followed Maynard to Cambridge he became great friends with the famously handsome young poet Rupert Brooke. Rupert would often visit Harvey Road, romantically reciting poetry by moonlight at the bottom of the garden, which was partly hidden from the house by a small orchard so that Margaret had to lean right out to watch from her bedroom window. Three apple trees still stand at the end of an immaculately kept lawn, but a new secret place exists in the garden now: the shed opens up to convert into a well-stocked bar. I imagine that Maynard, Margaret and Geoffrey, who went on to enjoy a lot of good parties, would all have approved.

Florence Keynes enthusiastically shared her passion for promoting social justice with all her children, but most actively with Margaret. Florence sat on the Cambridge Board of Guardians overseeing the provision of relief under the new Poor Law, and she would often take her daughter with her to visit the workhouse in Mill Road whose harsh policies and conditions she hoped to reform. The 'people in workhouses seemed to me to be undergoing a kind of punishment –', Margaret wrote in shock, 'punishment for being dependent on others'. Not surprisingly she quickly developed a sense of social responsibility to rival her mother's.

With their Cambridge family connections and shared interest in social welfare, it was inevitable that Eglantyne and Margaret would get to know one another. At the turn of the century everyone who was anyone connected with the university knew each other, and with so many large families mixing in the same circles it was not surprising that the Jebbs, Darwins, Keynes and Dimsdales were all, or would soon become, related through marriage. On one occasion Florence Keynes, serving as the first female Magistrate in the Cambridge Courts, tactfully excused herself from the Bench when Lady Darwin was being charged with dangerous driving, so as to avoid the embarrassment of one grandmother passing judgement on another within the same family. Florence and Maynard would also have known Eglantyne's uncle Richard, once an Apostle like Maynard, and well known as the University MP, and Maynard lectured Eglantyne's sister Dorothy when she was studying at his mother's old Cambridge College, Newnham, pronouncing her 'among the very ablest of the economics students'.[2] When Tye and Eglantyne moved to Cambridge in 1901 Margaret was still a schoolgirl, and although Eglantyne was soon introduced to Florence, Margaret would only have known her in the polite way that one knows one's mother's friends. Once the well-connected Eglantyne had proved effective at the COS a few years later, however, it was natural for Florence to place her rather directionless eighteen-year-old daughter as a volunteer within the organisation where she could keep a maternal eye on her, and where Eglantyne, now twenty-seven, might be able to provide some independent inspiration. Margaret made her first appearance in the COS office in 1903, but only started helping Eglantyne as a willing reader of her social survey in 1906. 'I am so grateful to you for your criticisms and advice. It *is* kind of you to take so much trouble for me,' Eglantyne thanked her. 'I wonder if you would mind calling me by my Christian name? I fear you cannot wish to, or you would have done so long ago ... But anyhow may I not sign myself, as I am, your affectionate, Eglantyne Jebb.'

The following year Eglantyne took on the launch and management of Florence's idea for a voluntarily run youth employment exchange called the 'Boys Employment Registry', or BER. Three years earlier as a member of the Cambridge Education Committee she and Florence had worked together to develop the idea of apprenticeships for boys leaving school at the age of twelve, most of whom became errand boys with no long-term prospects. The BER, which anticipated Beveridge's Labour Exchanges by two years, aimed to provide these boys with qualifications through further education where possible, but more often through apprenticeships in trades like building or boot-making. Eglantyne now became the registry's first Honorary Secretary. She was well supported in the role, with both Lady Darwin and Mary Paley Marshall on the committee, and the eminent mathematician Sir George Darwin auditing the balance sheets. But apart from a few weeks researching apprenticeship schemes in London, much of the early BER work was pure grind; going around petitioning various firms to take boys on in suitable positions.[3] It could be dispiriting work too, particularly for someone who always preferred writing policy to practical work, and had to force herself to make personal approaches. Nonetheless Eglantyne tirelessly applied herself to making the Cambridge BER an efficient and well-respected organisation securing boys permanent work in skilled trades. It is testament to her leadership and charisma that she achieved so much: few women, however respectable, championing unemployed and unqualified boys would have been able to change the entrenched attitudes among busy employers required to make the BER a success.

Early in 1908 Margaret, now twenty-two, became Eglantyne's trainee assistant at the BER, squashed in between the desks and filing-cabinets at the COS office at 82 Regent Street. It was now that Eglantyne described her young friend, at once protectively and patronisingly, in a letter to her sister Dorothy. 'She changes colour and assents in a great hurry to everything I tell her to do and, knowing how miserable she must be feeling inside, I am only asking her at present to do the easiest things,' Eglantyne wrote. 'She does a great many of these however most satisfactorily, and her mother makes me angry a little by expressing surprise in front of her.' Margaret had arrived at the BER with little self-confidence, nervous of raising her voice in public and scared stiff that prospective employers would snub her. She now bloomed under Eglantyne's guidance and soon began to idolise her new mentor, adopting as her mantra in times of uncertainty 'What would Eglantyne do?'[4] For her part Eglantyne appreciated Margaret's hard work, and was flattered by her evident admiration.

Over the next few months Eglantyne relied increasingly on Margaret as her erratic health began to cause concern again. That spring Margaret described her as pale, thin and ready to collapse. By the autumn her London visits to Dorothy and Charlie had become less frequent, the walking and riding breaks stopped altogether, and soon she was even forced to give up her much-loved horse, Estelle. Once again the doctors simply ordered rest. Mostly she accepted the prescription, but whenever her energy returned she could not resist the temptation to make a bid for freedom, sometimes walking in the fens where she claimed, to the exasperation of Margaret, 'that by dint of lying under damp hedges and lodging in draughty inns' she shook off her ill-health. Nonetheless after just eight months in the role Eglantyne resigned from the BER with the aim of returning to 'more congenial literary work'.

Eglantyne now exploited her ill-health as she had once used an uncomfortable college room: to protect her hard-won writing time. 'Of course she really rather enjoys not being able to see people ...' Margaret commented proprietarily. 'Contact with strangers makes her physically unwell.' Encouraged by getting a couple of articles published, that summer Eglantyne started work on her most ambitious social novel, *The Ring Fence*. Set in the Shropshire countryside of her childhood, the ring fence of the title is the high paling which surrounds the parks of two of its greatest landlords. Inside the fence is power, privilege and Toryism. Kept out: poverty, oppression and squalor. Written as an indictment of contemporary landlordism in the tradition of the morally enlightening Victorian social novel, Eglantyne's book is just about carried by its romantic plot, revolving around the passionate relationship between Hugh Overford, a selfish Tory landowner, and Frieda Jones, an idealistic advocate of cooperatives. As Eglantyne's literary confidante, Margaret enthusiastically compared her to 'a George Elliott or Jane Austin [*sic*], I don't know which yet'. But like much of Eglantyne's prose and poetry, although essentially inspired, *The Ring Fence* was rather laboriously delivered. Eglantyne fretted that it would be seen as both didactic and melodramatic, but she refused to edit it and was bitterly disappointed when it was never published. Margaret meanwhile had started her own social novel, *Vickery's Hats*, in which the eponymous hats symbolised the distinction between men and apes, and which broadly played off the acceptance of evolutionary Darwinism with a rejection of the callous ideas of social Darwinism. This too was destined never to be published, but Margaret at least had not given up her day-job.

Eglantyne had started preparing a rather reluctant Margaret to take over her role at the BER in December 1907. 'The courageous and conscientious way in which you set about working has often caused me a thrill of pleasure,' she flattered her friend. When it came to it the next spring however Margaret was at first shy of the responsibility, protesting that she enjoyed 'sheltering behind someone else's name'. She finally agreed a month later.

Taking Eglantyne as her example Margaret set high standards for her work, and demanded the same from her assistants, who included Eglantyne's cousins Gem and Eglantyne – the latter of whom Margaret found pretty and charming, but could not quite forgive for having Eglantyne's exact name. Where Margaret took a different approach was her personal involvement with the boys she was trying to place. Margaret loved children and knew all the boys on her books by name, often making personal donations for specific purchases. Occasionally she would even invite some over to Harvey Road for tea, and she would regularly make the effort to meet their families. 'Mr Rooke sits in a battered arm chair behind the counter' she described one visit to Eglantyne, an 'intensely interesting distraction is the proximity of Mr Rooke's head to a row of herrings – what will happen when he gets up!' But she also recognised the family's poverty, living in a house with walls so rotten that in some places she could see right through them, and she admired their dignity and happiness; traits rarely commented upon by charitable ladies.[5]

The BER now flourished under what Margaret Darwin called Margaret's 'spirited if unorthodox management'. Nonetheless, on a visit to the Darwin sisters in 1908 Gwen 'rather sand-papered' Margaret's pride by predicting what she and Eglantyne would be like at the age of sixty, and summing Margaret up as a 'philanthropist'. 'What a singularly vile word it is,' Margaret moaned. Philanthropy implied patronising charity, whereas Margaret and Eglantyne believed their work with the BER was at once pioneering and rooted in the enlightened idea of a social contract. Little wonder at Margaret's later pride when Maynard – who had already made the first annual subscription to the BER – praised her report on *The Problem of Boy Labour* as being 'extraordinarily good – so written as to be a most interesting and even moving document'. Margaret would run the BER for six years, and much of its growth and success, with over eight hundred boys on the books when she left, was due to her energy and devotion.

When Eglantyne left the BER in the spring of 1908, Margaret suddenly realised how much she would miss her. 'All the last year she has counted for more than anything else,' she confessed to her diary. Reading back it becomes clear that Margaret had already developed a bit of a crush on Eglantyne by January 1908 when she started inventing excuses, like borrowing a lamp or getting Eglantyne to sign a cheque, in the hope of catching sight of her. Soon her dreams were full of Eglantyne rescuing people, and she described her as 'a genius', 'looking very beautiful' and having 'infinite goodness'. 'I had not believed in such entire, unselfish goodness as there is in her …' she wrote in March that year, continuing:

> I hope no one but myself will ever read this, but if it should so happen that it falls into anyone else's hands, let them not smile, but know that all was said and meant in the utmost seriousness, and was of the utmost importance to me at least, and let them also remember that Eglantyne is not as other people and that she can do what others could not do.

Once they were no longer working together Eglantyne and Margaret developed a more equal relationship. Although Eglantyne was generally tucked away working on her novel, the two of them were writing regularly, and over the next year they often met in Cambridge. That July they spent a luxurious week in Yorkshire, where they went out walking and talking for ten hours at a stretch, and once eighteen miles to the sea and back. Later Margaret wrote miserably that she could never enjoy the same walks with anyone else. What they found so attractive in each other was not just a shared passion for social work but, underpinning this, an emotional and intellectual desire to find some higher meaning and purpose in life. It was a kind of spiritual affinity; in effect they were soulmates. 'Whatever happens I am yours,' Eglantyne wrote in November 1909, 'we'll keep our friendship unsullied and clear.' Writing of her love for Eglantyne a year later Margaret emphasised, 'it is based on so much too, my admiration of you, of your courage and unselfishness'.

However in 1910 Tye's health took a turn for the worse, and this, combined with the strain that she felt intensive social work had put on her daughter, persuaded her to leave Cambridge for the Swiss Riviera, taking Eglantyne with her. It was to Eglantyne's dismay, indeed almost despair, that these plans matured, as she had been looking forward to returning to some social work in the city – but as Tye's only unmarried daughter her responsibility was clear. 'Don't be miserable that you are leaving here. You don't know but you are unlike other people in that you don't need places and times to do your work,' Margaret wrote devotedly. 'You have done infinite good simply by being yourself. You yourself cannot understand. You say I cannot understand either, but I know that I am right. And it's not that I imagine it because I love you; it is because I love you that I know it …' Carried away with her own confession Margaret continued:

> wherever you are the world will be better for you. That you leave here is an incalculable loss to Cambridge, but Cambridge is after all only a little spot and we must not be selfish. Don't mind me saying all this, perhaps I can only hope that you will believe it. One thing is it is not all my own idea, many people realise that you can do wonderful, intangible, indescribable things. It is because you are good, true and faithful and unselfish.

But Eglantyne found she could do very little to make the world better from the health resorts of Switzerland, Austria and Italy between which Tye moved happily over the next few years. 'A hotel like this is for the rich rather what the workhouse is for the poor – the gathering place for the aimless and the homeless, the sick, the shiftless, the unfortunate,' she vented her growing frustration to Margaret:

The nicest are the sick, the ones I like least are the aimless; the shift-less are often eccentric but interesting, but the members of all these classes, if not idle by nature, are nearly always made so by the circumstances of their life. When I look around on them, and then think of you, I am indescribably thankful that yours is a rational workaday existence. It is the activities of life which make for the realisation of human unity.

For both of them their letters were now a regular source of much-needed comfort. 'I don't like to think of you going farther and farther away each day,' Margaret wrote that first long summer, 'though indeed the actual fact of your absence can't make me very sad because after all it's only a little veil over something so wonderful, I mean your friendship and love. I somehow believe it now and hug the knowledge and feel very glad.' And again a few months later she sighed, 'My own dear, beautiful Eglantyne, you don't know what a joy it is to get a letter from you ... I think you are as constantly in my thoughts as you were during the first two days. I love you very much and I belong to you.' 'It is indeed a red letter day for me when two letters come from you,' Eglantyne replied in one of her rare letters to Margaret that has survived, perhaps because it was left unfinished and might not have been posted. 'Your letters are like something very bright and shining and beautiful, and they make me feel as one feels when after a long cold numb day one warms one's hands at a leaping fire light in a quiet room ... Sometimes', she continued wistfully, 'I look at the second bed in the corner of my room and wish that you were sleeping in it. I should make you so comfortable and lend you my dressing gown and slippers.'

Eglantyne filled her lonely and 'useless' days by climbing in the Austrian Tyrol in long skirts and tightly buttoned jackets, and with slightly more abandon she learnt to ski and toboggan at Vermala, in the heart of the Swiss Alps, wearing a short skirt, putties and hoodie, all of which she sketched on herself in the margin of a letter to amuse Margaret. But with too much time and not enough company her letters soon revealed some painful soul-searching as she questioned her motives, and whether she was really needed to help set the world to rights. 'The hopes of the suffering children, the work of those who struggle with progress, is just as safe as before,' she decided rather miserably.

Eglantyne now recognised that what she loved in Margaret, and felt profoundly thankful for, was that unlike many of her friends who tried to 'forget and explain away anything that seemed absurd or uncomfortable' in her character, with Margaret she 'need not disown' her ideals. 'What they liked – wanted – was an intelligent appreciation of poetry, graceful companionship, anything but madness!' Eglantyne wrote, and yet increasingly she felt her passionate commitment to social service was like a 'madness running in my head'. Margaret, she felt, saw her as 'something I should like to be', and though 'far better than I am … not so different a person that it is hopeless for me to attempt to assume their clothing'. Little wonder that Eglantyne grew to care for the woman who released her from so much anguish by accepting, even admiring, her as she was. 'The reason I did not like going out into the world was that I didn't find God there,' she told Margaret, adding gratefully, 'I do not feel like that now … The love of a friend seems to have given me a clue to it … My darling you are wise and gentle and good and I love you more than I can say.' 'I am very happy, Eglantyne … [to] feel as tho' I'm some good to you,' Margaret responded happily. What is the pain of separation 'compared with the thrill of joy at the thought that you love me and that we truly belong to each other and that it can never be otherwise. I am devoted to you …'

In 1911 Margaret joined Eglantyne for three blissful weeks of climbing and conversation in the Tyrol and the Dolomites. Eglantyne kept a light-hearted record of their days on a series of post-cards. The first showed their Austrian guide, Alois Arnold, who Eglantyne told sternly she would never forgive if Margaret were killed. Alois laughed at them, and led them 'along the edge of precipices and across steep snow slopes' between mountain huts as they scaled the 11,520-foot Sugarloaf, Margaret repeating all the while 'Ich habe kein angst' (I am not afraid). It was a wonderful adventure in the clear mountain air high above the world, with enough risk to keep things exciting, and enough exercise to make the dry cheese they carried welcome at lunchtime and the straw mats in their shared cabin rooms comfortable at night. Margaret put a brave face on her return. 'In spite of missing you too much for words … you don't seem as far away as you have sometimes done', she wrote a month later, 'and often you are as near as anything. I can see you lying in bed like a carved figure and looking very beautiful.' Eglantyne found it harder to be alone with Tye again. 'I really seriously don't believe I should be able to live without you,' she despaired, adding in some confusion that she found her emotions both strange and foolish, and that she dearly hoped that 'someday … I shall come to love you better and therefore less dependently'.

Eglantyne's journal soon began to reflect her despondency as she described 'great rifted mountains … melancholy forests' and 'lowering skies'. At Oetz she was charmed by the silence and windless calm on the mountains before it snowed: 'the first flakes … slowly drifting down without haste, as it were, without purpose, upon the sullen, uncomplaining earth'. And the danger that had added to the frisson of her climb with Margaret was now evident in more depressing ways as she noticed 'ugly little paintings nailed against the trees', marking the tragic deaths of peasants killed while cutting hay or felling timber on the hillsides. Even so she could not resist a wry smile at the highly stylised pictures: 'evening clothes is the ceremonial dress of the country', she noted in her private journal, 'and the peasant for the purposes of death is disguised as a German waiter, and is pictured falling over a rock or being swept away by a torrent in decent black dress such as I can hardly believe he ever wore in life'.

Noticing her growing melancholy, Margaret worried that Eglantyne was not getting enough sleep, sent her tins of Ovaltine, and nagged her to spend less time on her novel or nursing Tye around the clock. 'Look here Eglantyne, it's madness,' she chastised her. 'You *must* have someone else to help you … You cannot possibly go on day and night. You'll simply get ill yourself.' But soon she recognised that Eglantyne's depressions were as much about frustration as exhaustion. Taking a different tack, she now argued that 'far worse than to be unhappy in the present is to lose faith in the possibilities of the future', and she responded to Eglantyne's blacker letters by teasingly comparing her to Florence Nightingale, whose biography she was reading. 'She had much more reason than you for depressions', Margaret told Eglantyne mischievously, 'because for ten years she could do nothing but enjoy herself.'

It was all very well for Margaret to tease Eglantyne: living in Cambridge and still working at the BER, her days were full and her conscience clear. But as well as BER news and requests for advice – Should she print extracts from the Factory Act for parents? Might they keep hens in the COS yard? – Margaret's 'often letters' to Eglantyne were also increasingly full of social gossip. 'I trust Margaret is enjoying herself in her quiet way,' her father once wrote home from a holiday in the Pyrenees with Maynard and Geoffrey. When not at the BER, everyone expected Margaret to be binding books and pruning roses, but now she was also beginning to enjoy a lively social life. Margaret belonged to an exciting intellectual and artistic circle, including her brothers, Bertrand Russell, Rupert Brooke and Ka Cox, Jane Harrison, Dorothy Lamb, Gwen Darwin and the French painter Jacques Raverat. 'What a place Cambridge was', Margaret Darwin enthused, for a time 'to be young was very heaven'. Margaret was one of the youngest, and increasingly in demand to lunch with Maynard, dine with the Stracheys and attend numerous Cambridge and London parties, often, as Eglantyne learned at intervals, wearing her favourite blue velvet dress with a silver trim.

Maynard proudly described Margaret to his on–off Bloomsbury lover, the artist Duncan Grant, as 'charming' and 'much more handsome' than their brother Geoffrey. Margaret had inherited a rather wild beauty and rebellious dark curly hair from her grandmother, but hers was also a forceful face, well fitted to present her increasingly strong opinions to the world: her childhood friend Ethel Glazebrook claimed she had the look of 'a bad angel'. Duncan Grant had been sufficiently struck to start a portrait in 1908, and two years later Gwen Darwin drew her in the gardens of Newnham Grange.[6] 'It is rather like; odd, but distinctly like,' Margaret wrote to Eglantyne while Gwen sketched. 'She lets me lie on the grass and move often, so it is easy work being drawn.' Gwen's pencil has caught Margaret looking up from her letter but deliberately gazing away from both artist and observer. With one dark eyebrow just slightly raised but lips firmly pursed, she seems to be almost visibly thinking about the absent Eglantyne, thoughts to which no one else is permitted access. Or maybe she is simply watching the rabbits, about a dozen of which were playing, she wrote, on the lawn. It amused Margaret that these clever people saw her on her own and could not guess how Eglantyne's friendship sustained her. 'We are so different yet in perfect sympathy,' she scribbled. 'It's like standing on a rock having you.' But Margaret's busy social life must have thrown Eglantyne's rather lonely existence on the slopes and in the lobbies of Spa Europe into sharp contrast.

A month later, in September 1910, Gwen announced her engagement to Jacques Raverat, and they were married the following June. Margaret, dressed as a gypsy, was escorted by her brother Geoffrey, 'looking lovely as a cowboy', to the celebratory party and later wrote to Eglantyne about dancing on the grass by the light of Chinese lanterns, and listening to Rupert Brooke recite poetry into the small hours. Going to weddings accompanied by her brother must have reminded Margaret of her own single status, but she was enjoying life and her thoughts were always with Eglantyne. 'You are my wonderful treasure which nobody but yourself can take away from me,' she gushed the same month … 'If you are my greatest happiness what can I do in return? I can love you, be happy with you, unhappy when you are unhappy, be faithful to you and try that you may never be ashamed of me Eglantyne – darling.'

That December when Eglantyne and Tye left for Oetz for another six weeks, Margaret's devotion reached new heights. 'My darling, no one, not even you, knows how much I love you,' she poured out her heart, continuing anxiously in another letter, 'Do you think you will get tired of it? I wonder – .' And on the 25 December she wrote 'to bring you what happiness [I] can on Christmas Day. It brings you love, I would give myself to you in my love.' Unable to give herself, Margaret instead started to send Eglantyne gifts: a copy of Shakespeare's sonnets that she had bound herself, and a hand-made puma belt. In November she chose a secret talisman 'which I shall wear until I see you … It hangs around my neck on a little chain.' In return Eglantyne sent a lucky charm, and then a coral necklace. After much plotting, in December they managed to share a room at a friend's house-party. In the new year Margaret wrote, 'I often dream about you, and last night I kissed you and hugged you in my sleep.'

Eglantyne and Margaret shared more than a close friendship or purely spiritual relationship. They arranged to share a bed when possible, and it is clear that sexual passion, if not physical sexuality, characterised their relationship. But intense female friendships were common at the start of the twentieth century, and sometimes encouraged as a precursor, and possible postponer, of heterosexual relationships. With lesbianism still not recognised in law or in polite society, active female sexuality was still automatically equated with heterosexuality, and romantic love and even emotionally and physically close relationships between women were usually accepted as 'pure'.

By 1911 however both Eglantyne and Margaret had realised that their friendship had crossed some line of social acceptability, and they started to be more discrete. 'I will say it inside an envelope', Margaret wrote conspiratorially, 'so that I can say "beautiful angel" out loud.'

Soon they were using pen-names, Eglantyne becoming 'Lulsy dear', 'My own darling Lulsy', and sometimes even 'naughty Lulsy', and Margaret signing off 'I love you most extremely specially, and I am, someone'. Later Margaret became Pollyanthemum, Polly or most often simply 'P'. Secure behind their pseudonyms, their letters now tentatively discussed friendships and marriage between women. There was no question that they loved one another and had committed themselves to a faithful relationship. In April 1912 Margaret wrote passionately of her 'frantic desire' to always be with Eglantyne, pledging that she would 'willingly give up the idea of children and everything else' were they able to marry. Never keen on the idea of children Eglantyne may well have considered her and Margaret's perhaps ethically 'higher form of love' as perfect. But by now Margaret had already met the man, a future Nobel prize-winner, whom she would later marry and have four children with. Eglantyne was about to be rejected again, this time in favour of a professor of frog anatomy.

Margaret met the eminent physiologist and Fellow of Trinity Archibald Vivian Hill, affectionately known as AV, in May 1912 through their joint membership of the Agenda Club, an organisation which aspired to make a practical, realistic and efficient business out of idealism. AV was an impressive figure, handsome, brilliant, and with a passion for scientific truth that was currently directed at the muscle mechanics of cats, and later giant Hungarian frogs imported for the purpose, but which he also extended to honesty, transparency and fair-dealing in all matters. Margaret was immediately struck by his combination of good looks, brains and social conscience. He is 'perhaps a little military ... 6ft in height with a very athletic figure and *I* think very handsome', she wrote to Ethel Glazebrook. 'Amusements – sailing, running and shooting ... he is very keen on social work and on the COS committee ...' 'I believe you would really agree with many of his views,' she told Eglantyne rather more cautiously. 'He is interested in the army without being jingo, Church but not bigoted, and a philanthropist.' In fact there was much that

Eglantyne would have disagreed with too. AV was humanitarian but also Conservative with both a big and small 'C'. Soon Margaret was politely arguing with him, 'Don't think me a fanatic. I am convinced that the majority of Conservatives are as honest in their convictions as are Liberals, but I think they are not in enough of a hurry ...' With equal tact AV wrote back, 'I wish you had written some more, as I am open to conviction.'

In May AV came to tea, in August he joined the BER committee, it would be dinner by the following January. Friends and relations on both sides encouraged the romance. His lot paid Margaret the dubious compliment that she need never be jealous because he had hardly ever looked at a woman before, to which Margaret responded wryly, 'perhaps that accounts for his present choice!' And Florence Keynes, possibly already with an eye to her daughter's increasingly intimate friendship with Eglantyne, was clearly just as keen on the match, informing Margaret in September that AV, just returned from a yachting holiday off Ireland, was 'bronzed by the sea breezes and looks more like a naval officer than ever'.

Although she liked AV, in 1912 Margaret was at the height of her passion for Eglantyne. In August, while AV was signing up for the BER, Margaret was sending Eglantyne her photo, and the next month she contrived to join her on a holiday to Killiney, the Jebb part of Ireland. Despite seeing AV more over the autumn, Margaret was still dreaming about Eglantyne in November, and at Christmas they were again discussing their 'marriage' and the possibility of buying a house together in Kennington, south London. Tye gave her blessing to both the house and 'marriage'. 'I believe she knows how much we want to be together and will help us,' Margaret wrote. Florence, who was perhaps more worldy-wise, was less accepting. 'Darling I felt rather horrid coming away this evening when you wanted me,' Margaret sent her excuses to Eglantyne as early as June 1911. 'But I asked mother and she said she *would* have thought it sentimental of me had I stayed!!'

Two days after Eglantyne and Margaret exchanged their 1912 Christmas letters discussing marriage, AV was a house guest at Harvey Road. 'Mother has a particular affection for AV Hill!' Margaret told Eglantyne, sidestepping the obvious reasons as to why AV might be hanging around, and why her mother might be encouraging him. Margaret continued to send Eglantyne passionate letters during the new year. 'P wants to kiss you vezy badly,' she wrote, and 'I want to kiss and hug you so much, and kiss you again and again.' But AV also cropped up in nearly all of Margaret's letters to Eglantyne in January 1913, writing her 'the most amusing letters' and discussing BER projects while she rode in his motorbike's wicker sidecar – affectionately known as 'Buster'. The most personal note Eglantyne gets by the end of the month is a reminder about the bill for her rather sad-sounding 'grey nightdresses'. Not surprisingly Eglantyne was getting ever more down in the mouth, leading Margaret to reprimand her 'You always seem to be in a state of lamentation when I am not with you.' It was a sharp turnaround from assuring Eglantyne that 'no dark and horrible fate can separate us', or worrying that the intensity of her love would bore her, just the year before.

Margaret was in a difficult position. By February AV was writing how her smile 'makes me happier than dynamos or Busters or whisky or frogs ever could'. She was nearly twenty-eight, and she knew that AV offered her the chance to have children, as well as financial security and social acceptability. Still clinging to Eglantyne while looking over her shoulder at AV, she wrote pathetically, 'I love you *vezzy* much.' Eglantyne rose above it, generously sympathising with Margaret and essentially giving her blessing. Probably Margaret was the only one left with any illusions when later that month AV rather sweetly proposed: 'perhaps we might promote a company for the advancement of humanity in which you and I will be partners, you to act as reformer of morals, and I as tinker of apparatus'. 'Of course I shall go and see what he means,' Margaret wrote to Eglantyne.

Having inadvertently walked in as AV proposed more formally to Margaret, Maynard described the scene to Duncan Grant, firmly implicating Eglantyne for Margaret's hesitation. 'Poor young man' Maynard wrote. 'He was practically in tears and had extraordinarily the appearance of having had his faced bashed in. Margaret was really calm and collected ... Tea had just been laid for two and their chairs were drawn up by the fire ... He was a pitiable sight and yet he's quite nice and really very suitable. Indeed it's not his fault that's responsible, but the fact that Margaret is more deeply entangled than ever in a sapphistic affair.'

Just how honest Margaret and AV were with each other will never be known, but three days later AV wrote to his mother, 'Margaret Keynes and I have agreed to promote a company by the title of Mr and Mrs AV Hill ...' Margaret meanwhile wrote to Eglantyne, saying that she was 'very lucky because she is going to get the best husband in the world, having already got the best friend and the best parents and brothers'. The engagement was official. 'She's in the highest state of elation,' Maynard updated Duncan, 'the family well satisfied, and even the sapphist not notably obstreperous. "She's much too sensible" Margaret said to me "to make a fuss."'

However sensible Eglantyne was, Margaret's desertion must have hurt a lot, and her face must have shown how bereft she was feeling at times. Margaret was not entirely insensitive to Eglantyne's feelings, and being so used to intimacy and honesty with each other, the two of them must have had some difficult conversations at this time. Eglantyne then wrote to reassure an anxious Florence about their resolution to continue their 'union' not through 'doing things together, but in the interest we will take in each other's different doings ... I ought to make my own life.' As good as her word, she immediately started making preparations for a trip abroad, this time alone and for work. She also dug out her diary, redundant while her and Margaret's letters had filled the last four years, and as coolly as she could, she evaluated her position. 'Many things have happened since I wrote …' she began:

> I have had Margaret's friendship – the greatest blessing of my life. Darling beautiful Margaret! How she has reconciled me to the world, to humanity, to life! It is she who has made me see and worship the good in human toils and interests and aspirations, just as I used to worship it in nature. She has interpreted life to me, through her I feel I can understand mankind as I never could before: it makes me realise a little more how Christ was needed to enable humanity to interpret mankind …

Margaret and AV were married on 13 June 1913. The day was overcast, but Ethel thought the wedding 'an ideal one'. A small notebook recording the presents lists an antique washstand from Tye, decanter and liqueur glasses given by Eglantyne's ever-fashionable aunt Carrie, and from Eglantyne herself, a sofa, to collapse on perhaps. Eglantyne had returned from her overseas trip just in time to join the dinner party the night before the wedding. In an emotional diary entry she revealed the extent of her personal turmoil as she realised they were thirteen round the table. Although she swore that she was not superstitious, she was alarmed to see that Margaret was the first person to rise from her seat after the meal.[7] 'I looked at her horror-struck,' she recorded later that evening. 'Her beautiful pale face had a faraway look – she smiled abstractedly and the terror of death clutched at my heart. It was not exactly that I feared for tomorrow or for the next day or for some time before the year was out. But some day I knew that no one would ever look again on that strange, significant face, so gentle, so proud, so brave.' It was not the usual response of a woman at her best friend's wedding, but it can be understood as the temporarily overwhelming grief of a disappointed lover. 'I love life, I love humanity, I love my relations, my friends, my pretty Margaret, and I can never forget that every day they are a day nearer the grave,' she continued in mounting anguish. 'Will all this beauty, this glory of joy be indeed extinguished in the night? Margaret's hair will turn to dust; pray heaven on that day I shall not be left to think "What's become of all the gold?" '

Eglantyne was not so much mourning Margaret as the end of their relationship, and six months later she was still lonely and grieving. 'I miss Margaret more and more … I miss her and I miss her, however things happen and wherever I am,' she poured it all out into her diary. 'This great affection of mine seems to shatter me and yet I do not believe it is wrong to feel it.' Once again her mystical belief in human oneness helped her to make some sense of her loss. 'Is the real separation perhaps not in death as we fear it but in life as we know it?' she mused. 'Are we born into differentiation – this terrible, walled-off, strangling, dark differentiation and do we die into unity again?' It was an idea, both around the importance of human spirituality and the essential unity of humankind, that was to become increasingly important to her.

Margaret meanwhile was enjoying her honeymoon with AV touring the Isle of Skye on 'Buster', where her greatest concern was how to fix the bike when she accidentally lubricated the belt with cream cheese. That December she resigned from the BER.[8] She was three months pregnant, and the first of her and AV's four children was born the following June; a daughter named (Mary) Eglantyne. 'Margaret looks very blissful and … admires her daughter very much,' Florence wrote to Eglantyne, who dutifully agreed to act as Godmother and opened a savings account for the baby. The two Eglantynes would see very little of each other however and, distancing herself even further, Margaret's clever and independent-minded daughter rejected her given name when she was teased at school and because, she later said, she did not like the feeling that she had been named to placate her mother's conscience over Eglantyne Jebb. Perhaps ironically she called herself Polly.[9]

Eglantyne and Margaret never lost touch completely, but their letters soon took on the polite interest of comfortable but distant friendship. 'I wonder how you are and all the children,' Eglantyne wrote rather dismissively in 1921. 'How nice of the children to be so nice! I shall love to see them some day.' They would never recapture their former intimacy.

Margaret had always been the more relaxed of the two about the unorthodoxy of their relationship. Her brothers were both bisexual, and as a young woman Maynard had brought her into contact with the Bloomsbury set who famously 'lived in squares and loved in triangles', and generally valued sexual tolerance. Despite her happy marriage it was clear to her children that Margaret later had some serious female admirers and hangers-on. Polly vividly remembered how much she hated to enter a room and find her mother sitting holding hands with another, often younger, woman who had a 'pash' on her. But when Margaret paid tribute to Eglantyne after her death, her focus was entirely ethereal. 'I feel it is a wonderful thing to have known so rare a personality, a person so little tied down by material things,' she wrote. 'In a way I think her friends cannot grieve very much at her death. Her body mattered to her so little, and her spirit must surely survive in some way.' Possibly then Margaret thought of her friendship with Eglantyne as in some way spiritual, without conceiving that it might have physical or sexual roots, but more likely she recognised that there was more to it.

Eglantyne for her part had always had intense feelings for her closest friends, women like Dorothy Kempe and Ruth Wordsworth at college, and had once rather disparagingly dismissed a fellow student at Oxford, 'you have affections, I have passions'. Her passion for Margaret was more intense than any previous friendship, but it does not follow that she necessarily saw it in different terms altogether. However the nature of pure love certainly caused her anxiety. In December 1913, six months after Margaret's wedding, Eglantyne tried to rationalise her emotional pain as existing only on a 'lower plane'. On the higher plane, she wrote, it is different. 'Here I am not unhappy, because she is happy and her happiness is enough for me. Here I seem to know she loves me still, for after all Love is a very different thing from the emotion it causes.' Although Eglantyne missed Margaret dreadfully, what she believed she craved was a union of the soul, not physical intimacy. How much she was perhaps deceiving herself about the nature of her feelings for Margaret is not really pertinent. She would almost certainly have been brought up in ignorance about homosexuality, the Christian position would not have given her any comfort, and unlike Margaret she did not move in circles where such things were discussed, so it is quite possible she would neither have recognised nor understood her feelings even had they been overtly sexual. The truth to Eglantyne was simply that she loved her friend on a 'higher plane'. 'Isn't there any love of man, except from love of God?' she returned to the question in a private journal the following year, before resolving her dilemma: 'it may seem that you care for the beauty of their face – but it is not true – you have unconsciously taken their beauty as a symbol of themselves'.

The ethics of biographical exposure are complicated. Attitudes towards sexuality have thankfully changed greatly since Eglantyne considered the nature of pure love. Today she might well have proudly considered herself gay, or she might have had less complicated relationships with many people and a completely different experience and understanding of love. Certainly however the most intimate and fulfilling relationship of Eglantyne's life was with Margaret, and even though it was ultimately not sustainable, her experience of love left Eglantyne a richer and more rounded person. Once she recovered her equilibrium after Margaret's marriage, she turned her back on personal romance, satisfied to dedicate her life to a new and selfless moral purpose. 'Of course it is very difficult when you see or write to a person every day,' Eglantyne confided in one of the most revealing and moving entries in her 1913 diary:

When you have grown accustomed to feeling their loving thought around you at every turn, when all the details of your life have awakened in them invariable interest and response – it is difficult then when this is missed not to feel a sort of frantic loneliness which would overthrow itself on human companionship wherever it was offered. After all people were never intended to live alone and I feel now as if I had been for years on a desert island, straining my eyes for the ship that does not come ...

I have one thing left that I want. I have some work to do.

Chapter 8

Relief in 'The Barbarous Balkans', 1913

This was the first time I had heard the phrase, shortly to become so familiar, 'without human feelings'.

Eglantyne Jebb, 1913

In the spring of 1913 Eglantyne travelled to the Balkans, a European war-zone, to oversee the distribution of aid for the Macedonian Relief Fund, leaving Margaret behind, in many ways permanently. This was Eglantyne's first direct exposure to the devastation caused by war and civil conflict. The miseries, suffering, fear and distrust that she witnessed, along with the terrifying deterioration of human empathy, would stay with her for the rest of her life.

Initially there had been some thought of Margaret and Eglantyne undertaking the journey together. 'I hope that [Margaret] hasn't been wearing herself out with Eglantyne's preparations!' Florence Keynes worried to Ethel Glazebrook early in 1913. 'Isn't it a blessing that she doesn't want to go too? I don't know what would have happened if it had not been for her engagement.' AV meanwhile could not understand what Eglantyne hoped to achieve from this dangerous visit and asked Margaret to dissuade her even though, he conceded, 'she will probably turn up all right again, in spite of her wild ways, and have lots of interesting stories to tell us'. Rather uncharitably he speculated that Eglantyne 'might be going simply out of pique that you had somebody who loves you more, if possible, than she does … Thank God I have finally prevented you from going anyhow.' With Margaret safely anchored at home, AV could relax. 'Please give [Eglantyne] my heartiest best wishes for her success,' he now wrote, adding rather disingenuously, 'I wish I were going too.'

It was Charlie Buxton, Dorothy's husband, who had first drawn Eglantyne's attention to the Balkans. Inspired by Gladstonian ideals of rights for small nations, and horrified by the repressive policies of the Turkish government of Macedonia, Charlie and his brother Noel had founded 'The Balkan Committee' in 1902 to campaign on behalf of the Christian populations living under Turkish rule. Operating from its office in George Bernard Shaw's London house under the presidency of the respected Liberal politician Lord Bryce, and with several friends including the journalist and MP Leonard Hobhouse and Charles Masterman – later head of national propaganda during the First World War – on its executive, the Balkan Committee enjoyed moderate early success. Responding to a massacre of Macedonian insurgents the following year Charlie and Noel set up the 'Macedonian Relief Fund', or MRF, as the independent relief arm of the Committee.

Macedonia has a long history of conflict. Until it became an independent country in 1991, the territory that forms modern Macedonia was ruled by a number of powers from the Roman Empire to the Republic of Yugoslavia. At the start of the twentieth century the Balkans had been under the rule of the Ottoman Empire for over five hundred years. Greece had won independence in 1829, and Serbia, which had gained some autonomy with two revolutions in the early nineteenth century, secured full independence with Russian support in 1877. With little industry or modern infrastructure Serbia, including modern Macedonia, was overwhelmingly agricultural, but Eglantyne found much of the scenery barren, with vast tracts covered with thorns and briars, and the land that was under the plough so insufficiently tilled that it yielded very little. At the same time Serbia's population was growing rapidly, more then doubling over the course of the nineteenth century to over two-and-a-half million in 1900, greatly increasing the pressure on the country and the region.

Charlie had first visited the Balkans to investigate the region's instability, with Noel and Charles Masterman, in 1906. He came away with a remarkably accurate impression of a group of 'small states with no mutual agreements', together comprising 'the danger point of Europe'. The following year Charlie's sister, Victoria, five years back from her adventures across Syria to Baghdad with Eglantyne's sister Lill, joined Noel on a similar fact-finding mission to Macedonia. Once back in England Victoria tried to generate some public interest and sympathy for the people of Macedonia by publishing an essay illustrated with photographs of atrocities taken by the European officers sent out since 1903 to inspect the local police but, like modern UN peacekeepers, without powers to prevent further conflict.[1] 'We publish these pictures with much reluctance,' Victoria wrote. 'We would gladly forget the horrid sights we have seen, and avoid harrowing our friends. But before evil can be conquered it must be faced, and to remove great miseries (such as those of Macedonia) it is above all essential that the public should realise them.'

The first photograph shows a father, mother and young daughter in traditional peasant clothes with loose white shirt sleeves, dark woven waistcoats, and pinafores over white petticoats. The daughter is barefoot and has rather pretty toes on show because she and her parents are all lying back on some picturesque hay-bales. Behind them a patchwork of fields fades into the distance. It is the very image of rural harvest-time in turn-of-the-century south-eastern Europe – except that this family have just been stabbed to death while working in the fields. The beauty and incongruity of the image, like a still from an art-house film, make it difficult to grasp the reality of the scene. Victoria's booklet contains six photographs of people who have been murdered, among them three peasants brought home to their wives, a couple left killed and mutilated in a field, and a schoolmaster hung from a tree with a white envelope containing the names of the intended next victims neatly slipped under the rope. The last picture shows a group of thirty-nine children at an Armenian orphanage at Monastir, now Bitola – an orphanage in part supported by the MRF.

In her accompanying essay Victoria argued that England was to a large extent responsible for the renewed conflict in the area, and therefore carried responsibility for the current situation. 'For the last four years, the newspapers have reported almost daily horrors from Macedonia,' she continued in a statement as pertinent today as it was then. 'By most of us these notices go unread. The facts given are so confusing, the situation apparently so complicated, the very names of the races concerned so remote and unfamiliar, that we turn away with a sense of relief that the completeness of our ignorance can be our excuse for lack of interest and of sympathy.' And like much modern campaigning material, Victoria's report ends with a thorough list of 'how to help', before her prophetic conclusion that unless reform is speedily carried out 'the bloodshed and anarchy that daily grows worse in Macedonia, will find their climax in war, which may possibly lead to a European conflagration'. Unfortunately few people, other than Eglantyne and those already converted on the Liberal left, either read Victoria's report, or were inspired by it.

The instability in the Balkans escalated rapidly. Alarmed by the Russian support that had enabled Serbia to increase both her territory and her regional status, in October 1908 Austria–Hungary successfully annexed Bosnia–Herzegovina with its population of nearly a million Orthodox Serbs. The invasion was naturally fiercely opposed by Serbia. The following year Bulgaria gained independence from Turkey, and in 1910 Greece adopted a more nationalistic military agenda; Albania led an insurrection in Kosovo; and Montenegro declared independence. While for many these national developments meant the restoration of the political, economic, cultural and religious freedoms suppressed by the Ottoman Empire, at the same time the region was descending into ever greater political rivalry and instability.

Events developed dramatically in late 1912 when the newly formed 'Balkan League' – a temporary alliance between Serbia, Bulgaria, Greece and Montenegro – declared war on Turkey. The aim was ostensibly to liberate Macedonia, although all the League countries also had their own, often conflicting, territorial claims to the area. The first months of the campaign saw great success with the Turkish administration driven out of Greece, Albania and most of Thrace, and the liberation of Uskub, now Skopje. Turkey's presence in Europe was soon reduced to a small region around Constantinople. But as the military front advanced through towns and villages across the Balkans, the human cost of the conflict began to escalate. Around one hundred and fifty thousand people left their homes in Macedonia and Thrace. Many of these were Albanian, mainly Muslim, some Catholic and a few belonging to the Orthodox Church. The Muslims were greatly resented for having lent their support to Turkey, and the Christians suspected of supporting Austria, a country with its own designs on Macedonia.[2] Thousands of Catholic Albanians were massacred by the victorious advancing Serbian army, and in a systematic programme of what would now be called ethnic cleansing, villages and crops were also destroyed. By the spring of 1913 food was scarce, and the homeless and hungry, many of them children orphaned or separated from their parents, were left without any support for the coming winter. A humanitarian crisis was unfolding in the centre of Europe.

Until 1912 Eglantyne had been following developments in the Balkans only from general international interest. Her own health, travel with Tye, writing and Margaret still claimed most of her time and attention. But that year Charlie and Noel decided they needed an emissary to organise the distribution of the MRF funds raised so far, and to report back on the effectiveness of the relief work being undertaken among both the Serbian victors of the war and the defeated Turks and Albanians. Already impressed by Eglantyne's experience in domestic development work, and recognising that with Margaret's coming wedding Eglantyne was in need of a diversion, Charlie asked her to undertake the mission on their behalf.

Eglantyne was now thirty-six and staring at a life of caring for Tye and local social work in Cambridge without Margaret at her side. Not surprisingly she leapt at the chance to channel her energies elsewhere. By January 1913 she was already busy raising additional funds for emergency relief in advance of her journey, which was to be undertaken as soon as there was a respite from the fighting. At first friends and family made sizeable donations, Tye leading the way with £50 – over £3,000 in today's money. But the fundraising soon proved hard going; much more so than collecting donations from reputation-minded dons for a memorial to Queen Victoria ten years before. 'It is very difficult to see how the need can be brought home to people,' Margaret wrote to Eglantyne. 'Are there any people who could give lantern lectures?' And again, 'It's very difficult to rouse people's imaginations where they think the countries more or less barbarous. Surely barbarians always live on nothing, they think.'

In 1913 it was rare for an English woman to travel alone around the UK, let alone to enter a war-zone in a region considered by many as 'barbarous', with or without a male escort. The exceptions were a few brave nurses who went out, either like the relief worker Mabel Annie Stobart offering medical support to the Bulgarian army in 1912, or more usually like Katherine Hodges with the MRF, and others with the International Red Cross, working among civilian populations. Serbia then had no national provision for the training of nurses, and the local middle-class women who volunteered were often so inadequately educated and experienced that the doctors Eglantyne later met complained that they caused more problems than they were worth, as 'when a man was badly wounded their only idea was to sit down beside him and cry'. Even in 1914, when the quota of foreign nurses had increased sizeably, the very presence of respectable women working independently in Serbia caused the peasants and soldiers no little amazement, and local children were fascinated by the nurses in their sensible English outfits, and especially by the stockings which lurked beneath their long skirts.

Eglantyne packed her long skirts too of course, but her modest selection of clothes was carefully chosen to be practical; little more than one spare outfit and a second pair of sensible shoes competing for space in her rucksack with her brush, sponge and soap, New Testament, notebook and seven pencils, one a modern 'ever-ready' design supplied by Dorothy. Her only luxury item was a Tyrolese brooch, perhaps bought with Margaret and taken as a memento of their climbing holidays, and even this would become a useful ice-breaker whenever Eglantyne met local women keen to find something to complement about her person.

Eglantyne's fold-out paper passport, 'adorned on one side with the flourishes of Sir Edward Grey's name ... and variegated on the other with the multicoloured stamps of the Balkan States', was issued on 18 February 1913, for entry to Bulgaria, Serbia, Greece and Turkey. Remarkably it still survives among the family papers once kept by Dorothy. For a while the survival of her papers was doubted even by Eglantyne, who was obliged to hand them over to an official at the start of her journey, travelling by train with the MRF nurse Katherine Hodges, through Bulgaria towards Belgrade. 'I was impressed at once by a due sense of their importance', Eglantyne confessed, and 'felt I could not be happy until he returned them; it was all our Bulgarian friend could do to convince me that they wouldn't be thrown out of the window'.

Eglantyne's fears proved unfounded, but they had been based on reasonable anxieties about the general disruption of war, and not from any particular concern about the honesty of Bulgarian officials. In fact Eglantyne was determined to stay non-partisan in keeping with the humanitarian nature of her mission. 'Even before I had left England I had made a secret resolution', she wrote in her MRF report, 'saying to myself "Beware of 'phils and phobes'." ' Securely entrenched in her bubble of impartiality she listened with interest, and sometimes horror, to those around her on the train. It was not long before her resolve to remain impartial was reinforced by the views expressed by a young Bulgarian officer returning to active service after leave: ' "They are not men!" he insisted. "Listen Mademoiselle! In the Balkan peninsular you will only find two races you will like. The Bulgars" ... he drew himself up, "and the Turks. The Turks are my enemies, still I recognise they are men. The Greeks are not, the Serbs still less. These people have not human feelings." ' This was the first time, Eglantyne noted, that she had heard the phrase 'without human feelings', which was 'shortly to become so familiar'. However in England she had already heard Lord Willoughby de Broke describe Albanians as 'wild, savage, wicked people'. Now, as she travelled around the Balkans, she came to appreciate how much religion was tangled up with race in politics and prejudice. To be Catholic in Serbia was understood to mean that you were not Serbian by blood, and you would naturally oppose Serbia. At Uskub a frail Catholic Albanian woman would breathe faintly into Eglantyne's ear, 'in her soft gentle voice', that the Serbs were 'wild people, people without human feelings', and even Eglantyne's trusted interpreter, whose name she Europeanised into Nicholas Pascal in an attempt to protect his Catholic Albanian identity, branded the occupying Serbs as 'wild people, people without human feelings'. Even on the last stages of her journey, travelling slowly home by train through Hungary, Eglantyne met 'a polite young man [who] began "Pardon me, Madam, but does not the cold

inconvenience you" ' as he reached to close a draft, before going on
to conversationally denounce ' "the people down there, the Greeks.
People without human feelings. Wild, wicked cruel people – and the
Serbs are just as bad." '

The repetition of the same or very similar phrases suggests that
part of what Eglantyne heard was the result of her own memory or
interpretation. However the essential impression that faith and
nationality had become the pretext for a process of dehumanisation
upon which fear, prejudice and sustained conflict depended was a
compelling truth that permanently influenced Eglantyne's outlook
and future policy work. For her distinctions of nationality and faith
had permanently lost their importance. Even the year she died
Eglantyne was still insisting that 'a leading characteristic of modern
thought is its insistence upon the unity of mankind'.

There was at first little evidence of war when Eglantyne arrived at
Belgrade to spend a few cold February days admiring the city while
waiting for her onward rail passes to be confirmed. Only the absence
of young men, various interrupted building projects around the city,
and the conversation carried out in front of a large map of the peninsular hanging in her hotel café betrayed the ongoing conflict, and
even that competed with a band playing Slav songs. Furthermore to
her surprise instead of territorial claims Eglantyne found herself discussing women's rights with her hostess, an Irish woman married to
a retired Serbian official who passionately claimed she would like to
see a few windows broken in Belgrade for *that* cause. Tucked away
discretely the evidence was there however, in the military hospital
where Eglantyne and Katherine Hodges distributed cigarettes on
their second day, in the impoverished civilian hospital, and in the
growing number of schools and nurseries for orphans, and
almshouses for war-widows. Provision might have been 'primitive'
in Eglantyne's eyes, but at least some welfare was being organised.

Eglantyne's general impression of security continued when she
arrived at Uskub, the ancient capital of old Serbia – now Skopje, the

capital of Macedonia – which was at that point many miles from the front. Perhaps thinking ruefully of Lill's adventures in Syria, Eglantyne had been privately relishing the idea of her personal danger far away from the increasingly claustrophobic comforts and company of Cambridge. Now she reported sulkily that she would 'have liked a little adventure', but 'everything was in absolute order, there were houses, shops, restaurants, poplar trees and no giraffes, just as anywhere else … no adventure to be had, and such are the disappointments of life'.

Slowly it dawned on Eglantyne that men saw action during war, but women and children 'suffer most because ingloriously. The soldiers are the "Heroes of Europe", but it is the thousands of sick and starving and helpless and deserted folk, whose misery is unrelieved by the sense of adventure and victory, who pay the price for war's arbitrament.' Thus Mr Peckham, the English Consul, was able to regale Eglantyne with the story of his part in the surrender of Uskub, involving raising a white flag made of a pillow-case strung on a broomstick, and of the gentlemanly codes of war that required the consuls to provide their pocket handkerchiefs so that they might be blindfolded for parley. The first thing he 'instinctively' did on arrival for talks, he told Eglantyne, was 'turn and shake hands with the soldier who had been leading him'. This cheery boys-own adventure was obviously not typical of the brutal conflict still taking place in the villages and countryside across the Balkans, but it was the first eye-witness account that Eglantyne had heard, and she was not overly impressed. The English, French, Russian and Austrian Consuls had in fact together played a significant role in ending looting, restoring order and ensuring that the army contractors continued to supply the city's military hospitals with food. But their authority was tentative. 'Anyone who disobeys this order', threatened a consular document arranging hospital supplies, 'will be severely punished as soon as authority is re-established.'

It was independent humanitarian agencies, like the MRF, who were providing civilian medical support and emergency relief. When

Eglantyne arrived ten thousand of the initial fifty thousand homeless, sick and starving refugees, mainly women and children, who had flooded into Uskub during the height of the conflict were still there and in desperate need of support. The MRF 'soup kitchen' consisted of a large cauldron standing out in an open field deep in snow, which released a thick volume of steam into the misty air as soon as the cover was removed. One of the thousands of the unemployed stood beside it ladling out so many spoonfuls into each tin mug or bowl presented by a shivering child. 'I don't think I ever saw a refugee child who wasn't shivering during the whole course of my journey, with the exception of those who had just finished their soup,' Eglantyne reported. Outside the house of the local MRF agent she found another shivering crowd, again mostly children. These were mainly Bosnian Muslim refugees who had come for the clothes doled out to them by the MRF before they started their long journey back home, a journey on which nevertheless, Eglantyne noted bluntly, 'two or three of them always died'.

This was the reality of war that Eglantyne now came to know; starving, displaced women and children, and the eternally inadequate provision of relief. She responded by taking a pragmatic view of the political situation, and focused on providing immediate humanitarian solutions. Avoiding the 'bottomless pit of political intrigue' which she felt hamstrung the consuls, she concentrated on gaining the support of the Serbian authorities for the distribution of MRF relief. 'My chief conclusion', she reported, 'was that the Servians [sic] were there, and had no doubt come to stay – and the same argument would also apply to any other government – there was only one thing to be done, and that was to make the best of them.'

The suffering that she witnessed, particularly of children, made a lasting impression on Eglantyne, but the distance she had yet to travel mentally was shown when in the evenings she found no irony in reporting with pleasure on the 'most delicious' dinner provided for her, or on the surprising needlework skills of Mr Peckham, the

British Consul, which were apparently exclusively employed in making curtains for his room. Nationality and faith aside, the poor were still, somehow, alien to Eglantyne, without the same level of human needs as her social equals.

Eglantyne came to like Mr Peckham but, still determined to be non-partisan, she was sceptical about his apparent anti-Serbian position. 'Fundamentally I could not help feeling that the chief fault of the Servians [sic] was that they had won,' she commented. 'The Englishman is ever and always on the side of the Bottom Dog. In fact as soon as a dog gets to the bottom it is at once glorified in his eyes by such a halo that he forgets that it is after all only the same old dog which he knew and disliked in the days of its prosperity.' She was also reluctant to believe the stories of atrocities that Mr Peckham cited, 'breathlessly and his cheeks flushed', against the Serbs, particularly about the fate of the five hundred sick and wounded Turkish and Albanian soldiers in the military hospital when the Serbian forces arrived. After dismissing the Croatian nursing sisters, Mr Peckham told Eglantyne, ' "a series of most extraordinary recoveries began to take place. The first day after the sisters were gone, eighty men were so well that they were able to leave the hospital, and the next day a hundred, and the day after more, till all the patients were gone, and where do you think they were? ... In the Vardar!" he exclaimed excitedly. "Drowned! *Now* what do you think of the Servians [sic]?" '

'I may say that I did not believe this story and that I do not now believe it,' Eglantyne asserted in her report. Eglantyne was well aware of the propaganda agenda attached to any conflict and she used this to justify her inability to give credit to such distressing rumours and reports. And yet knowing that bodies had surfaced in the river she was not able to entirely dismiss the hospital story. 'Outwardly I preserved an appearance of calmness', she wrote, but her faith in human nature under the pressure of war had been irreparably shaken. She now began to hear similar reports of the massacre of Catholic Albanians by Serbians in the area surrounding Prisrend, now Prizren in southern Kosovo, where she was headed next to organise relief. Mr Peckham asked her to investigate a list of the claims, including the disappearance of thirty Catholic mayors tied together and shot. Eglantyne consented, still half hoping to be able to refute the rumours.

Katharine Hodges now left for Salonika, today Thessaloniki in northern Greece, and a few days later, accompanied only by her interpreter Nicholas, Eglantyne travelled on to Prisrend by train. Breaking the journey at Ferisovitch, a small town with a particularly bloody recent history, Eglantyne accepted a lunch provided at the station by 'a kind young man who dealt in bombs'. Soon ingratiated into the local garrison she found herself invited to lunch by the Major, resulting in a Serbian escort to Prisrend in the Major's own car as the railway did not reach the town; hardly the entry she might have hoped to make into this predominately Catholic Albanian city.

Captain Dmitrovitch, Eglantyne's allocated escort, was the former Serbian Consul at Uskub, and the author of several books on the economic resources of Macedonia. Here was someone that Eglantyne felt sure could give her the information on atrocities that she had promised Mr Peckham. Taking the position that she wished to be able to refute reports of non-combatant deaths in the area, as made recently in the British papers, Eglantyne cautiously began to question the Captain. The conversation went very badly. She soon tried to drop the subject, but Dmitrovitch refused to let it go, announcing at every checkpoint 'Mademoiselle is interested in massacres.' Nicholas, her Catholic interpreter, sensibly kept as low a profile as possible in the back of the car, 'his vivid imagination', Eglantyne later wrote with considerable condescension, 'constantly picturing his head rolling on the floor at his feet'. Finally Dmitrovitch brought an Albanian non-combatant to testify to his contentment under the Serbian occupiers, which not surprisingly he duly did. '"Do you still believe in massacres?" the Captain demanded. The whole proceeding was so childish I could not think what he took me for,' Eglantyne wrote indignantly in her report, becoming ever more concerned that the Serbians really did have something to hide. Soon they left the valleys and low hills, 'bathed in purple mists', far behind and climbed the mountain pass that led to Prisrend. Arriving late that evening, Eglantyne and Nicholas were given rooms in the house of the widow of an Orthodox priest. Dmitrovitch then left them with these 'friends' and a promise to meet in the morning. It had become abundantly clear to Eglantyne that 'under hospitable pretexts he would never allow me to be left alone for one instant or given any opportunity to talk with the Catholic Albanians'.

Eglantyne always responded well to a challenge, and she immediately resolved to outmanoeuvre Dmitrovitch. Step one was to get Nicholas to deliver the letters to the local Catholic Albanians that she had accepted in Uskub, asking him to let the people to whom they were addressed know that she would be very glad to talk with anyone who might like to see her. Nicholas, Eglantyne later wrote with pleasure, was a 'born conspirator' and undertook his task with discretion as well as, although Eglantyne did not comment on this, considerable courage. Soon after lunch a prominent Catholic Albanian called Mr Mark called to invite Eglantyne to visit him at his house later that afternoon.

The most pressing task at hand however was to organise the distribution of MRF relief in the city. For this Eglantyne accepted Dmitrovitch's help to arrange a meeting with the Serbian General under whose authority Prisrend was administered. To her relief the General supported both her wish to see the poverty in the town for herself, and her plans to give alms with strict impartiality to those in need, whatever religion they professed. Having spent the morning touring the city, that afternoon Eglantyne went to the small room serving as a town hall to join the group of Orthodox, Muslim and Catholic representatives who had been nominated to act as the local MRF committee with the General's backing. During a discussion around the most effective type of aid and the criteria for relief to families, Eglantyne emphasised that 'no distinction should be made on religious or political grounds in the giving of alms, and that the work of charity was a work in which we should all unite in fraternal union whatever our differences'. It was her first official statement of the basic humanitarian position from which she would never deviate. Satisfied by the spirit of the committee that the distribution of aid really would be impartial – although she later also asked the Italian Consul to keep an independent eye on things – Eglantyne gave an initial £200 (worth nearly £14,000 today), shook hands with everyone present and left the room.

The Catholic representatives on the committee included both Mr Mark and another man to whom Eglantyne refers only as Mr Z in her report. Mr Z was a controversial figure. The Serbian Captain Dmitrovitch described him bluntly as 'a brute. Devoid of human feelings', but afterwards in Salonika Eglantyne heard Mr Z characterised as 'brave, self-sacrificing, generous, devoted'. Her own impression was that 'Mr Z's face was the face of a man who had it in him to climb any height or to sink to any depth, but the worst of it was it did not make you feel sure that he had climbed the heights. It was a face full of furious force.' Eglantyne recognised that this was the man who might be able to either finally refute or provide details of any Serbian atrocities, and although frightened by him she discreetly let him know about her appointment with Mr Mark later that afternoon. By this point Captain Dmitrovitch, who had struggled back into his galoshes, was hurrying after her, so seizing the moment she quickly arranged to go back to Mr Mark's house immediately to 'save him the trouble' of fetching her later.

'We set out together,' Eglantyne reported. 'When we came to where our ways parted Monsieur Dmitrovitch, who in absence of mind was taking his own way, recalled himself with a start and came ours. When we neared the house I am sure he was not invited to come in but in he came and walked up the stairs with us into a big sitting-room, luxurious in its simplicity. Nor did he behave very well. He stood about moodily, hardly speaking.' With her ever-present sense of social decorum and witty observation, Eglantyne made light of the situation as if it were an embarrassing parlour scene from a Jane Austen novel. In fact she must have been aware of the increasing danger she was putting herself into. After quarter-of-an-hour's polite chat with Mr Mark's wife over Turkish delight, the Captain suggested that they leave. Eglantyne politely deferred, and unable to remain in a Catholic Albanian house any longer the Captain felt obliged to leave without her. It was the moment everyone had been silently waiting for. Mr Mark quickly took his wife's place on the divan, and without further preamble Eglantyne asked, 'I wish to know if it is true that between five and six thousand people were killed at Prisrend before January.' Her report captures the scene as Mr Mark informed her that four of five hundred had been massacred:

> All of a sudden the atmosphere of the room had changed. Mr Mark's beautiful smile had gone. His head was sunk, a deep savage line appeared between his brows, a look of misery chased the genial light from his eyes. At the end of the room the men, who lived in the same house with him and who came in as soon as my guide went out, took up their places. There suddenly seemed quite a number of men with us. They kept a tense silence, watching and listening, and the air seemed charged with tragic passion.

Eglantyne's MRF report, still filed in the Save the Children archive, provides a vivid picture of the Balkans during a brief moment of calm between two wars, and also of her own evolving positions on the provision of relief, the importance of prioritising a humanitarian agenda, and the causes and consequences of civil as well as international conflict. In many ways we are lucky to have it. Dorothy later wrote that 'after 1914 neither she nor I ever had the possibility of writing down our experiences. There was no time or energy for anything which was outside the urgent necessity of the moment.' However Eglantyne herself admitted on the way home that she had 'not written down any of the information I wanted – only endless records of conversations'. The resulting document is often more like a private journal than an official report. Marshalled into eight untitled sections roughly by the places she visited, it follows a very conversational narrative and offers few statistics and little objective analysis of the situation. Wading through it is made slightly more confusing by the inclusion of two sections numbered 'five'. It was only on a second read that I realised this was not a mistake, but enabled the most explosive part of the report to be removed without trace, depending on the intended circulation. This was the section that covered Mr Z's testimony. 'Suddenly a step was heard on the stairs,' Eglantyne prefaced her second section 'five' dramatically. 'I had never heard it before but I recognised it at once; it was a violent step; it was Mr Zs!'

Between them Mr Z and Mr Mark quickly answered Eglantyne's questions. She was thankful to find that the numbers of those massacred were exaggerated. The individual cases, however, were horrific. She never discovered the fate of the Albanian mayors that Mr Peckham had referred to, but many of the Albanian civilian inhabitants of the village of Lumya, among others, had remained in their homes when the combatants retreated into the interior of Albania. Between thirty and forty were imprisoned by the advancing Serbians, she was informed, taken to Prisrend and shot without trial.

Eglantyne had only stayed at Mr Mark's house twenty minutes longer than Captain Dmitrovitch, but already her hosts were getting nervous: 'Everything is dangerous. You do not know how dangerous it is. Even you being here is dangerous ...' they told her. Without further delay she and Nicholas left Mr Mark's friendly refuge to continue talks at an unknown venue. 'I found myself outside in the street alone with Mr Z and Nicholas,' Eglantyne recorded:

Night was falling and we hurried along without speaking so as to avoid attracting attention. Presently we stopped before a door in the wall and Mr Z knocked loudly, impatiently, and I, noticing some soldiers further on down the road, crept into the shadow of the wall hoping to escape their observation. No one answered the knock and he knocked again still more fiercely and called in an infuriated voice. Then the door was flung open by a frightened servant, and before he had time to order me imperiously through I had slipped inside.

Waiting alone with Nicholas for a moment upstairs in a dark, panelled room with the blinds drawn at the windows, Eglantyne noticed the incongruous beauty of the deep relief carving on the ceiling. 'Hang on to this business,' she thought staring up, obviously terrified. 'Hang on, hang on. See it through.' Mr Z soon returned with a list of the names of the massacred men, the villages they had come from, and the dates that they had been brought to Prisrend. Quickly she began to copy, later relating: 'I thought only of spelling the words correctly, yet somewhere in the back of my mind I thought of the men too, – stalwart Albanian peasants who called to me across the grave; I thought of their confidence betrayed, their cheated hopes, the brutal capture, the fear, the anguish, their miserable days of waiting, their hasty, miserable death; I thought also of the wives and children ...' Fortunately the list was written in Roman script, mainly for concealment's sake as Latin characters would be unfamiliar to most of the population, but it helped Eglantyne to copy quickly, and soon she tore the list out of her notebook and put the pages, hastily folded, in an inner pocket.

It was night by the time Eglantyne left, Mr Z threatening her in the dark courtyard, 'Never, never tell anyone that it was from me you got the names.' Eglantyne understood that he was risking his life, but she was also scared by his roughness. Frightened too of carrying the list around in her pocket, that night she sewed it into her clothes. There were several sheets of paper, so they made rather a thick wedge. 'Afterwards, when the Servians [sic] extolled their virtues I used to feel it pressing against my heart,' she later remembered. 'How often I felt it there.' A few days later, taking her leave of Captain Dmitrovitch, again 'the names of the murdered men seemed to press against my heart till I could almost have cried out with pain'.

You could not make it up. A respectable Edwardian lady dives between Albanian safe-houses in Serbian-occupied Prisrend, in the company of a man she had only met that afternoon, had heard described as a brute and of whom she was personally terrified, in the hope of securing some evidence for crimes against humanity. Eglantyne had had her adventure, but it had turned out to be a deeply distressing episode that would fundamentally alter her understanding of human nature.

While writing categorically that these men were 'murdered', Eglantyne still refused to condemn the Serbs out of the context of war. She had noticed that the Serbs in Prisrend could 'not talk about the Albanians without shudders of horror', and felt it was likely that the Lumya Albanians were put to death 'under the blinding influence of panic ... to ensure [the Serbians'] own safety'. Hearing a man later describe war as drunkenness, under conditions of which any man may lose his head and become an animal, Eglantyne concluded that it was war itself, not any individual or race, that was the real enemy. As the rest of Europe began to gear up for the First World War this was a huge insight, and one that she arrived at independently from the contemporary pacifist movements led by groups such as the Quakers and more in tune with the sort of anti-war movements organised today. From now on international security became a fundamental part of her vision, without which relief, however essential, could only ever be a palliative measure.

'Having accomplished my mission both open and secret', as she put it, Eglantyne spent her last day at Prisrend having lunch with Captain Dmitrovitch, the General and thirty officers of the Serbian army, in an attempt to conciliate the powers that were. Dinner followed at the civilian hospital with Mademoiselle Petrovitch, the chief administrator, and a number of doctors. Eglantyne left for Monastir the following morning, driven as far as Ferisovitch by Captain Dmitrovitch. She then took a military train, sharing two seats in a horse-box while some officers sat on a tin trunk, and stretched over to show her photographs of their children and wives, or slept 'with their swords on the floor at my feet'. Eglantyne imagined their children probably also soundly asleep at that moment, and again felt unable to condemn any particular side in the war. Two days later she finally arrived at snow-covered Monastir, now the industrial and cultural city of Bitola in southern Macedonia.

Arriving in Monastir, Eglantyne was again confronted by a city overwhelmed by the influx of refugees; eleven thousand when she arrived. Most came from Muslim villages, or the Muslim quarters within the villages in the surrounding countryside, up to eighty per cent of which had been deliberately burnt during the conflict. Sometimes the houses were set on fire by their Christian neighbours, sometimes by soldiers, although visiting one village Eglantyne was told by the 'good Christians' still resident there that they had pointed out which should be burnt. Surveying the ruins she observed that:

> time had not yet touched to beauty the ghastly havoc or thrown any extenuating obscurity over the passion which had worked it; there was no moss upon the stones, no legendary halo about the day which saw them fall. The waste of human hope and effort recorded by those stone heaps which had once been homesteads, was unredeemed, uncompensated; the chaos of stones, charred and uncharred, was no more ugly than the miserable tale they told of purposeless suffering.

Over half of the refugees in Monastir were on the verge of starvation. Five thousand were being fed by the MRF, through the distribution of over a hundred thousand loaves of bread between January and April 1913, and the provision of a soup kitchen for two hundred children daily for a month between February and March. Monastir was at that time a city of fifty thousand inhabitants, and would have to absorb thirty thousand refugees before the end of the conflict. Exploring the city Eglantyne found eleven families sharing one house, and elsewhere thirty-two people living in just one room.

The result was starvation, accompanied by epidemics of influenza, bronchitis, pneumonia, typhoid fever and smallpox. Although there was considerable debate about whether it was justified – given that the provision of bread and soup was a more cost-effective way to reduce the death rate than medical support – the MRF also supported a hospital in the city. Here Eglantyne was warmly greeted by Nurse McQueen, the MRF's chief agent at Monastir who had started the hospital, and her friend Nurse Katherine Hodges with whom Eglantyne had travelled into the region a few weeks before. Both were remarkable people. Nurse McQueen was a Scotswoman and formerly national organising secretary for the Queen's Jubilee Nurses. Nurse Hodges would soon be attached to the first Serbian Unit of the Scottish Women's Hospitals during the war, and was later honoured by both Russia and France for her work as an ambulance driver. Two decades later she would still be driving ambulances, by then in the London Blitz.

When Eglantyne arrived at the 'rather austere' hospital her first feeling was a welcome sense of home conveyed by the presence of her two compatriots and a cup of tea served with the rare luxury of bread with raspberry jam. Her second was one of isolation. 'This was a lonely place for these two English nurses to live and work, month in month out,' she wrote, 'in this great barrack of a hospital, three days journey from Belgrade, here on the edge of this remote town in the mountains, far away from their friends and fellow countrymen.' The nurses slept in an unoccupied ward, two Turkish quilts dividing the room to try and contain the heat from a small stove. Sharing the room that night, Eglantyne found that 'the magnetism of the mountains kept drawing me out of the zone of warmth round the hospital stove to shiver in the icy blast which blew through the ill-fitting windows'. Nurse McQueen received a small wage from the MRF, but Nurse Hodges had come out entirely at her own expense. Both were working in these desperate conditions purely from a sense of moral duty and, in Eglantyne's word, 'love'. Eglantyne was indignant that they had so little support, and that limited funds meant that there were horrendous daily decisions to be made between investing in the prevention of starvation and the treatment of disease. Her anguish was heightened when the British Consul told her that just two pence a day could keep a man alive, and begged her to try to raise more funds on her return to England.

She left for home the following day. It was a long and tedious journey on slow trains crowded with soldiers going to or returning from leave, many of whom were ill and some clearly suffering from influenza. Few women were travelling, but Eglantyne managed to join the Russian widow of a Serbian doctor who was travelling with the Red Cross to distribute clothes to the sick and wounded, and a small party of Russian Red Cross nurses with whom she pooled rations.

Later she passed the time talking to a Serbian civilian who, having vainly sought comfort in both religion and socialism, was now planning to retire from community life altogether as a self-sufficient peasant even though he opposed property ownership as a symptom of capitalism. Eglantyne was also no socialist and 'tried to explain to him that the simple act of buying and selling which lay at the bottom of economic organisation was profitable to both parties, and that in my opinion instead of condemning wholesale our industrial system, what we should try to do was to obtain a fairer division of the advantage'. What annoyed her most however was not the man's wholesale condemnation of capitalism, but his rejection of citizenship. 'I seemed to see it all so clearly', she wrote:

> the man's passionate disgust with his present circumstances, and fervid aspiration after a simple blameless existence far removed from the annoyances and temptations of the world. He wanted to stand in the desert on a pillar of righteousness, and he was so much occupied in this project that the great spectacle of human life did not appeal to him; he had no time for it. His experiences of the struggles of the poor had left him, strangely enough, with no real love or pity for erring, afflicted humanity. The fact that other people also had their hours of

disillusionment and despair, their hours of ecstasy and rapture, left him cold, the urgent problems of the universe were nothing to him.

It was the antithesis of her own immediate response to the pain and misery, love and humanity she had witnessed in the Balkans. Her ideas were still far from fully formed, but already Eglantyne was linking active and responsible citizenship, irrespective of differences of nationality and faith, with the all-important development of international security without which no society could flourish.

Eglantyne was determined to continue her own active involvement with the Balkans, but on reaching Vienna she was too ill to go on. She had caught influenza, potentially fatal if it led to pneumonia, probably from one of the infected soldiers on the trains. Managing to find a cheap hotel near the station she struggled to her room but collapsed before she could even undress. She was soon delirious, moving in and out of consciousness, and tormented by the vision of Nurse McQueen having to close the hospital and end food distribution in Monastir. 'I must get back to England, I must get back. The people are dying, dying, dying,' she repeated feverishly over the next few days. 'More people are dead – I must get back, I must get back.'

Eglantyne got back to England a week later, still haunted by images of shivering lines of refugee children and the desperate need for more funds. She immediately urged the MRF to increase their relief work, and to organise in addition a scheme for the repatriation and resettlement of refugees; an idea that she would later develop effectively in Save the Children's programmes. But without further funds there was little that could be achieved. Determined to raise the necessary money, as well as the profile of the conflict in a region that most English people had still never heard of, that spring and summer Eglantyne undertook a demanding public speaking tour around England and Scotland. She raised a small amount of cash, 'a very tiny bit' she lamented, 'mostly given to me grudgingly by persons who said that we had so many starving people in England'.

Her PR work was slightly more successful. At the end of April, the *Glasgow Herald* published an article on Monastir where, she wrote, 'practically all the babies died. It was the children whom I pitied most.' Among the misery of starvation and disease, the most powerful image was that of thirty Turkish boys who had been abandoned at a boarding school when their teachers went to fight. When their food ran out the boys had simply gone to bed to die. 'It is easier to starve in bed, and you live longer,' Eglantyne explained bluntly, although in the event these boys were among the luckier ones found by an MRF agent. By the end of May, however, British public interest had waned again, and only the human interest angle of Eglantyne's journey secured any publicity. Articles like 'Where War Has Been Lady's Work in Macedonia' focused on the humanitarian work of Nurse McQueen at the Monastir hospital and with refugees across the Serbian interior as far south as Ioannina, now a Greek city, where she had witnessed 'the slow torture of gradual starvation'. Eglantyne continued to insist that more long-term relief was needed, and her articles would typically close with a call for donations to enable constructive work rather than just emergency relief.

But there was little response. It was with some bitter irony that Eglantyne later illustrated the shallowness of one of her fictional characters by her indifference to a newspaper article on the situation in Serbia: 'Angela read *The Times* out loud while the doctor was awaited,' Eglantyne wrote:

> She read one long article on Servia, and another on something else; neither article interested Mr Langham in the least, but it brought him some comfort to reflect that he was compelling Angela to think of something sensible for a few moments. She however had culti-vated the art of reading aloud without knowing in the least what she was reading about, and all the time she was narrating the intricacies of the situation in Servia, she was considering whether the new dress should be trimmed with embroidery or with lace.

Female nurses and doctors like Elsie Inglis who operated in the Balkans during the First World War would make front-page news just a year later when they returned to England en route to new posts or to raise funds through public lectures. But Eglantyne was just too early to capitalise on the propaganda machine promoting the romantic picture of war nursing, or on the wider public interest in Serbia as a nation. 'The hospital is closed now,' she ended her May article, 'but often I dream myself back across Europe.' Few others were yet dreaming with her. 'Miss McQueen's feeding continued for some little time', Eglantyne's 1913 report concluded bitterly, but 'a month or two later, war broke out between Serbia and Bulgaria … the country was devastated again, and I daresay all the people whom the MRF had saved through the winter perished in the renewed famine'.

For a while Eglantyne's sister Dorothy took over the good work, travelling to Monastir in Eglantyne's footsteps to offer assistance to Nurse McQueen. 'She is very jolly', the MRF team reported back, despite being given the job of 'searching out bad cases and looking after them'. The situation was still desperate and with limited resources the team still had to be appallingly selective. 'It was very difficult to know where and how to begin in such a large town and with such a mass of people,' one nurse wrote. 'So we judged best to work the district we are in as it is better to pull a few people quite through than to scatter the little doles broadcast. I hope you agree.' It is interesting that after her experience of teaching, unlike Dorothy Eglantyne never again undertook direct work with the beneficiaries of aid, as an assistant nurse or in any other role. In the Balkans she had seen her role very much as being in policy development, rather than service delivery, and this would remain her forte.

Eglantyne did however remember her debt to the many individuals who had helped her during her visit, and even made enquiries about the possibility of two Turkish clerks from Monastir obtaining British work permits, although without success. There is no record of what she did with the list of Lumya Albanians that she had

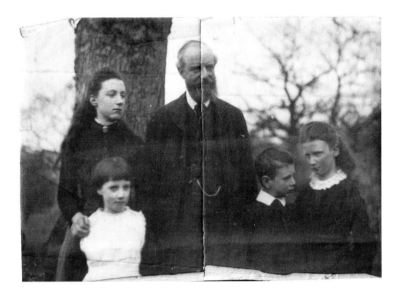

Plate 1 Arthur Jebb with, from left: Em, Dorothy, Gamul and Eglantyne, c.1889

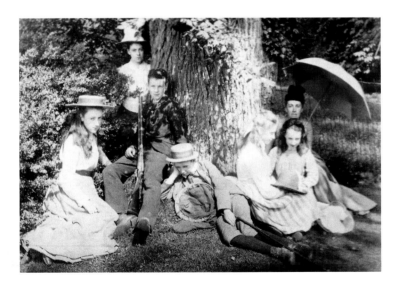

Plate 2 Tye with parasol, and all six of her children, from left: Lill, Em, Dick with rifle, Gamul with butterfly net, Eglantyne and Dorothy, August 1890

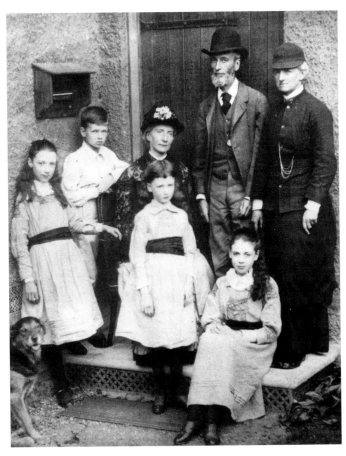

Plate 3 Adults from left: Aunt Nony, Uncle James and Aunt Bun, with children: Eglantyne, Gamul, Dorothy and Lill, at The Lyth, 1889

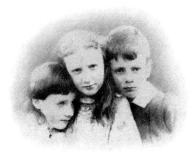

Plate 4 'The Covey of Partridges': Dorothy, Eglantyne and Gamul, *c.*1888

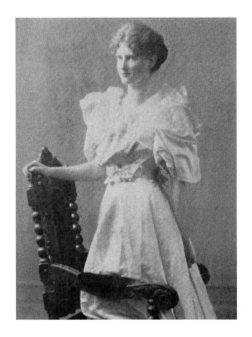

Plate 5 Eglantyne as an Oxford student, *c.*1896

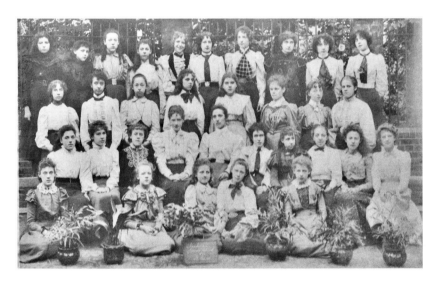

Plate 6 Eglantyne with her fellow Stockwell teacher trainees, 1899. Eglantyne is seated with her hands in her lap, third row from the back, fourth in the row

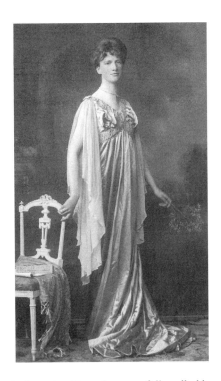

Plate 7 Eglantyne during what Dorothy scornfully called her 'worldly period', Cambridge, 1904

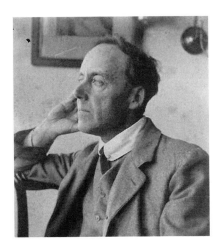

Plate 8 Marcus Dimsdale, about ten years after Eglantyne knew him, *c.*1913

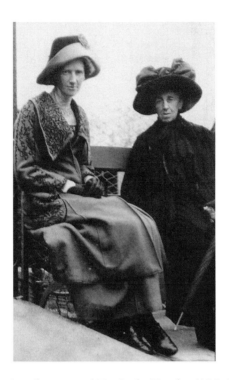

Plate 9 Eglantyne and Tye in the Tyrol, *c*.1904–1908

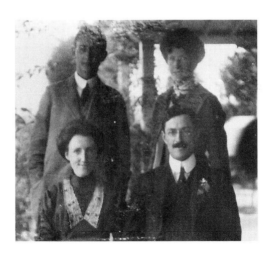

Plate 10 Tom Buxton (Charlie's nephew) and Eglantyne, standing behind
Dorothy and Charlie in Devon where Charlie was MP, December
1910. Charlie had grown a moustache to try to impress potential voters.

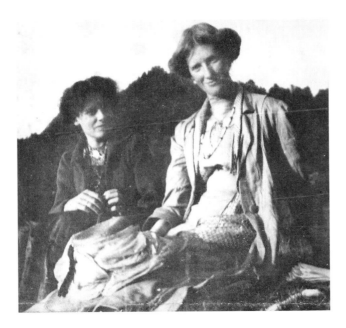

Plate 11 Eglantyne and Margaret, possibly in the Tyrol, 1911

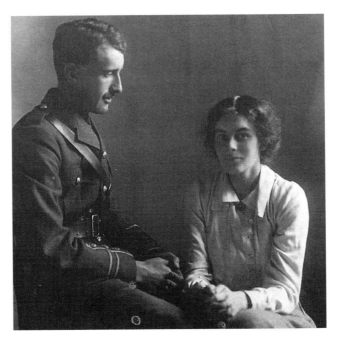

Plate 12 Margaret and AV Hill the year they married, 1913

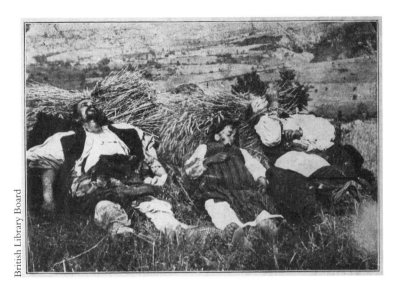

Plate 13 A Macedonian family stabbed while at work, from Victoria de Bunsen's *Macedonian Massacres: Photos from Macedonia, c.1907.* © British Library Board. All Rights Reserved (8027.a.29)

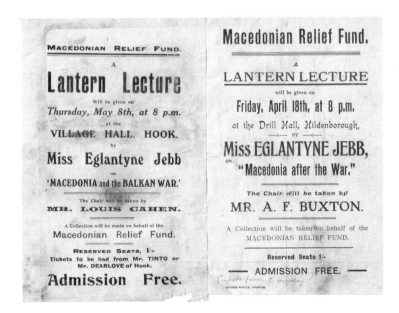

Plate 14 Fliers from Eglantyne's Macedonian Relief Fund fundraising and publicity tour, 1913

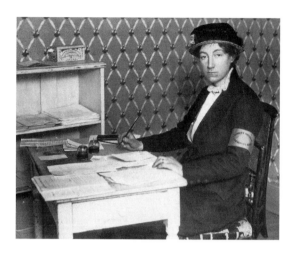

Plate 15 Lill as Director of the Agricultural Organisation Society (AOS), in her Women's Land Army armband, *c.*1916

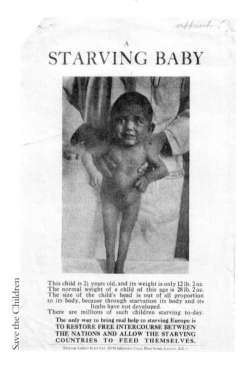

A

STARVING BABY

This child is 2½ years old, and its weight is only 12 lb. 2 oz. The normal weight of a child of this age is 28 lb. 2 oz. The size of the child's head is out of all proportion to its body, because through starvation its body and its limbs have not developed.
There are millions of such children starving to-day.
The only way to bring real help to starving Europe is TO RESTORE FREE INTERCOURSE BETWEEN THE NATIONS AND ALLOW THE STARVING COUNTRIES TO FEED THEMSELVES.

National Labour Press Ltd., 89/90 Johnson's Court, Fleet Street, London, E.C.4

Save the Children

Plate 16 The leaflet, showing a starving Austrian infant, that Eglantyne was arrested for distributing in Trafalgar Square, May 1919. The word 'suppressed!' is pencilled in Eglantyne's writing in the top right hand corner

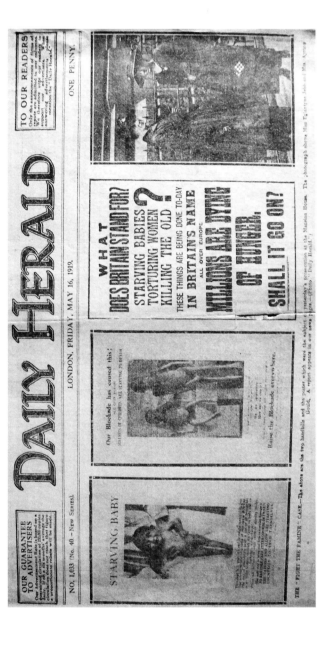

Plate 17 *Daily Herald*, 16 May 1919, featuring Eglantyne and Barbara Ayrton Gould outside their Mansion House court case, as well as the leaflets and poster they were arrested for distributing

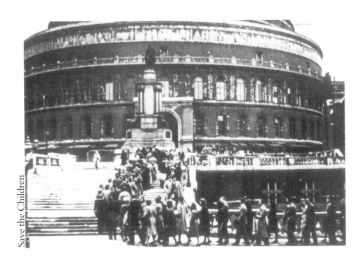

Plate 18 19 May, 1919, Eglantyne and her sister Dorothy launched the Save the Children Fund at a public meeting in the Albert Hall, which was packed to overflowing

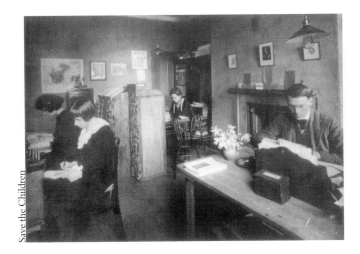

Plate 19 Save the Children's HQ in Golden Square, Soho, 1919. Staff and volunteers worked with leftover barrack room furniture and old shoe boxes. Eglantyne never wasted a penny that could be used for a child, and former workers recalled her retrieving errant pins from the office floor

"The Most Awful Spectacle in History."

MILLIONS OF CHILDREN NAKED AND STARVING IN EUROPE.

Every British Citizen Called Upon to Help— But it Must be To-day—To-morrow May Be Too Late.

WITH HUMAN DESTINY AT STAKE WILL YOU STAND IDLY BY?

Another Helpless Child is Dead—Another— and Another—While You Read—And Hesitate!

WE have won the War. We are justly proud. We are spending, on our well-earned amusements and our comfortable meals, millions of pounds every day!

And all the time, outside our very doors, a multitude of helpless children and stricken Mothers are perishing for want of food and clothes—not One Thousand, Two Thousand, or a Hundred Thousand, but MILLIONS! It is

2/- will Provide a Daily Dinner for One Child for One Week.

£1 will Feed and Clothe a Naked Starving Child.

£2/10s. will take an Ailing Child to Switzerland, where kindly Foster-Parents are ready to give it Three Months' Good Food and Nurse it Back to Health.

£100 will Feed 1,000 Children for One Week.

SUBSCRIPTIONS ON ACTIVE SERVICE WITHIN 24 HOURS,

Whatever you can give cannot be too small to be of value to the cause. Every penny you collect or subscribe will be immediately applied to the desperately urgent need of the starving and home-less. Within twenty-four hours your subscription will be doing active good, so perfect is the "Save the Children" Organisation—so eagerly helpful are its willing workers.

WHAT ONE PENNY WILL DO

The great call to our humanity and pity surely cannot fail to stir every generous feeling in our hearts. Nobody is asked to deny themselves. Pennies

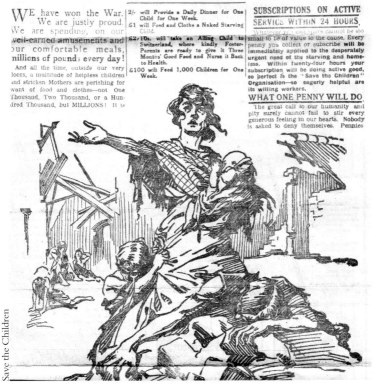

Save the Children

Plate 20 'The Most Awful Spectacle in History'; Save the Children fundraising advert, *The Times*, 4 March 1920

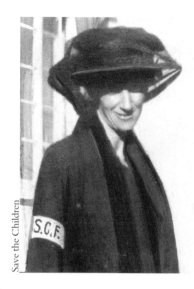

Save the Children

Plate 21 Eglantyne in Save the Children hat and armband, *c.*1920

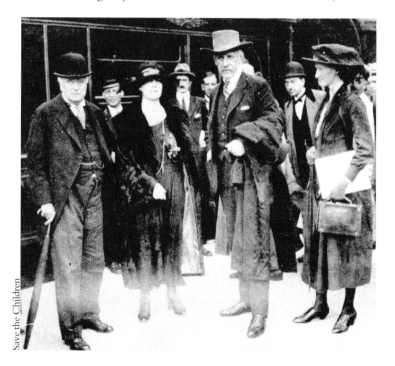

Save the Children

Plate 22 Fridtjof Nansen on his arrival in London at Victoria Station with Eglantyne, Lord Weardale (on left) and Ethel Snowden, 1921

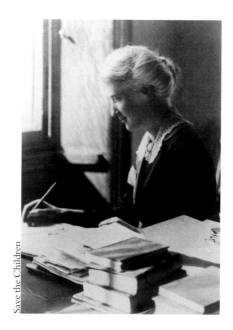

Save the Children

Plate 23 Eglantyne at her Save the Children desk, *c.*1922

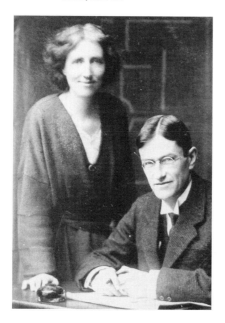

Plate 24 Dorothy and Charlie Buxton, 1922

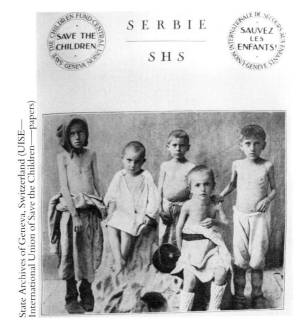

State Archives of Geneva, Switzerland (UISE—International Union of Save the Children—papers)

Plate 25 Bosnian Serb children as featured in the Bulletin of Save the Children International Union (UISE), 10 March 1920

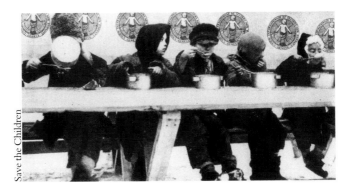

Save the Children

Plate 26 When news reached Britain of the famine in Russia, Save the Children was one of the first organisations to appeal on behalf of the six million children there who were suffering. By the autumn of 1921 they were running feeding programmes for up to 300,000 children every day

Déclaration de Genève

(Adoptée par le Conseil général de l'Union Internationale de Secours aux Enfants dans sa session du 23 février 1923, votée définitivement par le Comité exécutif dans sa séance du 17 mai 1923, et signée par les membres du Conseil général le 28 février 1924.)

Par la présente Déclaration des Droits de l'Enfant, dite Déclaration de Genève, les hommes et les femmes de toutes les nations, reconnaissant que l'Humanité doit donner à l'enfant ce qu'elle a de meilleur, affirment leurs devoirs, en dehors de toute considération de race, de nationalité et de croyance :

1. L'Enfant doit être mis en mesure de se développer d'une façon normale, matériellement et spirituellement.

2. L'Enfant qui a faim doit être nourri, l'enfant malade doit être soigné, l'enfant arriéré doit être encouragé, l'enfant dévoyé doit être ramené, l'orphelin et l'abandonné doivent être recueillis et secourus.

3. L'Enfant doit être le premier à recevoir des secours en temps de détresse.

4. L'Enfant doit être mis en mesure de gagner sa vie et doit être protégé contre toute exploitation.

5. L'Enfant doit être élevé dans le sentiment que ses meilleures qualités devront être mises au service de ses frères.

[Signatures of Eglantyne Jebb and various international dignitaries]

Plate 27 Facsimile of the Declaration of Geneva, signed by Eglantyne and international dignitaries, *c.*1924

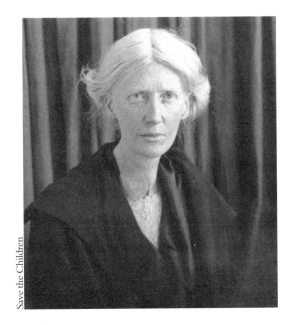

Plate 28 Eglantyne, *c.*1928

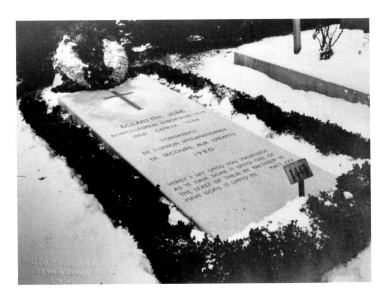

Plate 29 Eglantyne's grave in Geneva, December 1928

smuggled out of the country, and the atrocities are not mentioned in any of the press coverage I could find. Probably she gave the papers to Charlie Buxton in his MRF role, as he was well connected in diplomatic circles and would have been well placed to pass them on. She certainly filed her MRF report with him, but in order to protect the people mentioned it was never published.

Charlie and Noel continued to campaign actively both for diplomatic intervention and for the provision of relief to the Balkans, particularly to Macedonia. However when, in July 1913, Bulgaria declared war on her former Balkan allies in an unsuccessful attempt to annex the land that had been promised but not delivered after the defeat of Turkey, the region once again descended into war. Altogether approximately 122,000 people were killed in action during the Balkan Wars, with another 20,000 dying of injuries, and 82,000 from disease exacerbated by starvation.

In June the following year, 1914, Serbia found itself centre stage in Europe after the assassination of Archduke Franz Ferdinand of Austria on a visit to Sarajevo. Despite being allied with Russia, Britain, France and Romania, a year later Serbia was attacked by the Germans, Austrians and Bulgarians, heralding the start of the First World War. The MRF inevitably lost profile in the ensuing conflict, and soon stopped holding meetings. Charlie and Noel were in any case by then engaged on a diplomatic mission, supported by Lloyd George, Winston Churchill and Neville Chamberlain, to try to dissuade Bulgaria from forming an alliance with Germany. The British Secretary for Foreign Affairs, Sir Edward Grey, had cautiously ensured that the brothers travel in a private capacity however, rather than on official government business, and without his committed support, and unable to promise Macedonia to Bulgaria as her reward for remaining neutral, the brothers' negotiations failed. Nonetheless they still made headlines by narrowly surviving an assassination attempt by a representative of the Young Turk Party while they were attending the funeral of the King of Romania. Six shots were fired at point blank range. One broke Noel's jaw, prompting the *Berliner Tageblatt* to celebrate the closing of 'a mouth so full of guile and arrogance to everything that was not English'. Another pierced Charlie's lung but failed to reach his heart, its course having been slowed by a note-book in his breast pocket.[3] While recovering in hospital Charlie and Noel took the opportunity to discuss Herbert Spencer, John Stuart Mill and the ethics of political assassination with their captured assailant, Hassan Taksim, a young politician of high position. Noel also conducted 'a brief experiment in the psychology of political hatred'. Placing his (unloaded) revolver on the table he offered the unrepentant Taksim a second chance to shoot him. Taksim declined, leading Noel to conclude that 'our sense of one another had become too vivid; we were no longer abstractions to each other – the assassin on one side, the anti-Turk on the other. If every man's imagination penetrated the murky barriers of emotion, killing in war as in crime would become impossible.' It was a lesson in the importance of human empathy that Charlie took to heart, and would soon discuss with Eglantyne.

On their return, Charlie and Noel continued to highlight the 'supreme importance' of the Balkans region for international peace and security. The attempted assassination had lent them some profile and popularity: a street in Sophia was named Boulevard Brothers Buxton in their honour, and back in England they became, for a while, minor diplomatic celebrities. Capitalising on this in April 1915 they co-authored a book on *The War and The Balkans*, which proposed a European policy of concessions to try to secure peace. 'For the first time in history we are permitted to contemplate a state of affairs in which the gaunt spectre of Balkan hatred and of Balkan war will be finally laid to rest,' they argued. It was not to be, but they did not stop lobbying. Having almost caused riots during their election campaigning in 1916, Charlie and Noel were represented in the press as:

> a pair of mild-mannered men, yet wherever they go they arouse either civil or international war. At Bucharest they were nearly murdered by

the Turks, and in Bishopsgate the same impulse moved the Canadians. They did their utmost to win the Balkans for the Alliance, and had bullets only for their reward, yet now at home it is not bullets but brickbats. It is, I suppose, the inevitable judgement which must fall on a family that helped to liberate the negroes. But to speak seriously ... if only the people will let Mr Charles Buxton get his speeches off his chest they will soon find out how few people listen to them.

Like Charlie and Noel, Eglantyne had also moved from opposing ignorance and neglect in the UK to taking on a controversial international remit. But her experience of working with the poor in Marlborough and Cambridge had done little to prepare her for the 'horrors and terrors' of mass civil displacement, starvation and crimes against humanity created by the conditions of war in the Balkans. Desperate to maintain her fundamental faith in human nature, she progressed from naive disbelief to a compassionate viewpoint that blamed ignorance, prejudice and the brutalising impact of war itself for the fear and suffering that she had witnessed. In future she would focus on the prevention of international war and civil conflict through the promotion of relief, sustainable development and citizenship. Having been repeatedly asked 'And what do you think of your Balkans now?' after the outbreak of renewed fighting in 1914, Eglantyne wrote an article under the deliberately provocative title 'The Barbarous Balkans', almost certainly taken from Margaret's letter to her the January before, which set out her basic humanitarian response. Her two chief conclusions were that a nation should not be identified solely with its crimes, and that a wrong can never be made right by the essential righteousness of those concerned. 'I remember the words of a man "without human feelings", which unknown to himself I overheard,' Eglantyne ended: ' "With most of us civilisation is only skin deep. Place any man, – under circumstances of warfare, and you never know if he will not revert to savagery." And I cannot cast the first stone: I cannot say, "Events have now convinced me that all the Balkan races are equally barbarous." ... It is in war itself, not in its victims, that the barbarity lies.'

Chapter 9

Conversations with
the Dead, 1914–1915

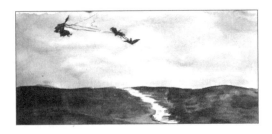

When you know for certain that death does not exist ...
you will find it the starting point for many great discoveries.

Eglantyne Jebb, 1914

'The dead cry out to be remembered' the great romantic biographer Richard Holmes has declared.[1] Although I never supposed Holmes meant this in a literal sense, the idea of biographers being haunted by the supportive or malevolent ghosts of their subjects is well established, and I couldn't help but be slightly disappointed that for me, whether I was sleeping in Eglantyne's childhood nursery at The Lyth or putting flowers on her grave in Geneva, the dead were always silent. For Eglantyne, however, the dead did cry out, in several countries and over many years, and she would come to find what she called her 'unusually close connection with the dead' in turns a powerfully liberating and painfully distressing experience.

A childhood sketch by Dorothy entitled, 'The Phantoms of Eglantyne's Brain'

Eglantyne had her first ghostly encounter in 1885 when she was only eight years old. Her three elder siblings, Em, Lill and Dick, had made a phantom arm by dressing an old stick in a shirt-sleeve and fixing it on an axle above a sofa so that by pulling a rope they could make it move. It was a crude but nonetheless effective device in a nursery where invention and imagination were everything. Lill then went to fetch Eglantyne, their 'victim', while Em, hiding in the next room, made 'piercing, fearful shrieks enough to frighten anyone'. Eglantyne did not know whether to believe in the 'ghoul' or not, but she put on a brave face and stood her ground even though her tormentors later bragged to an aunt that she was quaking down to her shoes. Although this was just a childhood prank, ghost stories were clearly a part of everyday life at The Lyth and Eglantyne's initial response, to accept the possibility that the 'apparition' was real and stand firm, was one that she never fundamentally altered.

As a young woman Eglantyne began to have more serious spiritual, or psychic, impressions. At the turn of the century her dead brother, Gamul, began to haunt her dreams and those of her younger sister Dorothy, and both of them came to believe that his visits represented something more transcendental than their own mourning process. Over the next few years Eglantyne became increasingly fascinated with the idea of a spiritual life, but at the same time she was tormented by inner spiritual difficulties. Then in 1914, as the First World War claimed lives across Europe, she began to hear new voices speaking to her from 'the other side'. Rather marvellously this time not only did she answer; she also diligently noted everything down.

Spiritualism had first caught the public imagination in the late 1870s. At a time when so many died young from disease or in childbirth, direct communication with departed loved ones was an attractive alternative to the more formal consolations provided by the established Church. To many the church already seemed to be responding inadequately to the growing social problems associated with the industrial revolution when Darwin's theory of evolution shook the literal authority of the Bible in the 1860s. This was an age of huge scientific advances. The laws of physics were being mapped out, and new technologies like the invisible power of electricity and the captivating processes of photography were being harnessed for the first time. If such previously unrecognised and seemingly miraculous physical laws and forces existed in the world, then the current boundaries of human knowledge seemed insufficient reason to rule out reports of spiritual, psychic or paranormal experience. 'At present I am inclined to think that it is a deliberate imposture,' Eglantyne's self-possessed Aunt Carrie wrote in 1874. 'But I have not evidence enough for an induction [proven conclusion].'

Studying Moral Science at Newnham College in the first few years of the new century, Eglantyne's sister Dorothy found herself discussing psychic phenomena with her friend and tutor Jane Harrison. Dorothy and Jane were among those following the open-minded research being carried out by the first Principal of Newnham, Nora Sidgwick, an eminent mathematician whose results of a 'census of hallucinations' were strikingly positive.[2] 'Mrs Sidgwick and many others among psychical researchers think themselves now within measurable distance of a great discovery of some force in a sense as finite as electricity – though far less within the scope of our intelligence,' Dorothy wrote enthusiastically to her mother and Eglantyne. Many other young academics, like Marcus Dimsdale's Cambridge friend the writer Arthur Benson, followed the scientific investigations of the Society for Psychical Research. 'The whole thing is strange of course, but no stranger than wireless telegraphy,' Benson wrote in 1906: 'Face to face with the impenetrable mystery, with the thought of those whom we have loved, who have slipt [sic] without a word or a sign over the dark threshold, what wonder if we beat with unavailing hands against the closed door? It would be strange if we did not, for we too must some day enter in.'

This renewed interest in spiritualism reached its height as mortality figures began to climb during the First World War: in 1914 there were 145 active societies affiliated to the National Spiritualists Union, and by 1919 the number had grown to 309. 'The War came, and when the war came, it brought an earnestness into all our souls and made us look more closely at our own beliefs and reassess their values,' Sir Arthur Conan Doyle, the Sherlock Holmes author, champion of spiritualism and a neighbour of Tye and Eglantyne's at Crowborough in Sussex, wrote in 1914. The establishment press and clergy might criticise the revitalised movement for 'preying' on the emotions of the bereaved but, like many, the creator of the great rationalist detective found considerable solace in spiritualism with its alleged proof of existence beyond the grave, giving 'a call of hope and of guidance to the human race at the time of its deepest affliction'. By 1914 Eglantyne had already experienced the death of a close brother and the trauma of war and civil conflict in Macedonia. Although Tye disapproved of spiritualism it was almost inevitable that Eglantyne, convalescing in Crowborough with the leisure to spend time thinking, would give some consideration to this fashionable and comforting diversion.

Eglantyne believed she first saw a spirit soon after the start of the war in 1914. One evening, travelling by train, she joined a girl in an otherwise empty carriage. After the train started moving however she noticed another 'figure' who urged her to speak to the girl. At first Eglantyne was reluctant, not wanting 'to engage in conversation, and … at a loss as to how to begin', but after some hesitation she opened by commenting on the dimness of the light in war-time trains. The girl soon got talking about how sorry she was for the relatives of the men who were then dying so fast, but Eglantyne had seen that the third figure was a youngish woman, so she steered the conversation round to sympathy for people who had also lost other relations. At this the girl thawed, confessing her grief at losing a close sister. As Ruth Wordsworth later repeated the story: 'Eglantyne, never telling her of the apparition, talked quietly to her about the unseen world, and her own belief that those who had passed from sight were much more united with us than we generally recognised. '"And" as she put it "the curious thing was that she believed me and received comfort!"' Although Eglantyne served more as the medium than the recipient of spiritual support in this story, it was a hugely significant moment for her in that it opened up both the possibility and potential value of spirit communications in her own mind.

But Eglantyne's very personal spiritual experiences also had their roots in religious mysticism, and her desire to develop her own direct awareness of spiritual truth and an intimate relationship with divine reality, or God. Mysticism was enjoying a revival at about the same time as spiritualism, and for many of the same reasons. 'The world in general is perhaps more tolerant of mysticism at the present time than at any previous period,' Tye wrote in a long manuscript, because, 'science, which a few decades ago, was expected to clear up everything for the man of common sense, has opened up such vast, such undreamed of abysses of wonder, and speculation that even the most materialistic and superficial of worldlings is brought to pause'. After Gamul's death Tye had joined the Catholic Apostolic Church, a small Christian sect that respected personal spirituality. Soon she was converted to mysticism, explaining that 'all religion is the Spirit of Love' and mysticism 'something indistinguishable from the purest religious consciousness'. Eglantyne, who was always studying her own religious and spiritual feelings, was greatly interested in and influenced by her mother's evolving beliefs. Unlike some of her sisters, she understood and supported Tye's conversion because Gamul's death had also coincided with, and perhaps prompted, her own discovery of mysticism while at college. Her first transcendental impression of the unity of humankind and the world had been inspired by her college study of mystic revelations, and was followed a couple of years later by her 'vision' of the face of Christ in the schoolroom, which she believed to be a profoundly significant Divine message.

Over the next ten years Eglantyne kept notes on her uplifting transcendental experiences. However as her health deteriorated, forcing her to cut back on her Cambridge social work, she became increasingly tormented by thoughts of her own worthlessness, and her moments of mystical reflection became less positive. In 1911 she wrote a convoluted paper, full of repetitions and crossings out, on what she called the 'Psychic Life', defined as an intermediary life-stage when a person's interests move from the 'egoistic, material world' towards the spiritual one, but before 'spirituality of thought and conduct' is attained. 'The ideal life is a life of dignity and useful-ness' she scribbled between blots in scratchy black ink. She would, she pledged, commune with God and replace selfishness with love as a 'modern mystic'. But Eglantyne's aspirations to lead this noble 'psy-chic life' were frustrated by her fears of failure, and that her ideals might prove 'ridiculous ... betraying my dearest hopes'. Torn between self-conceit and self-punishment she decided she must learn to embrace failure and humiliation if she was to benefit from the spir-itual lessons they might afford. It was clearly not an entirely healthy proposition.

Seeking reassurance about her spiritual difficulties Eglantyne sent her notes on the 'psychic life', along with the manuscript of her lat-est novel, to Margaret Keynes. 'What a terrible thing it is to be a genius!' Margaret supportively replied on cue. 'It is the way with all artists as well as writers, they can't do as they would and so they often despair. But that is a different thing from thinking that your work is valueless. How could anybody's work be worthless when they are striving, straining every nerve after truth?' Although keen to support her adored Eglantyne, Margaret did not share her faith. 'When I talk about religion I always discover how very little religious I am. I really have no faith,' she confessed, continuing rather more pointedly, 'I am inclined to say a great deal of religion and religious emotion can be accounted for as superstition and imagination.' However much Margaret loved Eglantyne, she could only offer her limited sympathy with regard to her spiritual distress. She was completely unable to accept mysticism, and like her mother and Maynard, she could be very disparaging about spiritualism. 'Professor Barrett of psychic fame came to lunch yesterday and told us his latest and unpublished experiences,' Florence Keynes wrote dryly to her husband in September 1912. 'He did not strike *me* as especially gifted with powers of quick observation.' Little wonder then that after Margaret's marriage to AV in 1913 Eglantyne chose not share any more of her developing spiritual impressions and meditations with her former dearest friend and confidante.

'My friends cannot fight my battles for me,' Eglantyne told herself in another manuscript she called *The Soul's Roadbook*, written in 1913. This seventy-six-page typed essay was an attempt to steer herself away from her spiritual difficulties to a place of 'courage, patience, hardihood, peace and joy'. Its opening gives a bleak picture of where she was coming from: 'From time to time in life I am much beset and tormented by the distress occasioned by certain spiritual difficulties,' she wrote. 'These difficulties are not many in number but very formidable, in as much as they often threaten the wreck of my happiness. They have stood like giants in my path, emerging at unexpected times and falling upon me mercilessly.'

1913 was the year that Margaret would marry and Eglantyne went to the Balkans, returning only to learn of renewed conflict in the region and of war escalating across Europe. The bulk of the year was spent on her miserable Balkans publicity tour, continuing to serve on various local district visiting committees and COS meetings to allocate grants to the 'deserving' Cambridge poor, and – as the last unmarried sister – looking after Tye. None of this was satisfying or rewarding work. The movement towards war had dissipated public interest in Macedonia and Eglantyne realised she was not going to raise significant further funds. She also knew that many of the people she had befriended in the Balkans were likely to be killed in action or die from starvation or disease as a result of the renewed conflict, and she began to feel that even her relief mission had been essentially futile. Unable to raise the funds for the causes she believed mattered most, she was intensely frustrated to see local charitable committees distributing grants in ways she believed would only perpetuate domestic poverty. 'I wish to say "You would do better if you gave this money to the Devil" but I am silent and smile,' she vented her frustration in her *Roadbook*, continuing with at least a little of her old dry humour: 'A fire rages in my heart, until I wish there were a sword in my hand that I might kill them all – poor old ladies!'

As the year dragged on, and Margaret's December wedding loomed, Eglantyne became increasingly depressed by her sense of failure. 'My conscience has always sought to pull me one way, while all the rest of me struggled to go the other,' she made her fictional Frieda Jones despair at one point. Now Eglantyne again felt the draw of giving up all her good intentions, which seemed in any case to result in so little, but she could not in good conscience go through with it. 'I cannot prevent a yearning often arising in my heart for the life which I see my girl friends lead: so quiet, so respected, so sheltered,' she confessed. 'I think such a life is right for them: why then this conviction that if I lead it I should be damned?' She prayed fervently for the strength to love service for its own sake, but set herself such painfully high standards that she was bound to fail. 'At night I sometimes give way to the constantly recurring temptation to pray for death,' she now wrote in her *Roadbook*. 'When I have turned out the light I often shed tears to think that I must wake again. This desire for death shows me how little indeed I have died to the selfish affections of my lower nature. For I am prompted simply by the wish to escape from the personal pain of living ...' Two pages later she was faltering again: 'What Christianity taught was self-sacrifice, even unto the laying down of one's life. And now still when the question comes, as it comes again and again: "Canst thou lay down thy life for

thy brethren?" I feel my heart reply: "No, I want my life for myself." '
But by the end of the year she was back chasing the 'ideal life' of service. 'If we lose our life, spending it for others, lavishing upon them
our strength, our power,' she reasoned, 'we find our life.'

The problem was that Eglantyne was now in no position to lavish
her strength on anyone. She was thirty-seven, often exhausted, thin-
ner than she had ever been, and the silver was starting to show
through her trademark red hair. Still plagued by doubts and insecu-
rities about her abilities, responsibilities and direction, her introspec-
tive and rather circular meditations in her *Roadbook* were no longer
enough to move her forward – what she needed was external
support, guidance, sanction, and above all in the short term occupation, as her elder sister Lill recognised.

By 1914 Lill had built on her pioneering work promoting farming co-operatives to become a Governor of the national 'Agricultural
Organisation Society', or AOS as it was known. Remembering
Eglantyne's editorial skills on her book, *By Desert Ways to Baghdad*,
Lill now found her sister a position as Editor of the AOS weekly, *The
Plough*. Eglantyne had once been quite interested in farming co-
operatives. In 1902 she had travelled to Denmark to observe the
schemes that Lill so admired in practice and, appreciating the principle of collective rather than competitive working, she had even made
co-operative small-holdings one of Frieda's key interests in *The Ring
Fence*, started around 1908. Now she threw herself into her AOS role
with her usual commitment, soon acting, she half-boasted half-
moaned, as 'not only the editor but the entire staff as well – journalists, clerks, typists, office boy, all rolled into one'. According to her
cousin Gem, now a civil servant for the Board of Trade in the
same building, Eglantyne 'turned a drab little periodical into … a
most attractive guide to a new moral and economic order'.
Eglantyne enjoyed the work, and it would have lasting value for her;
supplying many of the ideas on land use and farming practices that
she later employed in Save the Children's early programmes with the

resettlement of refugees. But she was also exhausted by it, often feeling unfit to do anything after eleven in the morning.

Eglantyne's 'chief ally and helper' in this demanding role was a decorated army officer who had served in the Boer War and was now secretary of the AOS: Colonel Henry Lionel Pilkington. Pilkington is at once the central but a very shadowy figure in this story. At fifty-six, almost twenty years older than Eglantyne, he was described in appropriately military terms by their mutual friend Maud Holgate as 'a very distinguished man in mind and bearing'. Like Eglantyne he had witnessed the devastation of war, and he had also known personal tragedy: following a breakdown his wife, Louisa, had been committed to an asylum where she died. Perhaps these histories created some natural empathy between him and Eglantyne. Intellectually they certainly valued each other, and at the AOS Eglantyne and Pilkington formed a close and lasting friendship. It lasted even beyond his unexpected death following a short illness in the spring of 1914.

At the start of March, although feeling somewhat stronger and glad to have the distraction of work, Eglantyne had been temporarily dragged away from London, inwardly kicking and screaming, for another restorative holiday with her mother in Locarno, on Switzerland's Lake Maggiore. It was here that she learnt of Pilkington's sudden death from septic pneumonia. To her great sorrow she had not been around either to be a support during his illness or a mourner at his funeral. For some weeks she replayed the key scenes from their friendship through her mind, dwelling particularly on their last meeting. 'I seemed to remember every look, every gesture', she wrote in a private journal a week after she heard the news, 'especially … the kind of impression which his presence made, the feeling it stirred in me'. She kept her feelings closely guarded however, commenting only to her friend Dorothy Kempe that 'he will be a very great loss to the AOS'.

Eglantyne soon missed Pilkington so much that she started to feel he was in some way still with her. Still in Switzerland, she caused concern by insisting on climbing the deeply snow-covered mountains without a guide, and otherwise locking herself in her room. Once back in London she picked up her editorial work, but the woman who could climb the Swiss peaks unassisted found the office exhausting, and soon she was working mostly from home and sometimes from bed – and she was lonely. 'I nearly killed myself entirely writing in bed in order to let the printers have copy up to time,' she moaned pathetically to Margaret. Two months later Tye insisted that Eglantyne join her in Crowborough, which was then enjoying a growing reputation as a health resort. It was here that most of the discussions between Eglantyne and Pilkington's 'spirit' took place over the course of 1914, through what turned out to be a particularly dull winter, and into the wet spring of the following year.

'I went into my room …' Eglantyne's fantastic journal, *Conversations with the 'Dead'*, opens dramatically, 'but I had locked my door, for fear I should cry':

> He came to me, and said: 'Why are you unhappy?'
>
> 'I am so sorry that you are dead.'
>
> He burst out laughing. 'Dead, dead, dead! I wish you wouldn't use that word. Why, I am much more alive than I've ever been before. You are much more dead than I am!'

To a modern audience this seems a remarkable introduction to a work of non-fiction. Psychic or spiritual experiences by the recently bereaved, biographers or anyone else, are the preserve either of the truly spiritually sensitive, the fraudulent, the gullible or the insane. Either Eglantyne's discussions with Colonel Pilkington, deceased, were indeed real communications with the spirit world, or the manuscripts of their almost daily conversations record an enormous self-deception. Even to Eglantyne at first it seemed too good to be true, and she admitted she was very aware that her 'conversations' might emanate from her own 'vivid imagination'.

Modern psychology was just emerging in 1914 as Freud's work began to expose and interpret the relationship between the conscious and the unconscious mind. Eglantyne may or may not have been familiar with Freud's ideas, but she would certainly have been well aware of the concept of the unconscious mind.[3] Coleridge and other writers had recognised the 'insensible' and 'involuntary' aspects of the self manifest, for instance in dreaming, since the early 1800s, and by 1907 Frederic Myers, one of the founders of the Society for Psychological Research, had noted that the 'idea of a threshold ... of consciousness; – of a level above which sensation or thought must rise before it can enter into our conscious life; – is a simple and familiar one'. Eglantyne referred to deliberately attending to her 'conscious intelligence', which she believed mediated her discussions with Pilkington's spirit, and recorded that 'it was some time' before she 'could feel certain ... when I was listening to him and when I was simply inventing the answers I expected'.

With a series of unpublished novels behind her, Eglantyne was used to inventing characters and dialogue. When they spent their month convalescing together in Dartmoor in 1907 Ruth had commented that 'Eglantyne never held herself responsible for what any of her characters did. Sometimes looking rather awed at their behaviour she would just say that *they did it*, and that was that. She evidently watched it happening and couldn't stop it. She threw her whole self into the story.' And the devout Anglican Maud Holgate, who having known Pilkington in life was one of the few in Eglantyne's confidence about their spiritual discussions, felt that given 'in writing her novel Eglantyne might so brood over a character as to produce unconsciously the answers which would emanate from such a character', then her spiritual conversations probably resulted from a similar process. Nonetheless Maud conceded that Eglantyne 'was gifted with such unusual spiritual perceptions that the probability of their being *real* "conversations" ' struck her forcibly when she was reading them. Concerned that Eglantyne was becoming obsessed with what she considered at best a morbid habit, she urged her friend to stop consciously seeking the conversations. Eglantyne, not appreciating Maud's want of sympathy, simply stopped updating her friend. 'One can never really know the exact truth', Maud concluded, 'but I am sure that she was herself convinced that she was being answered by her friend and I feel that it was a sacred thing to her.'

Having had psychic impressions of her own, Dorothy was more willing to believe in the authenticity of her sister's spiritual experiences – however even she felt that to some extent the conversations might have been an end in themselves. Dorothy knew that Eglantyne was addicted to exploring her thoughts and experiences through writing, and she would later introduce a posthumous edition of Eglantyne's poetry with the comment that Eglantyne wrote simply because she could not help doing so: 'her inner experiences did indeed leave her no peace till they had found an outlet in rhythmic words'. As had happened after Gamul died, for a while Eglantyne's almost constant stream of prose and poetry dried up when she heard the news of Pilkington's death. Possibly words, even pulled into poetry, did not seem sufficient to capture all she felt, or perhaps it was just too painful to set her living emotions into the concrete of completed verse. Certainly Eglantyne's ability to express herself in poetry and novels, or through the 'conversations', seems to have been mutually exclusive. Once she returned to writing verse and fiction from 1915 she put her spiritual journals aside – although perhaps her new writing filled the gap left by Pilkington's absence rather than usurping him.

Wherever they came from, Eglantyne's spiritual conversations gave her the chance to discuss her anxieties and aspirations with a trusted friend in absolute privacy, and at times and places completely at her own convenience. Furthermore Eglantyne had admired Pilkington in life, but after death he could provide support and guidance from the higher, spiritual, plane that she had long aspired to reach. With so many good reasons to suspend her disbelief,

Pilkington's spirit had soon persuaded her to accept the reality of his presence without the accompanying sensual experience of his being there physically. 'It would be a mistake', she wrote, 'to crave the vivid consciousness which, as he had explained ... was pseudo-consciousness.' Not for the first time Eglantyne found herself equal to a serious leap of faith, telling Pilkington 'I ... treasure my religious views even in opposition to my intelligence.' For Eglantyne 'real intercourse' now for a while became the spiritual interchange of thoughts; worldly social intercourse by comparison was 'unreal'.

It is perhaps ironic that Eglantyne's most complete novel is set firmly in the real world, and more than once ridicules upper-class spiritualist 'sensitivities' by contrasting them with society's evident insensitivity towards the material suffering of the working classes. Meanwhile her main non-fiction journal revolves around her conversations with a spirit. But in fact *The Ring Fence* and *Conversations with the Dead* explore the same themes – the nature of truth, love, private responsibility and public service – simply from opposite ends of the fact–fiction spectrum. It was these issues, rather than the literary medium, that really interested Eglantyne.

Eglantyne and Pilkington had a large agenda to cover and the result was over one hundred pages of often circular conversations in the first manuscript alone, revolving mainly around the nature of life after death, spiritual truth, selfless love, the problem of individualism, and the general superiority of the spiritual and intellectual above the material, physical and emotional. Worried that she was not grasping all that Pilkington meant to convey, Eglantyne often added caveats to her accounts of their discussions. '*Note*', she wrote at one point, 'these conversations are, as I feared from the first, rather difficult to remember.' And later, 'Simple, however, as were the things he said to me, I did not find it at all easy to follow his reasonings.'

Many of the subjects Eglantyne and Pilkington covered were not unique to their discussions, but reflected wider contemporary debate in spiritualist and mystical circles – and indeed in society more broadly. Individual versus collective responsibility, for example, was a much broader social debate that had already played itself out in the development of Eglantyne's social and political thought, and inevitably individual versus collective consciousness found itself at the centre of much spiritualist discussion. At one point Pilkington told her that 'if we are conscious of individualism, it is limitations of which we are conscious, and these limitations baulk us'. The idea was that all people were essentially 'one with spiritual life' but that individual consciousness created a mistaken belief in independence and private self-interest. The prolific spiritualist writer Evelyn Underhill – at least one of whose books found its way on to Eglantyne's shelves – later took up this theme in her classic 1929 book *The House of the Soul*, arguing that 'Christian Spirituality knows nothing of ... individualism.'[4] Eglantyne was already fascinated by the relationship between the individual and the universal, the particular and the general, and the idea expressed in the *Conversations* that people are 'subjected to differentiation ... in order that we might enter into a closer unity' would later be reflected in her concept of all individual children having universal human rights.

However although in theory Eglantyne was already advocating that all peoples were equal, her discussions with Pilkington were still framed by Western cultural bias, and were at times overtly racist. 'Easterns' and 'Orientals' were not culturally creative, Pilkington informed her, because creative power was associated with the practical ability which these peoples lacked. Even the great poet Rabindranath Tagore had only been able to emerge in India, he went on, 'at a time when the West has given stimulus to the commercial development of his country'. It was an unlikely position for a disembodied spirit supposedly bringing a message about the unity of human consciousness to take, and provides an insight into some of the crucial issues that Eglantyne still had to resolve.

Most of Eglantyne's discussions with Pilkington's spirit however focused on her overriding personal preoccupation: how to return to an active, meaningful and moral life. As well as her unreliable health, social conventions had placed two further obstacles in the way of her embarking on a vocation: firstly any faint hope she might still have for romance, and perhaps now more significantly her overriding duty to look after Tye.

Eglantyne was very concerned about the nature of true love. She had never wanted children of her own but typically formed very close and monogamous friendships, from Dorothy Kempe at Oxford to Margaret Keynes in Cambridge, and she clearly longed for a soulmate with whom to share her inner life. Her rejections in turn by Marcus and Margaret had left her feeling emotionally crushed and deeply lonely, but it was her relationship with Margaret that caused her the greatest anxiety. She had already tried to persuade herself that true, selfless love existed on a 'higher plane', and that the psychic life she strove for 'probably despises all sensuous indulgence'. Now she took the opportunity to explore this idea further:

Eglantyne: Isn't there *any* love of man, except from love of God?

Pilkington: There is only the love of man's lower nature, which is not love at all, though it often passes under the name. This is, however, absolutely the deadliest injury which you can inflict on anyone.

Eglantyne: I should have thought that people often began by loving their friends in the wrong sort of way, say first for the beauty of face and feature and then that gradually their love purified itself …

Pilkington: It doesn't matter so much what you love, or seem to love about them, what really matters is how you love … selfless love is, equally invariable, love for the best that is in them, for their spiritual being. It may seem that you love them for the beauty of their face, – but it is not true, – you have unconsciously taken their beauty as a symbol of themselves.

By translating the feelings inspired by Margaret's 'beauty' to a higher, spiritual level, Eglantyne was able both to make sense of her devastation at the end of their relationship and at the same time see her emotions as morally irreproachable.

Although she had already started to reject the 'sensuous', Eglantyne's romantic aspirations perhaps only finally died with her less-complicated feelings for Colonel Pilkington. Maud Holgate later told Dorothy that Eglantyne had been attracted to Pilkington, and Eglantyne's immediate response to his death, brooding over the feelings he had once stirred in her, seems to confirm this. 'Your friendship with me has always been a matter of conscious intelligence,' his spirit told her early on in their conversations, to which Eglantyne responded ruefully 'I interrupted him with a denial but he stuck to the point.' It was hard for Eglantyne to let go of her emotions for Pilkington in order to develop the purely intellectual or spiritual relationship with him that his spirit now advocated. At first she argued that she would prefer to keep her emotional 'memories', even at the cost of her own pain, than allow them to become indistinct, but Pilkington explained that she 'must go on from something lower to something higher, and … be willing to abandon the lower, material side, understanding that its pleasure was not real happiness'. The development of this relationship, literally from the physical to the spiritual world, encapsulates how Eglantyne would view all ideal relationships from this point on. There would be no more thoughts of romance or emotional friendships at the same level of intimacy as that with Margaret. ' "Thy Kingdom come" did not merely mean for me that the slums should be tidied up,' Eglantyne told Pilkington's spirit in March 1914. 'The coming of the Kingdom meant for me the redemption of the Body.'

Eglantyne's mourning process for Pilkington, perhaps also representing grief for the end of her romantic hopes, continues this theme. 'It's just shock you are suffering,' Pilkington assured her at their first interview, 'it's partly physical.' Eglantyne found great comfort in the knowledge that she could continue to talk with Pilkington, perhaps even more intimately than she would have done had he lived, and not long later she wrote that while she 'was still lamenting his death ... what I had called "anguish" had disappeared – the stab which recollections brought'. Within a few weeks she believed that death was simply a 'transmutation' to a spiritual level of existence, and she was able to write confidently that 'when you know for certain that death does not exist ... you will find it the starting point for many great discoveries'.

In this way Eglantyne's 'conversations' were clearly cathartic, like many spiritualist communications between the bereaved and their departed loved ones. But at the same time they were also a determined and deeply sad assertion of her personal physical denial. Perhaps thwarted love is too often credited with being the motive force behind women's achievements, but it seems that Eglantyne's frustrated sexuality really was a significant factor driving her passion for her cause just a few years later. Released from her anxieties about any past stray affection, the requirement to mourn Pilkington, and indeed even the need for future personal physical fulfilment, Eglantyne could now concentrate on planning her life's route towards the higher, spiritual plane to which she so aspired.

Eglantyne's shift towards examining her elusive vocation is the clearest component of her *Conversations*, and was also very much in keeping with the spiritualist tradition of championing active social reform. 'The influence of these conversations upon me has been to make me feel that to be united with God you must be united with life ...' Eglantyne breathed a great mental sigh of relief. 'Power of life must manifest itself in action ...work ... is the purposeful manifestation of the Divine Will.' Now she simply had to narrow down what it was that she wanted to do. Perhaps thinking of her responsibility to look after Tye, Pilkington reassured her that 'in working, as in everything else, one should try and get away from the personal aspect'. After discussing agricultural co-operatives and slum work, neither of which continued to inspire Eglantyne, he advised her to take a broader perspective on politics and her own goals. 'Your scale of values is wrong …' he argued, 'you should stand above [circumstances] mastering them instead of being mastered by them'. It was advice that resonated deeply with Eglantyne's desire to expand her focus away from the personal sphere. His next comment also held a profound significance for her: 'If only you had any faint conception', he told her, 'of the way in which the slightest use of spiritual power would sweep away your difficulties like leaves before the wind.' When Eglantyne finally found her cause in the global promotion of children's welfare and rights a few years later, her visionary perspective, combined with her belief in her spiritual mandate, not only inspired those around her but enabled her to reject the possibility of failure.

Although Eglantyne's recorded 'conversations' with Pilkington's spirit dried up after the spring of 1915, she maintained her interest in spiritualism and the unconscious mind throughout her life. In 1918 she had a number of 'dreams and psychical experiences', many of which revolved around Gamul whom she 'distinctly associated …' with the effort to promote life', and that year she also produced two more half-Freudian half-spiritual journals. Her *Book of Dreams* records a visit from a spirit standing at the head of her bed who 'galvanised' her by sending a violent sensation through her body, much like an electric shock, leaving her 'tingling through [her] fingertips' as she quickly recited some psalms. Afterwards she felt a great improvement in her health, although she was unsure how much this could be attributed to the apparition. 'I was very glad to feel myself in touch again with someone on the other side' she noted, before admitting to feeling 'vexed to think that I could have given way to my imagination'.

However by October 1918 Eglantyne's psychic impressions had become focused around 'terrible images'. Her occasional visions of the deaths of friends and relatives, most vividly illustrated by her prescience of Margaret's death at her wedding party in 1913, were now occurring more frequently, and her next private journal,

Experimenting with Dreams, recorded her attempts to exert some self-control. 'How often have I not imagined my relatives dead', she wrote, 'and wondered whether I had any psychic means of testing the mental image.' Her last recorded spiritual impression of 1918 was of a small girl ambiguously telling her that 'too much light blinds'. Perhaps she had decided that experimenting with the spirit world was at best a mixed blessing. In any case she now refocused her attention on the material world, and Save the Children – a resounding assertion of the value of life – was founded the following spring. Yet Eglantyne continued to be plagued by disturbing dreams and images. In 1925 she vividly recorded one dream in which she experienced the 'psychic' impression of watching someone drown himself, and in 1928 she recorded waking to see 'an evil thing, half woman, half animal' leaving her bedside. As she grew increasingly ill that year she even feared that 'the powers of evil' were coming to 'take possession' of her, and she would be 'killed now by this evil influence coming from the other side'. Her relationship with the spiritual had turned out to be unmanageable and at least as distressing in the long term as it had initially been supportive.

None of Eglantyne's later psychic experiences were as sustained, or held the same emotional weight with her, as her post-mortem discussions with Colonel Pilkington however. Once she had accepted their psychic validity she attached huge significance to them. 'I could see that she lived for that daily talk and all it meant to her,' Maud later wrote to Dorothy. 'What a tremendous help they were to her in preventing her from becoming "self-centred" and leading her to be indeed a channel of God's will and to be used by Him for great work.'

In fact Eglantyne and Pilkington's 'conversations' served a number of purposes. As a cerebral exercise they provided a practical outlet for Eglantyne's frustrated intellectual energies and a creative way to externalise her otherwise inarticulate thoughts and concerns when poetry and prose temporarily deserted her. As informal therapy, she was able explore her ideas and anxieties mediated through the alter ego of her spirit friend and so unrestricted by her conscious sense of probity. In this way she could resolve conflicts around her unfulfilled sexuality, and make positive sense of the grief brought by the rejections and deaths of those she loved. But above all the conversations provided her with a positive spiritual mandate for undertaking the public social role she craved.

Eglantyne yearned to live a life of moral purpose and social value but feared that her Cambridge projects had been parochial and her relief work in the Balkans futile. Margaret had married at the end of 1913, Pilkington died the following spring. Eglantyne felt lost and lonely. Although often painful, her spiritual examinations led her to the idea that life passed through several phases, from the material to the psychic, and then on to the spiritual, and she began to believe that it was only in her current incarnation that she was isolated; in the wider context she was part of a greater, shared, spiritual reality. It was a belief that gave her great comfort, and enabled her to reconcile herself to gaining personal emotional fulfilment through a life of public service.

'What is it that really matters?' Eglantyne asked Pilkington's spirit towards the end of one of their conversations:

> The chief thing that matters – perhaps the only real thing because it sums up everything else – is fidelity to one's ideals. In every political idea there is some truth. The question is should we actualise the truth or not, shall we make it reflect itself in our policy, or leave it as an unrealised aspiration?

What really matters about Eglantyne and Pilkington's conversations, where their real significance lies, is in what they reveal Eglantyne believed represented fidelity to her ideals, and what needed to be prioritised in her policy for her own life. Eglantyne's personal, mystical brand of spiritualism enabled her to see her life not as lonely and fractured, but as part of a greater, common experience. As such it made sense for her to realise her personal and social aspirations through a public vocation touching the lives of the many rather than just the few. However, as many female social pioneers had found before her, accepting a call to a higher purpose was not the same as finding opportunity and direction, and Eglantyne still had many obstacles to overcome before her hopes for living a meaningful life in the material world could be realised.

Chapter 10

Surrounded by Action, 1914–1916

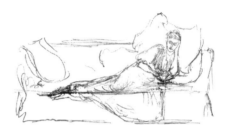

In idleness it seems impossible to be happy.

Eglantyne Jebb

This is 'the most bloody awful time of all bloody awful times …' Margaret's young husband AV wrote home despairingly in 1916. Between 1914 and 1918 Eglantyne's life, in common with that of everyone in Britain, was overshadowed by the First World War. 'I have absolutely no cause for personal grief –', she wrote firmly, 'I who have no near relation at the Front.'[1] But Eglantyne knew many young men who went off to fight for their country, and she shared the grief of her friends who lost husbands, brothers and cousins, as well as the profound shock of the whole nation at the escalating horror and human cost of the war. For Eglantyne's three sisters, as for many women, the war was an unprecedented call to, and opportunity for, greater public action. By

Eglantyne propped up on a couch, drawn by Tye, undated

now Em, Lill and Dorothy were all married with children, but nonetheless each either energetically supported the war effort or tried to influence national policy in another direction. As a result Tye's family scrapbooks, still carefully preserved at The Lyth, are bursting with cuttings recording the very different wartime activities and achievements of her two elder and her youngest daughters. Only Eglantyne, who had recently been so active in the Balkans, was quiet; caught up in a painful struggle of her own as she rather mutely witnessed the war escalate and her hopes for peace and a more equitable international society fall apart around her. Surrounded by action at every level, her own apparent uselessness added to her misery, and she finally cocooned herself away to brood on human nature, the horror of war and the deficiencies and injustices of the world in general.

Eglantyne's apparent paralysis was perhaps all the more surprising because war had always aroused the strongest emotions within her. As an imaginative nine-year-old she had developed a deeply romantic view of the glories of battle, inspired by the poems of Tennyson and family stories of Cavalier Jebb ancestors standing beside King Charles on the field at Chester.[2] Hours were spent investing her family with military titles and duties, planning campaigns and waging war on the ground staff at The Lyth, which generally involved leaping from yew trees while yelling helpful commands to the gardener like 'tear their eyes out Neddy-boy'. If she stopped to consider it she might have realised that the Charge of the Light Brigade in the Crimea and the Battle of Rowton Heath at Chester – if you were a Royalist – were both famous defeats. More poignantly her French–Alsatian governess, Heddie Kastler, had often entranced her with stories of the cruel Prussian occupation of Alsace-Lorraine after the 1870 war. For the fiercely romantic young Eglantyne however it all only added to the tragic appeal of vain human struggle expressed through noble warfare.

By the time she was herself a struggling twenty-three-year-old schoolteacher however, the in many ways disastrous Boer War had brought some of the brutal reality of conflict home to Eglantyne. 'Do you find that your feeling on the subject of war changes as you grow older?' she challenged Dorothy Kempe in 1899. 'I recollect that when I was a child the idea of fighting filled me with positive glee, and [now] the delight that children take in the idea of English victories quite puzzles me, while the absence of the slightest horror connected with the actual fighting and killing makes me rather ill.' Nonetheless she accepted the premise of the war and undertook her patriotic duty by knitting soldiers' balaclavas, mittens, socks and – as her skills were less than perfect – footless stockings and scarves, although not without some blithe misgivings. 'I wonder how on earth they are going to carry all the things presented by the daughters of England, without resembling the knight in Alice in Wonderland,' she wrote. 'Does it not contain a fresh danger to our arms? "The English army, having fallen lame on a march, were ..." etc. ... I can only stretch my imagination so far as picturing a disgusted Tommy throwing it away with "d- the thing!" after a valiant effort to drag it over his head ...' The following year she wrote a full if rather comical report of the return of one 'solitary hero' to Marlborough, greeted by the town crier, the national anthem and 'an unhorsed wagonette of somewhat funereal aspect, mounted however with a Union Jack'. And three years on, still soldier-watching, she told Dorothy of her frustration at 'longing to be in the thick of every battle', while having to confess pathetically 'that the only soldiers I have seen were two ... pointed out to me walking along the bit of road we can see from the dining-room window'.

It was not until she witnessed the impact of conflict in the Balkans ten years later that Eglantyne replaced her gentle patriotism with a passionate antipathy towards all war. With the start of what was known, for a while, as the Great War, she and her younger sister Dorothy both became committed pacifists; a hugely unpopular position to take when so many families were losing their loved ones in the fighting. It is 'curious that as small children she and I were such little *Nazis* in our love of soldiering and advocation of martial heroes!' Dorothy later looked back, when with the onset of war in 1914 'we recognised pacifism as inseparable from our religion; inherent in all we loved most and believed most intently'.

When Britain declared war on Germany at the end of a sunny bank holiday weekend in August 1914, *The Times* reported that the 'demonstration of patriotism and loyalty became almost ecstatic'. Huge numbers believed the government that the war would be 'over by Christmas', but within a year much that had been taken for granted, from the aims and duration of the war, and the acceptable levels of losses that might be sustained, to the structure of society at home, had come to be fundamentally questioned. By the Armistice in November 1918, over eight and a half million soldiers had been killed. The total of deaths including civilians reached over twenty million internationally. In Britain alone over five million men, most under the age of forty, had been mobilised to fight. More than one in eight never returned home.[3] 'Youth alone, it seemed, had the task of trying to save civilization from the catastrophe which had befallen it,' Vera Brittain wrote after losing her brother, fiancé and many of their closest friends. This loss of what became known as a 'generation' of young men was also that of a generation of young women now unlikely to marry and have families of their own.[4] For Eglantyne, already considered an old maid at thirty-eight when war was announced, any last thoughts of marriage could pretty well be forgotten. The 'sacrifice of youth' must have been poignantly brought home to her on many levels.

Yet in other ways the war was unexpectedly liberating for British women, giving them unprecedented opportunities to move into the paid labour market or take up positions of public authority to fill the vacancies left by the men called to serve. Between 1914 and 1918 an estimated two million women replaced men in employment, and the accepted perception of what women were capable of changed irrevocably. In 1918 graduate or propertied women over the age of thirty were finally granted the vote. 'The war revolutionised the industrial position for women,' the suffrage leader Millicent Fawcett wrote that year, 'it found them serfs and left them free.'

Many women also spent the war overseas as nurses and relief workers, often being inspired to great acts of courage and crossing boundaries both social and geographic that they would never have considered in the security of peacetime. The vision of these women was far ahead of the male establishment whose attitude in 1914 was summed up by Sir Frederick Treves, Chair of the British Red Cross, when he told nurse Mabel Annie Stobart that there 'was not work fitted for women in the sphere of war'. Stobart, who had already worked as a nurse in the Balkans in 1912, was undaunted and continued to serve in the region, financially backed by Charlie's brother, Noel, serving as Chair of the Balkan War Relief Committee. And when the British War Office rejected an offer of help from the Scottish doctor Elsie Inglis, famously writing 'My good lady, go home and sit still,' Inglis independently raised fourteen Scottish Women's Hospital units for France, Serbia, Greece, Salonika, Russia and Romania.

For a while in Macedonia Eglantyne had lived and worked alongside some of these courageous women, like Katharine Hodges who became attached to the first Serbian Unit of Dr Inglis's hospitals. But Eglantyne did not offer her services now. She had welcomed the adventure of overseas work when it was focused around the organisation of relief, something she had a skill for, but was less enamoured with the idea of hands-on nursing; the personal rarely appealed to her. Now even the value of her relief work seemed negligible given the seemingly irresistible movement towards aggression, war and despair across Europe. For some time nothing seemed to hold any promise or consolation. Meanwhile Eglantyne's sisters and closest friends all responded very differently to the extraordinary circumstances of the war, endeavouring to make meaningful contributions to the war effort, relief work and international political debate.

Lill had consolidated her position as a national authority on rural reform and agricultural production as a Governor of the AOS, where for a while in 1914 she sheltered Eglantyne in the editorial office. As well as helping to develop the Women's Institute movement in Britain, Lill now also set about establishing a new organisation that would later become famous as 'The Women's Land Army'.[5] The announcement of national conscription in 1916, making agricultural labourers liable for military service, inspired her to propose 'a Government Land Army on semi-military lines'. Once the Cabinet had approved the principle Lill threw herself behind the recruitment of 'land girls'. 'Have the women of Britain awakened sufficiently to the fact that ultimate victory and the position of England after the War depends as much on them as on the men who are actually fighting?' she sent out her call to action in *The Times*.[6] Within a year over nine thousand women were digging the fields and shocking the nation by wearing breeches. Lill turned down the offer to become Director of the women's branch of the Board of Agriculture, but in August 1917 she was honoured with an OBE for her founding role in the Women's Land Army. By the following year there were thirteen thousand women working on the land.

Em had long before fallen in love both with the country her mother came from, and with an Irishman, Beverly Ussher, and by 1914 she was living a quiet family life at Beverly's estate in County Waterford. The first years of the war did not touch her much, but in 1916 she and Eglantyne, who was visiting for a few months, were shocked by the brutality of the British suppression of the Easter Uprising and its violent aftermath. Em had great sympathy with the cause of Irish independence and, inspired by Eglantyne's attempts at social fiction, she now began a novel of her own to highlight the injustice of British rule in Ireland, incidentally usurping Eglantyne as the family storyteller.[7] Em's previous publications had been limited to botanical teaching observations and a guide to public schools. Her novel, *The Trail of the Black and Tans*, was in a different league altogether: an action-packed adventure centred around the resistance work of a selfless young brother and sister, the wonderfully named Joanna and Shaun Cromwell, it concluded with several dramatic deaths and the lesson that no side ever has a monopoly on decent people. Provocatively dedicated to 'men who desired truth at all costs, and who pursued it with unflinching courage …' rather excitingly the novel had to be published anonymously in 1921 – Em chose the fantastic pseudonym 'the Hurler on the Ditch' – for fear of reprisals such as having her house burnt down. The book went on to become a bestseller although – or perhaps because – it was by then a slightly historical subject, the survivors of the Easter Uprising having convened the first Dáil and established the Irish Republic in January 1919.

Dorothy and Charlie spent the war, and the rest of their lives, as tireless campaigners for peace and international justice. After their valiant but futile diplomatic mission to Bulgaria, Noel Buxton continued to serve as a Liberal MP, but Charlie became a founder – and significant funder – of the 'Union of Democratic Control', a political pressure group set up to oppose the war and the way in which its members believed the government had railroaded British involvement through. Other founding members included Ramsay MacDonald, who resigned as Chair of the Labour Party when it supported the government's war budget, the Labour MP Philip Snowden, Bertrand Russell and the feminist Maude Royden, a contemporary of Eglantyne's at Oxford. Prefacing a collection of essays promoting international political co-operation, Charlie wrote that their 'one predominant aim' was 'securing that a world catastrophe such as the present shall never recur'. His own position was neatly summed up in a leaflet he wrote for the 'Women's Peace Crusade', privately published by Ethel Snowden, Philip Snowden's politically active wife:

When the lives of millions are at stake it is criminal to neglect to examine fully every possible opening for ending the War on just and honourable terms. There have been many such opportunities which have been missed ... Real Statesmen would have used these opportunities either to secure our aims without further fighting, or to make it quite clear to the peoples of the Central Powers that we are not continuing the war for the purposes of aggression ... Another opportunity will occur – shall it be lost?'[8]

But however diplomatically worded, any criticism of the war policy was unacceptable to many, and Charlie's publications quickly caused public outrage. In 1916 he consolidated his unpopularity with a lecture tour to promote a negotiated peace. 'I have heard him speak before', one Mr Glover of the 'Anti-German Union' reported, 'and he ought to be hanged by the neck until he is dead.' Later that year he published his lectures under the title *Shouted Down: A Practical Permanent and Honourable Settlement of International Disputes*. He was soon expelled from his local Liberal Association, but continued to be an effective thorn in the government's side.[9]

Disgusted by the continuing war policy, in 1917 Charlie and Dorothy joined the Independent Labour Party, the only political party to oppose the war – although even it had not run a public peace campaign. Soon rejecting the Church of England's stance on the war, they also joined the Society of Friends. 'You will be interested to hear that Charlie and Dorothy are now Quakers!' Eglantyne wrote to Tye that February, focusing on the spiritual rather than the political implications of their decision. 'I am very happy about it ... It seems to have brought into Dorothy's life a sense of spiritual fellowship which she never had before. When it was settled that "rapt" look which she sometimes wears informed me that something very happy indeed had happened to her.'

Dorothy however, like her husband, had increasingly been focusing on politics. When the international suffrage movement was put on hold for the duration of the war, many seasoned female campaigners turned their attention to influencing the war policy. Soon the 'International Committee of Women for Permanent Peace' was advocating the settlement of disputes between countries in an international forum in which women could play an equal part. Rejecting the idea that the war was inevitable, over a thousand women from both belligerent and neutral countries defied all obstacles to meet at an International Congress in the Netherlands in April 1915. Of the 190 British delegates only twenty-four women judged non-militant by the authorities were given permits to attend, the others having their passports refused or cancelled. The Congress opened six days into the Second Battle of Ypres, in which one hundred thousand men, including the husbands, sons and brothers of many of the delegates, would lose their lives. The women meanwhile together developed principles on the basis of which they believed the slaughter could be stopped and a permanent peace constructed. They then demanded an end to the war, urging the USA and Sweden to begin a mediation process. 'Folly in petticoats', screamed the British *Sunday Pictorial*, while the delegates were described as a 'shipload of hysterical women' by *The Globe*, and as 'pro-Hun Peacettes' in the *Daily Express*. 'Women peace fanatics are becoming a nuisance and a bore,' the *Evening Standard* threw in its pennyworth, and *The Times* opened a long leading article with the words 'The Women's International Congress, which met at The Hague last week, was of course a fiasco.' So 'why', asked the journalist Evelyn Sharp, who had been refused a passport, did it 'devote a whole column or so to talking about it?' Inspired by the principles of the congress and disgusted by the subsequent press coverage, Dorothy joined the 'Women's International League for Peace and Freedom' that grew out of the congress in October 1916, soon meeting many well-connected women like Maude Royden, Kathleen Courtney, Emmeline Pethick-Lawrence and Ethel Snowden, who would become allies in her and Eglantyne's own campaigns.

Even Margaret Keynes, now Mrs AV Hill, had a more active war than Eglantyne, and she was stuck in Cambridge, looking after what was soon a family of four young children. Despite the domestic demands on her Margaret took a lead role in securing local accommodation for over a hundred Belgian refugees within the first year of the war. AV meanwhile had put his research into amphibian muscle mechanics on hold while posted in charge of a unit of mathematicians carrying out experiments in anti-aircraft gunnery on the south coast. Florence Keynes, in 1914 the first woman to be elected to Cambridge Borough Council and busy with numerous war projects of her own, released his sixty large Hungarian frogs into the river at Reach, where they flourished, producing a now quite sizeable population in Romney Marsh. Maynard's national service had started in the immediate run-up to the declaration of war when the Treasury summoned him for advice on an early August Sunday. Wary of train delays AV drove his brother-in-law up to London in Buster, his idiosyncratic motorbike sidecar – although Maynard alighted as they drew near to Whitehall, having felt 'it would be incongruous to approach the august portals of the Treasury on a pre-war London Sunday afternoon in this conveyance'. The following year Maynard entered the Treasury for the duration of the war, 'advising and trying to prevent panic' in Margaret's sisterly assessment, and gaining huge respect for his leading policy role at the centre of the inter-allied economic effort.

Eglantyne meanwhile was notably absent. In 1915 she had slowly withdrawn from her London-based AOS work to live increasingly with Tye at her newly built house, Forest Edge, in Crowborough where she squirreled herself away in her room talking to Colonel Pilkington's ghost. After years of frustration at being removed from her pre-war Cambridge social work by Tye's wish to travel round Europe, her lack of activity now that women in general, and she in particular, had greater opportunity to contribute to the public life of the nation than ever before seems deeply ironic. But Eglantyne was temporarily not fit for service.

Those closest to her had always believed that despite Eglantyne's love of horse-riding, cycling and climbing she had a 'naturally' weak constitution which inevitably failed her when she pushed herself too hard. This was certainly Tye's opinion when she insisted that her emotionally fragile daughter stop teaching at her miserable Marlborough school, or accompany her on tours of Swiss health resorts. And for some years even Eglantyne had admitted that all was not well. 'I am always very tired …' she had confessed to her diary as she withdrew from the Cambridge Boys Employment Registry in 1908, 'I often feel sick. I have pains which are probably neuralgia. I can hardly keep my eyes open, it is a great effort to do any work.' But Eglantyne also recognised that half of the problem seemed to be in her head. 'I should not mind all this if I could only keep good,' she continued, 'but when I am tired my worst characteristics come out … I have exalted ideas of my own cleverness … Although I have a vague idea that somehow or other I am a genius – a genius in general – I am an imbecile in every particular and do my work very badly.' Time and again Tye and the doctors prescribed rest, but enforced unemployment only frustrated Eglantyne, exacerbating her blacker moods until she wrote desperately to Margaret 'in idleness it seems impossible to be happy'. Margaret saw how closely Eglantyne's physical health corresponded with her state of mind. 'You know when you get thoroughly run down like that you are absolutely certain to get miserable feelings back,' she wrote in 1911. 'Darling do allow that when you are tired out you get despairing sort of feelings.' The following year she was more direct, writing 'Sweet, you have got a nervous breakdown and you must accept the fact and take miserable feelings merely as one symptom … Mother doubts if great brains and strong physiques ever go together, but it is very hard luck to have to realise your limitations.'

Eglantyne was never one for accepting 'limitations', and at first she tried to defeat her illness through positive mental attitude. 'My fatigue is a fatigue habit', she self-diagnosed, 'and as such should surely be subject to a mind cure. I must experiment in order to try and get stronger.' In a typical burst of optimism and energy she had never questioned having the stamina for her Balkan relief mission in 1913, but back in England with war escalating, and herself again increasingly redundant, her depression returned with force, and not for the first time she began to have suicidal thoughts. In 1902 she had rather romantically considered drowning her grief in 'the darkening marshes' outside Cambridge after Marcus Dimsdale had married Elsie. Overworked and exhausted in 1908 she admitted to herself, 'I have arrived at that stage when, in my heart, I don't really seem to want to get better. I don't know why. My comfort seems to be to hope all the time that I may fall ill or have a bicycle accident or something.' In her 1913 *Soul's Roadbook* she had written overtly of her 'desire for death', and now again, in 1914, her lowest year, she began to pray for an 'escape from the personal pain of living …'

Eglantyne's swings between debilitating depressions and renewed bursts of confidence and energy clearly followed a pattern, but to say that she suffered from some kind of bipolar disorder adds little insight into how she would have understood her own condition or been diagnosed and treated at the time. The causes of mood swings are hugely involved, ranging from genetic disorders and organic ill-health, to personal loss and international tragedy. All of these factors may have played a part with Eglantyne. However during 1914 her condition deteriorated significantly, and the next year she developed a visible goitre – a swelling of the thyroid gland – and she was finally diagnosed with a thyroid disorder.

The thyroid is the largest gland in the neck, and is often described as being shaped like a butterfly with left and right lobes that wrap around the trachea. Eglantyne's damaged thyroid fluttered nervously around her throat, sometimes gripping a little too tightly and in its panic producing excess or insufficient hormones to regulate her body's metabolism. The influence of such extremes or fluctuations can be far reaching and quite critical to the normal functioning of the body, affecting heart rates, body weight, energy levels, mental processes and morale in the short term, and if left untreated impacting on the cardiovascular system and other major organs. Eglantyne may have suffered from hyperthyroidism – an overactive butterfly – a common condition that is still difficult to diagnose, and that could have contributed both towards her periods of hyperactivity, rapid heart rate, and at times nervous and over-agitated behaviour, as well as her more sustained periods of exhaustion and weight loss. The Irish physician Robert Graves who discovered overactive thyroid disease, commonly known as Graves' disease, suspected that severe emotional stress could trigger the symptoms, and commented on the stressful events in many of his patients' lives that came several months before the development of hyperthyroidism. This corresponds with Eglantyne's dramatic responses to stressful events, like Margaret's marriage and Pilkington's death, with a period of exaggerated mental anguish and physical frailty. However in 1915 understanding about thyroid disorders was still limited, and an operation would have been seen as the best treatment for an obtrusive goitre if rest and fresh air could not effect an improvement. By now Eglantyne was so thin and frail that she had to rely on a bath-chair to get out of the house, and it was probably in an attempt to avoid surgery that she agreed to move in permanently with Tye at Crowborough.

Eglantyne had supervised much of the construction work on her mother's Crowborough house, but she was not particularly pleased with the result, reporting bluntly that it looked hideous from the road. Nonetheless there were wonderful views across the High Weald from the back, and the rooms were big and airy; 'as for the attic' Eglantyne wrote, 'if the Germans land on the South coast, we should be able to quarter a regiment there'. Here she and Tye received many visitors, including Lill, Dorothy and Gem, and close friends like Ruth who was recently back from five years in Japan and had been a passenger on the *Lusitania*'s last voyage that May. Most guests carefully avoided depressing discussions of the war. Gem, described by Eglantyne as 'looking more like an old tramp than usual in an old mackintosh coat which I had given her about six years ago, after having worn it out', would sit and recite Wordsworth, Milton and Keats for several hours. With Lill and Ruth they discussed the growing Women's Institute movement, Tye finding it pleasingly reminiscent of her Home Arts organisation twenty years before. Dorothy's talk was more political and agitated. 'Lill and Dorothy are so far apart in their opinions that they refrain from entering on debateable territory when they are together,' Eglantyne recorded with interested amusement, continuing perceptively, 'I come about halfway in between, Dorothy shooting into space, Lill striding along on solid earth, I fuming somewhere in between.'

It was impossible to block out all news of the war, and in any case, this was not what Eglantyne wanted. Trying not to be a complete recluse she had invested in a stout white horse to pull her bath-chair through the woods and over the commons, and she called him Tommy, the generic name for a common British soldier.[10] Even on these very local excursions she would occasionally come across signs of the war, such as soldiers digging trenches and practising man-oeuvres at, appropriately enough she noted, an old Roman camp. Then a visit from Lady Darwin who had lost her only son, Erasmus, in April 1915, filled Eglantyne with helpless compassion: if only they could talk about it instead of making polite conversation, she wrote miserably.[11]

Eglantyne made little reference to the war in her private corre-spondence between 1914 and 1917 however. Removed from the detail of daily news and discussion, she turned her mind to the ques-tion of who, or what, had caused the war. In late 1915 she wrote a paper which stepped back even further to ask 'Who Makes War?' It was a theme that would come to dominate cultural as well as politi-cal debate in Europe over the next forty years.[12] Eglantyne's thoughts did not yet contribute to this public debate, which is a pity because in many ways her fresh emphasis on shared humanity and human responsibility, rather than what we might call 'blame culture', was quite visionary. Unlike many, Eglantyne did not blame men,

Germans or any other particular social group for creating war, and equally she did not exonerate women, self-proclaimed 'Christians' or even 'pacifists', who might often condemn international conflict, she wrote, 'only to advocate war between classes'. Instead she championed the need for a new collective responsibility to redress human hatred and embrace brotherly love at an individual level. 'Let us have the courage to face the truth' her passionate paper declared; 'It is not particular nations or classes or statesmen which are the makers of war; it is not Kings or Emperors, it is not militarists, it is not the armament makers, it is not the scare-makers and the Press: it is you and I. They are the puppets of destiny: we are the creators of destiny.'

However while Eglantyne might bravely criticise misguided 'Christians', hers *was* essentially a religious analysis: it sat well with the New Liberal concepts of citizenship she had already adopted, but was notably devoid of any political or economic inquiry and would not have suited Charlie's anthologies of anti-war essays. Eglantyne's faith was firmly planted in the moral re-armament of the individual long before that idea had been developed into the international religious movement of the late 1930s. It was a position that both reflected and reinforced her growing belief in common humanity and the importance of individual citizenship linked to broad social repsonsibilities. From now on her very personal faith and her public social policy would remain firmly aligned. Nonetheless she made no protest at the series of government war policies that restricted civil liberties, and she did not advocate international negotiation, call for public protest, or even promote her own ideas around individual moral responsibility. Despite all her passion, her standpoint reflected a moment of fundamental introspection and passivity.[13] She simply did not have the physical stamina to navigate her illness and engage actively with public life.

Eglantyne was relieved to find that her tiredness and depressions had a physical cause, feeling that the knowledge armed her to combat them more effectively. 'The trouble about my complaint is its extraordinarily depressing effect,' she told her aunt Bun. 'The fits of depression which have been such a tiresome trouble to me all my life have no doubt had this physical basis ... The sane wholesome facts of daily life should be a corrective to the distorting images of illness yet I did not know how to focus my mind on them.'[14] Now that she finally had a diagnosis she should have been focusing on her physical health, but in this she also proved fairly ineffectual. She had promised her doctor to take her pulse but her watch had no second hand; she was to keep a record of her weight but she only had a machine for weighing letters and she hadn't shrunk enough for that; and she was to measure the girth of her neck but found it varied depending how she tilted her head. In August 1915 she visited her doctor in London, who recommended radium treatment, or X-rays, which were more expensive and would take longer. Not surprisingly she opted for the radium, but then she postponed even that so as to spend more time in the Sussex countryside. Soon she was not strong enough to tolerate an operation even should it have been deemed necessary.

That autumn Eglantyne's doctor recommended she spend the winter recovering her strength in the Scottish Highlands. Delighted with the prescription, she quickly decamped to an isolated cottage at Tomatin, sixteen miles from Inverness and more than a thousand feet above sea-level. Here her only neighbours were a few hard-working women whom she occasionally visited by ski or toboggan, commenting loftily that they 'don't belong to any class except the great class of humanity ...' – although she couldn't resist also noting that 'the absence of teeth labels them with a wholly fallacious class badge'. Meanwhile indulging her well-established sense of romantic melancholy, once referred to by her uncle Richard as 'divine despair', Eglantyne celebrated the 'splendid desolation' of her surroundings, describing one windswept view with evident delight as 'grim almost to tragedy'.

Eglantyne had always been torn between her need for society and solitude, work and withdrawal. 'Seclusion is to me a heaven on earth,' she once confessed, and now she revelled in the remoteness of her snowy cottage, free from both obligation and reprobation. 'Never all day the voice of a human', she wrote in a moment of relief; 'who would not be a hermit?' Just a few years earlier she had been sharply dismissive of a Serbian civilian she had met whose only ambition was to remove himself from society as a self-sufficient peasant. 'I seemed to see it all so clearly', she had reflected disparagingly; 'the man's passionate disgust with his present circumstances, and fervid aspiration after a simple blameless existence far removed from the annoyances and temptations of the world ... the urgent problems of the universe were nothing to him'. But now she did not let it bother her that her hermit's life in the remote highlands of Scotland hardly sat well with her own highly developed ideas on active citizenship and social responsibility. 'Indeed I think one of the best things one can do for the country is to forget it sometimes, and attend to the nearest claims instead,' she wrote to Margaret.

The closest Eglantyne got to work at this time was beginning a new social novel, *Confessions of a Kleptomaniac*. Sadly no manuscript survives but Eglantyne used the word kleptomania in terms of social theft; the unnecessary accumulation of material wealth at the expense of those with greater need.[15] Now in her simple cottage, divested of most of her possessions, she tried to live out her ideals, experimenting with living on 6d a day through a strict diet of lentils, oatmeal, peas, turnips, potatoes and rice. She kept a notebook on her project, with careful tables listing the prices of 'all articles used', as well as telling descriptions of her performance. 'The bread I ate was of varying date,' one entry read, 'some more than a fortnight old.' She also cheated, recording that 'the milk I had made my meals much more pleasant, especially as my half pints were singularly large ones. It is a very economical plan to buy milk from people whose quantities are double the average size.' Even this was a short-lived experiment however. 'I have a good Scots lassie called Jessie who comes to help me every morning except Sunday,' she was soon writing to Bun, even boasting, 'I have nine cookery books, I have made gooseberry tart, and Jessie says my scones are as good as her mother's.'

By early January 1916 the snow had melted enough for Eglantyne to collect firewood from the moors. The final thaw arrived that April, bringing with it her first visitor, Charlotte Toynbee, who discussed her writing projects and took her on a tour of Inverness.[16] Soon it was time to return to England, where for a while Eglantyne picked up her work with the AOS, watched Lill's project with the Women's Land Army gain momentum, and prepared herself for the thyroid surgery that was now unavoidable.

Eglantyne's operation took place on 14 August 1916. She pronounced her consultant, James Berry, to be 'an old fashioned surgeon', and he certainly looked the part with his serious face and neatly pointed beard, although his crumpled eyes behind round glasses were not unsympathetic. Had Eglantyne felt up to it they would have had plenty to talk about, as Berry had a particular interest in south-eastern Europe and had volunteered with the British Red Cross in Serbia during the war. He was also an expert in thyroid surgery, and later became one of the foremost consulting surgeons and lecturers on clinical surgery of his day.[17] For her own part, Eglantyne was now forty years old, uncomfortably thin with soft, almost translucent skin, heavily greying hair and a goitre in her neck that Berry described as 'the size of a small orange'. After the operation he noted that there was no 'naked eye' evidence of Graves' disease, and it is possible that the tumour was benign. In any case the surgery that Eglantyne underwent under Berry's supervision was deemed a success, and she was quickly dismissed to convalesce with her eldest sister, Em, in Ireland.

She returned home towards the end of 1916, at first staying with Tye but as her strength and energy returned increasingly gravitating towards Dorothy and Charlie in London. She was devoted to all her family, but she and Dorothy were the most in tune in terms of faith and politics. Now Eglantyne began to take a keen interest in a new project of Dorothy's which aimed to promote a more humanitarian understanding of Britain's enemies, and with it the possibility of a negotiated peace. Despite regular relapses in her health she would never again retire from society or active social service. There would be no more long luxurious weeks devoted to writing or walking in the countryside, but she would also never again suffer the intense frustration of having time on her hands without the energy or occupation to make use of it. Meanwhile her few years' sabbatical had enabled her to digest her social priorities. Unlike Dorothy, Eglantyne did not wish to make an overtly political contribution to the world, but something purely humanitarian that reflected her belief in the spiritual oneness of humankind, and focused on the promotion of individual responsibilities to create just and peaceful societies. As an American delegate to the International Women's Congress of 1915 wrote: 'In the distress of mind that war breeds in every thinking and feeling person, there is a poignant relief in finding a channel through which to work for peace.' Dorothy was about to provide Eglantyne with that channel, but Eglantyne had already found the humanitarian message that she hoped to promote.

Chapter 11

Found in Translation,
1917–1919

I've an increasing suspicion,
Although hitherto I have hid it.
God will not let us off scot free
When we say that the Government did it.

Eglantyne Jebb, 1919

'I am beginning to loathe the newspapers', Beatrice Webb wrote in her diary in August 1914, 'with their bombast and lies about atrocities, or their delighted gossip about the famine and disease in "enemy" countries.' Despite widely reported war-fever many politicians, social analysts, pacifists and feminists in Britain were privately horrified by the blatantly propagandist tone and jingoistic reporting of the war in the press. It was Eglantyne's sister Dorothy, however, who was to take on the British newspapers. Exasperated by the biased coverage of the Women's International Congress, growing hysteria about German war crimes, and the lack of reports on dissent with the war policy, Dorothy decided that the best way to restore some balance to the public debate would be to publish extracts from the newspapers of enemy and neutral countries. Her aim was to promote a negotiated peace by showing both that these countries had a case for consideration, and that they were far from single-minded in the pursuit of war.

It was a fantastic idea in both senses of the word: the British press had never been more strictly controlled than in 1914. Frank revelations of military mismanagement and incompetence dispatched by *The Times* correspondent William Howard Russell and the photography of Roger Fenton during the Crimean War fifty years earlier had revolutionised war reporting, bringing the realities of conflict, both good and bad, home to readers with unprecedented immediacy. Then at the turn of the century the widely reported disasters and domestic policy implications of the Boer War had been hugely damaging for the government, contributing to the dramatic Conservative defeat in the 1906 general election. The Liberals had learnt the lesson and the first organised British press censorship, including a ban on photography, came in with the First World War.[1] Given this consistent move towards control over newspaper coverage, the government was not likely to accept a proposal from an obscure female pacifist to reproduce and circulate uncensored and probably inflammatory articles from the enemy press.

Despite historically advocating peace and non-intervention in foreign affairs, in 1914 the British Liberal government under Herbert Asquith accepted the necessity of declaring war on Germany. In order to sustain the war effort the Liberals were now obliged to appeal to a spirit of nationalism that they had previously found distasteful, and promote the encroachment of the State upon the rights of its citizens that they had always championed so highly. This volte-face was evident in the very first government measure of the war, the Defence of the Realm Act, which was rushed through Parliament in August 1914, conferring unprecedented authority on the state and its agencies to control the lives of ordinary people. A whole range of restrictions followed, ranging from press censorship and food rationing to conscription and the introduction of passports. All of these measures would affect the way in which Dorothy and Eglantyne viewed the progress and impact of the war, their own commitment to Liberal principles, and their right, even their duty, to protest when they believed the moral position of the government they had hitherto actively supported became untenable.

Dorothy's great bugbear was not press censorship per se, but the deliberate vilification of the German people, now 'the enemy' in the press, to help justify the war. One of the main foreign policy goals before the war had been to maintain a balance of power in Europe. Years of favouring Germany to counterbalance the strength of Britain's historic enemy, France, had made German culture very fashionable in Victorian and Edwardian Britain. Many upper-class homes like The Lyth kept German governesses for their daughters, or sent them to Germany for six months' 'finishing'. Em had studied portrait painting at Dresden, and Margaret Keynes had had a less productive sabbatical in Wittenberg. Dorothy and Eglantyne meanwhile had formed close bonds with their German governess, a hardworking woman whose 'quiet eyes, half grave, half humorous' Eglantyne would later remember in her 1918 poem, 'To my old German governess, dying in consequence of the Blockade'.[2] The sudden reversal of British allegiances and growing hostility towards Germany, which intensified with the two countries' naval rivalry, therefore ran directly counter to the sisters' experiences and the traditional cultural associations of many people in Britain. By 1912, when her own children, Eglantyne and David, were six and two, Dorothy was getting increasingly concerned about the security of German nationals living in Britain, and she invited a German family to live with them. Within months of war being announced she had moved her family into a rented flat to make their more spacious house available for German women stranded in London. This was the start of what was to become Dorothy's lifelong crusade for justice for Germany, and for oppressed minorities within the country under the Nazi state.

Dorothy's concerns about the security of German people stranded in Britain in 1914 were not without foundation. The Allied propaganda machine rapidly proved highly effective in portraying the enemy not as a modern nation, but as the 'Hun', a brutal race who could not be trusted. 'England was … blockaded against the truth,' Charlie's secretary Mosa Anderson wrote. 'We were presented with a picture made very plausible by means of clever quotations from German jingoistic writers, of a Germany thirsting for world hegemony and united, man, woman, and child, in their ruthless savagery.'

By the end of 1914 xenophobia was rife in both Britain and Germany and a plethora of 'atrocity stories' in which enemy soldiers were demonised started to hit the press in both countries, filling the vacuum left by lack of real news about progress with the war. In Britain shopkeepers with German-sounding names were hounded and their premises sometimes smashed, long-trusted German governesses were accused of espionage, and there were even reports of dachshunds, the German breed of dog, being destroyed in the patriotic frenzy. A sense of humour may have been evident when in 1915 the German Kaiser at Madame Tussaud's was moved from the royalty rooms to the Chamber of Horrors, but national security measures were far from light-hearted. Soon even naturalised Germans in Britain faced compulsory registration, and many were interned. Dorothy was the only woman to officially visit the camps for German men to keep an eye on conditions, and for a while, as Eglantyne worked for the AOS, Dorothy ran a handicrafts class in an internment camp under the auspices of the Society of Friends. It was unpopular work that set many tongues wagging, but nothing compared with the idea of deliberately promoting 'enemy propaganda'.

Although it was considered distinctly unpatriotic, if not seditious, through Charlie's political network Dorothy managed to extract permission from the new Prime Minister, David Lloyd George, to regularly import twenty-five newspapers from neutral and enemy countries. Soon even papers from Austria and Germany started arriving through her and Charlie's north London letterbox. Looking back at this astonishing result Dorothy could only explain that prompted by a 'psychic premonition' she had applied immediately for a lifting of the ban in her case and 'was amazed, – or at least my friends were, – to receive the necessary permission by return of post'. The War Office undertook a daily review of the foreign press, but circulation was closely restricted. Even the MP Philip Snowden was refused a copy of the official review in 1918, on the grounds of the 'necessity of economy in paper'. 'I think the writer might have invented a more plausible and somewhat more accurate reason for his refusal,' Snowden wrote dryly to Charlie. But possibly the Board of Trade – who signed off Dorothy's approval in 1915 – was not unwilling to have extra 'intelligence work' undertaken voluntarily, and did not expect Dorothy's private print-run to generate much interest.

Dorothy, however, was planning on making an impact. She quickly turned the spacious attic of her and Charlie's Golders Green home into translation HQ, roped in as many friends as possible to work as translators, sold her mother's car to pay for a short-hand typist, and from August 1915 – just as Eglantyne's health was forcing her to give up work – Dorothy started anonymously publishing extracts from the papers in a weekly leaflet she called 'Notes from the Foreign Press'. Things quickly snowballed, and soon she was supervising a major operation with large teams of voluntary linguists and specialists in current affairs translating over a hundred papers a week imported from France, Germany, Austria, Italy, Russia, Hungary, Romania and Finland, and carefully representing a balance of royalist, socialist, conservative, republican and independent editorials.

Dorothy's stated aim was 'to supplement the English press in providing information as to the points of view held in other countries, both allied and enemy, in connection with the war'. The unofficial intention was to provide a balanced picture of events to influence both public opinion and statesmen, and ultimately help to shorten the war. This was a hugely daring pacifist venture at a time of relentless pro-war and anti-German propaganda, and as such it was widely criticised by the established press. It was therefore a courageous act on the part of Charles Kay Ogden, a second-hand bookseller and editor of the intellectual university weekly the *Cambridge Magazine*, to publish the translations from October 1915. Ogden gave eight regular pages, more than half of each issue, over to the translations for the remaining years of the war. At a cost of just 1d, but with unique international coverage, the *Cambridge Magazine* soon developed into a leading anti-war publication.

Ogden was known as CK by his friends, and rather daringly as Adelyne More to his readers and even Dorothy in occasional letters, although in fact his pseudonym was a play on 'add-a-line more' in editorial comment rather than a gender reference. He was a charismatic and pleasingly eccentric character; a rationalist intellectual who dedicated his life to the questioning of orthodoxies and pursuit of knowledge. Dora Russell, for many years a social activist alongside her husband Bertrand, knew Ogden from their days together in the 'Cambridge Heretics Society', which met at his flat throughout 1910 for wide-ranging debates in which authority in all matters of religion and belief was rejected. 'Ogden presided with his usual impish provocation of argument ...' Dora remembered. He was 'a small man with a round head thinly covered with fair hair, the forehead of an intellectual, gold-rimmed glasses over grey eyes, [and] a round pink face with the complexion of a baby. There was something gnomish about him ...' He was certainly idiosyncratic, sometimes asking people to join him in putting on a mask so they could 'talk in terms of ideas and not in terms of personalities', and typically sporting an artificial cigarette with a bulb at the end which could be made to glow red when he wished to feel more at ease talking with smokers after his own health forced him to quit. Disliking fresh air and exercise he would hold court in stuffy rooms, refusing to open the windows but setting up an ozone machine instead, the artificial substitute always being immensely preferable, he would regularly tell his audience, to the real article.[3]

Dorothy and Ogden knew each other both through their Cambridge connections and indirectly through Charlie's Liberal networks, as Jane Harrison, Rupert Brooke, Francis Darwin, Bertrand Russell and Gilbert Murray all submitted pieces for Ogden's magazine. Other regular contributors included Thomas Hardy, George Bernard Shaw and Arnold Bennett, all of whom would later lend their public support to Dorothy and Eglantyne's work.

Part of Ogden's motivation for publishing the translations was that he was inherently supportive of freedom of speech and information. Early issues of the magazine had been dedicated to debates from the university's most progressive societies, including the Heretics, and supporting controversial issues such as women's rights and suffrage. But he was also fundamentally opposed to the war which he viewed as 'a lot of nonsense, something he could not have imagined would be embarked upon by intelligent people'. From 1914 he focused the magazine on war and the defence of civil liberties, reporting on the tribunals of conscientious objectors, meetings of the Union of Democratic Control, Charlie's lecture tours – which led to a series of scandals – and from late 1915 adding Dorothy's translations.[4] So aligned were their interests that Charlie and Dorothy even contributed towards the costs of the magazine from July 1915.

Eglantyne joined Dorothy's team in early 1917, and being fluent in both French and German she soon took over the French, Swiss, Italian and Russian papers with twenty-three volunteers working to her, including journalists like Henrietta Leslie, the popular novelist Ethel Sidgwick – the daughter of Arthur Sidgwick under whom Eglantyne had studied at Oxford – and Charlie's secretary Mosa. She also brought in new translators, at first rather clunkily developing the tactics for inspiring and flattering people to come on-side that would later prove invaluable to her. 'I am telling myself that you will probably … be too busy to undertake it', she wrote to one potential recruit, 'so that I may not be disappointed when I have to leave the work to someone less intelligent.' She was rarely refused, and the team kept growing.

Eglantyne was now officially living in the house next door to Dorothy but often staying over to get the work done. Mosa was struck by her 'idealistic, poetic nature', and although she recognised that Eglantyne was still 'in very poor health' she also saw someone 'intensely vital, with an eager, questing mind and an intense interest in the world'. Finally back on her feet after much sisterly support Eglantyne was desperate to make up for lost time. 'It was a combined effort, rather than anything I did for myself, which saved me from permanent invalidity,' she would write to Margaret in 1918. 'I'm hurrying up now to try and do something for somebody before I die!' Like Dorothy, she had found a renewed sense of purpose in the press project and, acutely aware of the need to seize the moment, the pair of them now worked obsessively, often late into the evenings, only breaking to catch the 11pm post.

'You are not like other ladies,' David Buxton, now eight and feeling the fallout from Dorothy's devotion to the project, told his rather pleased mother, 'more like a working woman … more like a man.' Dorothy was not like other ladies, rarely letting herself be distracted by the needs of her children, the limits of her volunteers' time and good-will, or the expectations of society. She found the disruption caused to her work by 'miserable "holidays" … exasperating'. Children's toys, hockey sticks and the general paraphernalia of normal life were all 'banished and their place occupied by neat piles of papers', she wrote proudly to Ogden, and when David was ill with flu and a temperature of 102, she simply scribbled a note along with her weekly submission, 'he wants me all the time … the *Cambridge Magazine* (my part) as you may have noticed – shows symptoms of flu too'. Never having shared Eglantyne's ability to laugh at herself, Dorothy now became increasingly puritanical and demanding. 'What fools the PO [Post Office] people must be,' she griped once on a postcard on which ironically – or perhaps deliberately – she had stuck the stamp upside-down. Another time she complained to Ogden about his own staff, suggesting:

Either (1) he drinks
       (2) is an utter fool
       (3) is hopelessly overworked.
The last is no doubt the explanation – combined with a dash of (2).

Although she worked some minor miracles in the area of press free-dom, Dorothy's tireless dedication to the translations came at a price. 'From 1915 onwards our house in the garden suburb … became a political and editorial office – a hive of industry, where, however, any normal domestic or social life was virtually unknown,' David looked back from the 1970s. 'My mother, who had a formidable constitution, laboured day and night … but the long-continued overwork and overstrain told upon her and she developed a form of epilepsy, horrifying, especially to her two children. And of course, though devoted, she was hardly available as an effective mother to those children.'

Eglantyne and Dorothy had long ago chosen to prioritise their work before their health, family life and social position; for them the needs of suffering humanity always came before those of individuals, particularly themselves. But if Eglantyne visited Tye and Bun less often, she still wrote to both regularly, drawing great strength from their correspondence. And Dorothy took off those days she could to look for birds-nests and pick primroses with her children, managing to inspire as well as intimidate them. Young Eglantyne and David Buxton would grow up at once rather resentful and extremely proud of their mother and aunt's achievements, which had their beginnings in this war work.

From the start Dorothy laid down strict guidelines to ensure that the translations avoided military subjects, and could not in any way be, or be laid open to charges of being, damaging to Britain's war work. Instead they focused on the aims and causes of the war, its eth-ical conduct, support for peace, and the developing idea of a League of Nations. Articles covering anti-war debate and demonstrations showed that there were moderate peace-seeking voices in Bulgaria, Holland, America and elsewhere, and even a growing peace movement for a settlement on terms tolerable to the Allies in Germany and Austria-Hungary.[5] 'It ought to go without saying', the *Berliner Tagblatt* wrote in November 1915, 'that the German people … long for an end of this monstrous slaughter.' It did not go without saying, but now that it was repeated in English, MPs like Philip Snowden and Charles Trevelyan could start to press for a negotiated settlement in the Commons.

Other extracts showed that the hard-line parliamentary speeches reported in the British press supporting the destruction of Germany by among others Runciman, Sasonoff and Asquith – who, the Prussian press reported, 'foams with hatred and rage' – were only hardening German resistance and increasing support for their intransigent military leadership. 'There remains much that is impossible and shameful in these terms,' the German *Kölnische Volkszeitung* commented on peace discussions in Britain in December 1915: 'even the most peace-loving must say to himself: it is hopeless to deal with such people, and there is only one way to bring him to his senses, i.e., to go on fighting.' More bluntly the *Vossische Zeitung* wrote, 'if the enemy do not give up their foolish intention to humiliate and annihilate Germany, it will not be Germany's fault if more blood is shed and the desire for peace on earth and goodwill at Christmastide remains but a pious wish'.

Dorothy and Eglantyne were also both keen that the translations had a humanitarian agenda, looking at the treatment of prisoners and, above all, the impact of the war on social and economic conditions in Europe. Agricultural production had been greatly reduced when farm workers went to fight, and the closure of borders combined with the general breakdown of European transport systems during the war was hampering the distribution of those resources that were available. By 1915 there were already shortages of food, medicines and fuel, and it was clear that the British economic blockade was effectively cutting off supplies not only to enemy armies but to civilian populations across central and eastern Europe.

By 1916 shortages had reached crisis levels in many countries, and the translations revealed a horrific picture of the suffering being caused. At first detailed accounts mainly came from the neutral papers of Sweden and Switzerland. Across Europe the elderly, women and children were starving to death; people in Finland were eating the bark from trees; Romanians were dying of cold with no fuel; and in Belgium, Luxembourg and Poland children were 'searching dustbins like starved dogs'. Diseases that followed starvation like typhoid and tuberculosis were rife, and mothers were reportedly concealing the bodies of their dead children so that the rest of their family might benefit from their bread rations. Soon similar reports started to emerge from Austria. The Swiss doctor Frédéric Ferrière of the International Red Cross reported that most of the population of Vienna were 'slowly starving to death', weeping mothers killing the babies that they could not feed and malnourished six-year-olds 'so thin and small that they looked like children of two'. Then in November 1917, despite tight German press censorship, *Kölnische Zeitung* published a landmark report on starvation across Germany revealing appalling levels of infant and child mortality as new mothers no longer had the milk to either breast- or bottle-feed their babies.

To anyone reading the translations it was clear that the war, directly aggravated by the economic blockade, was creating a humanitarian crisis across Europe on an unprecedented scale, which was neither morally justifiable, nor in the long-term interests of a safer and more stable Europe. Furthermore the British government seemed to be ignoring the growing movement for a negotiated peace, even within Germany and Austria, which held the potential for an earlier end to the war on terms acceptable to the Allies.

Sadly however, domestic circulation of the *Cambridge Magazine* was hampered by the refusal of many booksellers to stock it; when Dorothy met Ramsay MacDonald at a party in 1916 he told her that he had been trying in vain to get hold of it for a month. As a result she promoted private subscriptions and the translations quickly became required reading among opinion formers, reaching a circulation of over twenty thousand between 1917 and 1918 ranging from diplomats in the USA to a Russian proletariat musician who wrote to Dorothy, 'I weeped [sic]. I could kiss you for thankfulness.' General Smuts in South Africa, one of five members of the British War Cabinet, told Charlie Buxton that he read the *Cambridge Magazine* thoroughly before circulating it around his staff – 'He was enthusiastic about you', Charlie wrote to Dorothy, 'and said, "she must be a great woman!" '

Hundreds of politicians and social activists read the translations in Britain too. One MP who preferred to remain anonymous told Dorothy how much he valued the translations for supplying 'a gap in the home press which is probably intentional. The more we can realise the feelings of other people now hidden from us behind the smoke of war, the better.' Other subscribers irked Dorothy, as she wrote to her friends, by complementing Charlie on 'how *his* [sic] work was bearing fruit'. Many more, like the Liberal academic Gilbert Murray, wrote to Ogden. 'You realise of course that I do not agree with all your views about the war ... and I daresay there have been phrases and articles that have made me angry,' Murray, who was not a pacifist, told Ogden in March 1917. 'But I think on the whole it has been a courageous and brilliantly conducted paper of considerable social utility.' Soon Ogden was receiving dozens of letters of encouragement from well-known MPs, academics and clerics, which he quoted at length, if anonymously, in special issues.

Numerous celebrities also lent their public support. In October 1916 an elderly Thomas Hardy allowed Ogden to publish an advert in *The Times* quoting his praise for the magazine, which, he said, he read every week, 'turning first to the extracts from foreign newspapers, which transport one to the Continent and enable one to see England bare and unadorned – her chances in the struggle free from distortion by the glamour of patriotism'. In the same spread Jerome K. Jerome –

also too old to serve but volunteering as an ambulance driver for the French army – said that the translations should be compulsory reading to ensure 'more clear thinking and less shouting', and adding:

> The *Cambridge Magazine*, the only paper that for the last two years I have read with any interest. It is the only paper that any man who cares to think for himself can read with any satisfaction in the present time. It is the only paper from which one obtains the undoctored truth and undistorted fact. There are only two methods that occur to me, of teaching the actual position of affairs. One is to compel every adult civilian in Europe to spend three or four months in the fighting line, the other is to compel them to read '*The Cambridge Magazine*'.

George Bernard Shaw, Sir Arthur Quiller Couch, Eden Philpotts, Arnold Bennet, John Galsworthy, and the poet – later Poet Laureate – John Masefield among many others also lent their names to the magazine in the hope of raising its readership and encouraging public support for peace. Even the young Jewish Italian artist Amedeo Modigliani wrote to Charlie from France to express his support. 'It would please him very much if you could make some reference to him', Charlie wrote to Ogden, 'as he is very keen about the magazine.' Dorothy was a little bemused, writing rather disingenuously to Ogden that she was 'incorrigibly illiterate' and had never read Shaw, 'nor anyone else I ought to have; – not even Shakespeare – so there!'

There was also opposition to the translations. Unfortunately when she clipped it for her scrapbook Tye cut off the name of the publication that printed this tongue-in-cheek article:

> Lines on the Cambridge Vice Chancellor's lament to the *Morning Post* on his inability to suppress that pernicious print, the *Cambridge Magazine*:
>
> Oxford (by sound historians we are told)
> Burnt Milton's writings in the days of old.
> The times are changed and Cambridge now takes her turn;

No Milton being obvious to burn,
In distant reproductions of the scene,
Our Council burns 'The Cambridge Magazine' –
But no! in vain analogies we patch;
They'd like to burn it but can't find a match!

But many criticisms were very serious. Some people resented giving space to the sufferings of the enemy while there was so much loss at home. Others, like the composer William Sterndale Bennett, objected specifically to the pacifist implications of the translations on behalf of serving soldiers. Making enemies was convenient too, Eglantyne decided wryly, it saved valuable lobbying time later. A year's worth of press scrutiny had not only given her and Dorothy detailed knowledge of the situation in Europe, but also a valuable insight into the processes of political advocacy at home.

Ogden also faced increasing criticism for his editorial line during the war, his personal popularity not helped by the fact that due to rheumatic fever he was unfit for military service. A concerted attempt to discredit him, ending in physical threats towards the end of 1918, led to his and the magazine's defence by twenty-two college lecturers including Maynard Keynes. But not all academics were so supportive. Dr Rouse of The Perse School in Cambridge refused to sign an appeal condemning the threat of violence against Ogden, writing, 'I beg to inform you that you richly deserve all you got. Cambridge is no place for people such as you, nor, indeed, is England. You might feel more at home in Germany.' Rouse's letter was boldly reproduced in the *Cambridge Magazine*, but the night that the Armistice was announced Ogden's Cambridge premises were wrecked and not long later he was attacked by some patriotic Cambridge undergraduates. 'I am so sorry to hear that you are going through such an extremely dreary and depressing time,' Dorothy wrote to him that December, 'but you have weathered bad storms before, and as your courage and pertinacity never failed you, so may they not do so now.' Ogden finally stopped publishing the translations in 1919, when he left Cambridge to live next door to Maynard Keynes in London's Gordon Square.

The Armistice was signed with Germany on 11 November 1918. Just twenty-four hours later, capitalising on his popularity, Lloyd George announced a general election with himself leading a 'National Liberal' coalition of Liberals and Conservatives. It was the first election to be fought on the grounds of universal male suffrage and with a limited female vote, reasons which were later cited for a general dumbing down of political debate. In fact much of the election rhetoric simply reflected and responded to ongoing anti-German public sentiment, as in the famous election speech by the Conservative politician Sir Eric Geddes who pledged that, 'the Germans, if this Government is returned, are going to pay every penny; they are going to be squeezed, as a lemon is squeezed – until the pips squeak. My only doubt is not whether we can squeeze hard enough, but whether there is enough juice.'

At the end of December the National Liberal coalition won a massive landslide, retaining Lloyd George as Prime Minister. It was, the Labour MP John Robert Clynes wrote, an 'election won on hate'. The defeat of many Independent Liberals, including Charlie, contesting Accrington, ended the Liberal majority in the house and Lloyd George's once-moderate talk of a righteous peace was replaced by a call to make Germany pay for the entire cost of the war as the political and economic penalty for devastating Europe. 'Britain', he declared, must be a land 'fit for heroes to live in'. German industrial capacity 'will go a pretty long way …' and Britain must have 'the uttermost farthing', and 'shall search their pockets for it'. Searching pockets involved plundering the defeated countries of whatever of their wealth or resources remained while continuing the economic blockade as a means of forcing through punitive peace terms. 'I feel physically sick when I read the frenzied appeals of the Coalition leaders – the Prime Minister, Winston Churchill and Geddes – to hang the Kaiser, ruin and humiliate the German people, even to deprive

Germany of her art treasures and libraries,' Beatrice Webb scrawled in her diary in December 1918. 'These preliminaries of peace have become almost as disgusting as the war itself.' Germany, Hungary and Austria faced disorganisation, economic ruin and now also continuing famine.

In January 1919 Lloyd George took his reparations agenda to Versailles, where he started to hammer out peace terms with the American President Woodrow Wilson, Italian Prime Minister Vittorio Orlando and French Premier Georges Clemenceau, who was even more intent on destroying the German economy and political system. As the British Deputy Chancellor Maynard Keynes was also present, pressing claims for a just and realistic settlement and advocating an unpopular regeneration programme which including lifting the blockade, raising a loan to feed starving Europe, limiting German economic reparations and launching a credit programme to kick-start the continental economies that could then produce and purchase their own supplies and provide a long-term market for Britain. He was frustrated at every turn, reporting that 'the fundamental problem of a Europe starving and disintegrating before their eyes was the one question on which it was impossible to rouse the interest of the Four'. Maynard estimated that in order to meet Allied demands Germany would be required to pay £400 million over forty-two years, 'double the highest figure that ... any competent person here or in the United States has ever attempted to justify'. It was an impossible request for a country devastated by war, and in effect a death sentence for the German population. That May Maynard's closest ally, General Smuts, described the pair of them sitting together in the evenings after a good dinner: 'I tell him that this is the time for Grigua's prayer for the Lord to come himself and not to send his Son, as this is no time for children ... And then we laugh, and behind the laughter is Hoover's horrible picture of thirty million people who must die unless there is some great intervention.'

Having failed in all his aims Maynard resigned from the peace conference, depressed and ill, at the end of May. 'I wish I could talk to you about the whole miserable business,' he replied when Austen Chamberlain pressed him to reconsider. 'The Prime Minister is leading us all into a morass of destruction. The settlement which he is proposing for Europe disrupts it economically and must depopulate it by millions of persons ... How can you expect me to assist at this tragic farce any longer.'

None the less Maynard was probably the most influential early critic of the continued blockade, and his scathing account of the peace settlement on practical as well as moral gounds, published in his book *The Economic Consequences of the Peace* in the autumn of 1919, reached a huge international audience. The right-wing press now presented him as a pro-German sympathiser and one reader of the *Saturday Review* suggested he should be given an iron cross, but he was hailed as a visionary in many countries. Margaret proudly gave Eglantyne a first edition copy of her brother's book, which she dedicated to her friend in pencil inside the front cover. It is impossible to know whether Eglantyne found the time to read Maynard's great work, but she already shared his concern not just that the peace terms were protracting the famine in Europe, but also about the impact this would have on the political perspective of future generations. 'Never in the lifetime of men living has the universal element in the soul of man burnt so dimly,' Maynard closed *The Economic Consequences of the Peace*. 'For these reasons the true voice of a new generation has not yet spoken, and silent opinion is not yet formed. To the formation of the general opinion of the future I dedicate this book.'

'I shall never forget the sense of crisis which pervaded the household,' Charlie's secretary Mosa wrote when Eglantyne and Dorothy heard of the decision to continue the economic blockade after the Armistice. For four years Dorothy had devoted all her energy, private income and every available moment to promoting peace through her press translations, and since she had joined her sister's team early in 1917 Eglantyne had also worked round the clock despite her recurring exhaustion. Both had risked private and public censure with the sole motive of promoting an earlier end to the slaughter of young men in the field and the starvation of the elderly, women and children left behind. The idea that the blockade could now be continued as a political tool to enforce British authority after peace was declared seemed beyond comprehension. Eglantyne explored the possible reasons in a 1918 poem:

> Now, over our afternoon tea, dear friend,
> Let's consult together why
> We're starving sixty million people, between us,
> You and I …
> Is it to make them accept terms of peace
> which they otherwise wouldn't?
> Or is it that we may get hold of some markets
> we otherwise couldn't?
> Do we want the food – though it's more than
> We could eat – for our own poor nations?
> Or do we simply want to reduce
> The enemy population? ...
> Perhaps it is to punish sin? The fact is I
> Want to know the what to say
> When asked what my motives exactly
> Were, by God, at the Judgement Day.
> For I've an increasing suspicion,
> Although hitherto I have hid it.
> God will not let us off scot free
> When we say that the Government did it.

Maynard however offered a cynical but frighteningly plausible view as to why the government was essentially to blame: 'The blockade had become by that time a very perfect instrument':

Its authors had grown to love it for its own sake; it included some recent improvements which would be wasted if it came to an end; it was very complicated and a vast organisation had established a vested interest. The experts reported, therefore, that it was our one instrument for imposing Peace terms on Germany, and that once suspended it could hardly be reimposed.

Dorothy had been hoping to wind down her work after the war, but now she decided to keep publishing the foreign news translations, focusing on French and German assessments of the peace terms. With depressing prescience the French *Populaire* was arguing as early as December 1918 that 'the seeds of future wars' would be sown 'with both hands' if the new Germany was treated as a continuation of the old regime, but few round the negotiating table were listening. From 1919 to the end of 1921 Mosa Anderson took over the editorial work, publishing the translations in the *Guardian Weekly*. By then however it had long been clear to Dorothy and Eglantyne that although the reports might continue to build public support for less punitive peace terms and an end to the blockade, a much more focused lobby was required if lives were to be saved immediately. 'It has been a great wrench for me to give up the *Cambridge Magazine*,' Dorothy wrote to Ogden at the end of December 1918, 'I never thought that I should find other work that seemed even more urgent.' But now she and Eglantyne together launched a new campaign.

Armed with their knowledge of conditions in Europe gleaned from the press translations, and inspired by a sense of life and death urgency, at the end of 1918 Eglantyne and Dorothy quickly joined like-minded contacts from the Women's International League to form a new single-issue political pressure group: the 'Fight the Famine Council'. Lord Parmoor, a Liberal peer who had opposed the war, accepted the role of Chair. Lady Kathleen Courtney, whom Eglantyne knew from her Oxford days, and Dorothy from the Women's International League (and who was now Parmoor's sister-in-law) supported him in the role, and the rather formidable-looking Marian Ellis, a leading member of the Society of Friends and for a number of years President of the Women's International League, joined Eglantyne to serve as the two Honorary Secretaries. Dorothy, who was still editing the foreign news translations, took charge of information gathering, beginning by keeping detailed case-books of the situation country by country. Charlie's brother Noel agreed to act as Treasurer. Charlie, although preoccupied with vainly fighting a seat in the general election, also joined the Famine Council and as usual opened up his address book.

Eglantyne, Dorothy, Kate and Marian worked ceaselessly through December, approaching an impressive list of potential supporters, mainly independent journalists, authors, liberal-minded politicians, economists, academics, churchmen and several of the celebrity endorsers of the *Cambridge Magazine*. Although not everyone they contacted was convinced, they secured an impressive line-up: Ramsay MacDonald, Philip Snowden, Maude Royden, Gilbert Murray, Olive Schreiner, Leonard Woolf, Jerome K. Jerome, thirteen Bishops and several Deans all signed up as Council Members. Asquith, the former Liberal Prime Minister, and Sir William Beveridge, then at the Ministry of Food, also gave their backing, and Maynard agreed to lead an economic sub-committee. Not long after Charlie's friends Sydney and Beatrice Webb, H.G. Wells, George Bernard Shaw, Seebohm Rowntree, Margaret McMillan, the pioneer of British nursery education, and C.P. Scott, Editor of the *Manchester Guardian*, among many others were all signing Famine Council petitions.

Eglantyne and Dorothy were keen to escalate their campaigns but Parmoor felt they should wait until new reports on conditions in Europe emerged from sources like the American Relief Administration, which was headed by the future US President Hebert Hoover. 'On the other hand ...' Marian argued, 'the situation becomes more critical every day ... I feel desperately anxious about the whole matter, and as you know, Lord Parmoor, though admirable, is just a little slow.' In the end unofficial campaigning started before the Famine Council was publicly launched, and with Marian's encouragement Parmoor put his name to letters in the British papers, reaching an audience in the UK and on the continent, and also met US President Wilson on his visit to London to support the formation of the League of Nations, all before December was over.[6]

The Famine Council was formally inaugurated at a public meeting held on New Year's Day 1919 at Central Hall, Westminster – a venue that had been regularly used for suffrage meetings as it is just across the road from the Houses of Parliament. Its stated objectives were overtly political: to end the blockade through the collection and promotion of reliable information on conditions in famine districts, and to secure an international loan to get Europe's economy going again. To supplement the press campaign a series of leaflets were published, ranging from economic reports and political analysis to more provocative titles like 'Death of a People' and 'Shall Babies Starve?' designed to win public sympathy. Speeches were made in Parliament, and in February 1919 Winston Churchill, formerly an ally of Charlie's but now Britain's Secretary of State for War, wrote to *The Times* that the blockade was 'repugnant to the British nation'. Contact was also established with the Pope who sent his apostolic blessing to the Famine Council officers and suggested co-operation on relief, but Parmoor was keen to keep the Council focused on political action. Eglantyne and Dorothy meanwhile undertook speaking tours, mainly round influential London drawing-rooms, arguing that economic collapse in Europe was against the long-term interests of Britain, that famine itself creates international instability by promoting anarchy and revolution, and that it was in any case morally wrong to let the innocent die, whether victor or vanquished.

The government however, Churchill not withstanding, was not persuaded and still carried the popular support of the country. The

British people had been taxed beyond endurance by the horrors of the war and were now preoccupied with their own sorrows and plans, and still intensely hostile to the countries that had taken the lives of so many young men. As a result most people were quite unable to grasp the horrors that were being inflicted in Europe each day that the blockade continued, and many – believing that the reports Dorothy and her team translated about the suffering were exaggerated – were angered by the apparent efforts of the Famine Council to sympathise with the enemy and redirect attention and resources from Britain to Europe. The government was also irritated by the campaign and Ethel Snowden later talked of the constant fear of arrest.

Nonetheless by March 1919 the Famine Council had organised a resource centre for pooling information on the famine, a major publicity drive, and a second public meeting to call for the end of the blockade and immediate measures for relief, again to be held in Central Hall. The meeting, on 12 March, was well attended, leading to a series of regional spin-off events. To Eglantyne and Dorothy's delight the resulting petitions, submitted to 10 Downing Street on 2 April, contributed to getting the blockade lifted from some countries, although not the worst hit: Germany, Austria and Russia. However, it now became clear that, even where the blockade was raised, food supplies were unable to reach the majority of the starving populations because of their lack of purchasing power and the general breakdown of European transport systems.

'His Majesty's Government are fully conscious of the very serious situation existing in Central Europe', Lloyd George eventually told the House of Commons in December 1919, 'and … are taking all possible means to alleviate the difficulties.' But this public statement of good intentions did not lead to pursuing the basic policies that the Famine Council had already been pushing for a year: the complete end of the blockade, revision of the peace terms and provision of immediate relief and long-term investment. 'The machinery for starving Europe could not rapidly be changed into machinery for feeding Europe' Eglantyne admitted, but no headway would be made until the Allied policy of what she summed up as 'submit or starve' was overturned.

The Famine Council continued collecting information and lobbying to end the blockade, and then for a revision of what Parmoor summed up as the 'harsh and unjust' terms of the Paris Peace Treaties, on and off until 1921. But by April 1919 Eglantyne and Dorothy had already decided that political lobbying was not achieving enough; children were starving across Europe and if lives were to be saved money was needed for immediate famine relief. Could it be right, they demanded in a privately published leaflet, that 'our enemy's child was dying, but no cup of water must be handed to him without cash down'? 'Paris is very self-important,' they continued prophetically:

> It believes it is making a new Europe, that it is writing history with a large and firm hand, but history is being made elsewhere. It is being made in 1,000 hospitals, in innumerable humble homes all over Europe. The cry of the child for bread is hushed in a nameless grave, but surely his voice will waken again. It will resound down our century. All shall hear it. It will become a voice of thunder which shall send statesmen and politicians, Parliaments and Churches to their doom.
>
> Our spurious patriotism, our moral indolence, all that tissue of pretences which we call 'civilisation' has destroyed the child, but the child in its feebleness and its pain may perhaps have destroyed this 'civilisation'.

Chapter 12

Save the Children, 1919

Surely it is impossible for us, as normal human beings, to watch children starve to death without making an effort to save them.

Eglantyne Jebb, May 1919

Almost lost among the many fascinating and disturbing documents in the Save the Children archive is a rather crumpled leaflet headed 'A Starving Baby' above a photograph of an Austrian child: a young girl whose physical development has been arrested as a result of malnutrition. The girl's seemingly huge head and intelligent face look jarringly out of place above her baby-like body with its tiny arms and feeble, tapering legs. Pathetically unable to support herself she is held up for the camera by an anonymous nurse. There is something monstrous about this child, like a circus curiosity or a hybrid monkey-mermaid, and in some ways she is a freak; not born of nature but produced by British, Liberal, post-war economic policy. The caption beneath the photo reads:

> This child is 2½ years old, and its weight is only 12lbs 2oz. The normal weight for a child of this age is 28lb 2oz. The size of the child's head is out of all proportion to its body, because through starvation its body and its limbs have not developed. There are millions of such children starving to-day.

Marked in pencil, in the top right hand corner of the leaflet, is the single word 'suppressed!' This is Eglantyne's unmistakable writing, neat but hurried, the exclamation mark recording her personal indignation at the British government's decision to restrict public awareness of the human cost of their policy to continue the economic blockade to Europe. For photographs to accuse, and possibly alter conduct, they must shock. The photographs of starving Austrian children that Eglantyne reproduced on her leaflets might not now pass Save the Children's image policy guidelines, which aim to preserve human dignity and avoid the patronising presentation of pathetic, anonymous victims of war or natural disaster solely to pull heart – and purse – strings. But in 1919 when the children of Germany and her allies were the direct victims of ongoing British economic policy Eglantyne decided there was a moral obligation for the British public to confront these photographs, disturbing as they were, because after months of parliamentary lobbying with the Fight the Famine Council it seemed to her that only popular pressure would persuade the government to lift the blockade, and so end the needless starvation in Central Europe. Although she had only hurriedly produced a small print run, Eglantyne's 'starving baby' leaflets were soon at the centre of the public controversy which led to the launch of the 'Save the Children Fund'.

Eglantyne was arrested for distributing her leaflets in London's Trafalgar Square on a cool, cloudy day in April 1919. She was forty-three, and instead of mellowing into a graceful and accepting middle-age like her mother, who had long ago settled into her invalid's sofa, Eglantyne was once again full of the social indignation that had driven her before her thyroid condition had sapped her strength. Now she was back, this time enthusiastically exhibiting her born-again passion for human empathy and social justice in the heart of London.

Trafalgar Square has been London's principal site for political protest since the Chartists assembled there to demand electoral reform in 1848 soon after its construction, and was regularly used – against the wishes of the authorities – by the suffragettes, Labour, socialist and pacifist demonstrators in the years before and during the war. Beatrice

Webb recorded sauntering through a 'mixed crowd of admirers, hooligan warmongers and merely curious holiday makers' in the summer of 1914 to watch anti-war demonstrators 'gesticulating from the steps of the monument'. Now, in April 1919, it was natural for the former women's suffrage activist and Famine Council supporter Emmeline Pethick-Lawrence to choose the square as the venue to address an anti-blockade meeting before marching down Downing Street with protest banners. She was accompanied by the thirty-one-year-old secretary of the Women's League, Barbara Ayrton Gould.[1] The next week Barbara was back in the square, now helping Eglantyne leaflet the pedestrians rounding Nelson's Column and visitors to St Martin-in-the-Fields and the National Gallery. Although Trafalgar Square is never empty the war had reduced the passing trade for protestors since Beatrice Webb's visit. There were fewer holiday-makers, and although the National Gallery had stayed open throughout the war – despite closing for a few months in early 1914 after a suffragette slashed the Rokeby Venus – visitor figures were nonetheless down as sixteen of the twenty-eight exhibition rooms were still being used for storage by the Ministry for Munitions. Perhaps because there were not so many passers by to leaflet, one account has Eglantyne and Barbara chalking up the pavements to get their message across. If true it was probably Barbara, the seasoned suffragette, who brought the chalk, although Eglantyne had never been above making a dramatic statement and might well have enjoyed adding her own writing to the paving in the square. Chalk-dust aside, Eglantyne as usual looked the epitome of English dignity; thin but proud and naturally elegant, dressed in rather unfashionable dark clothes of good quality durable fabric, slightly fading auburn hair pinned up under her hat, eyes and attitude brilliant. The sight of the two women – Eglantyne with her head held high, leather-gloved hands still distributing her wodge of shocking leaflets as she was escorted away by police, followed by the defiant younger Barbara – must have caused quite a stir among whatever post-war crowds were in the square that afternoon.

Eglantyne and Barbara's arrest seems a rather heavy-handed response to the efforts of two female pamphleteers with no previous record or particular notoriety in a traditional site for public protest. Barbara and Emmeline had made little public impact with their demonstration the week before, and she and Eglantyne were unlikely to generate significant popular support through a couple of cold spring afternoons spent handing out leaflets, however shocking the images reproduced. However the Famine Council had been gaining increasing political backing in Westminster, along with the Union of Democratic Control becoming a key rallying point for parliamentary dissent against the war and post-war policy, and in particular Lloyd George's aggressive economic repatriation agenda that was exploiting the continued blockade. Eglantyne was still the Honorary Secretary of the Famine Council, and her 'starving baby' leaflet was just the latest piece of their increasingly sensational publicity to try to shift reluctant public opinion in support of this parliamentary trend.

Understandably so soon after the Armistice, the popular feeling in the country was that now was a time to celebrate peace and focus on domestic recovery, not to question the less comfortable premises and consequences of the war that had cost so many lives. The war effort had revealed considerable hardship in Britain including the malnutrition among poorer communities that had led to the introduction of national food rationing just a year earlier. As a result after the Armistice there was a great resurgence in domestic charitable giving, as well as major state investment particularly in maternal and child welfare programmes through the Ministry of Health, created in 1918. Foreign aid, however, especially to countries that had been at war with Britain just months earlier and were now being targeted by the British government for economic repatriations, was simply not on the public agenda.

The situation was not helped by the British press, who seemed determined to believe that the miseries of the country's former enemies were exaggerated, and were quick to find reasons to dismiss reports of suffering. In January 1919 the estimates made by Herbert Hoover, as Chair of the American Relief Administration, that between four and five million children were starving in eastern and central Europe received staggeringly little coverage given both the weight of the claim and the authority it came from, and the Famine Council faced similar difficulties with a hostile press. Determined to influence the public agenda Dorothy set up a 'Famine Information Bureau' under the banner of the Council that March, collecting reports from a range of agencies to verify the situation beyond dispute. Perhaps unsurprisingly the government's 'Official Committee for Relief in Europe' was 'unable' to provide Dorothy with any figures regarding the numbers of children in need of attention and aid. Forced to get their statistics elsewhere, the Council lost considerable public confidence after being attacked in the papers for having taken the apparently unsupportable line of meeting German experts for an overview of conditions in Germany. 'We must have figures …' Eglantyne wrote to Dorothy in exasperation, 'it is the only way to combat political influences. It is the only way to prove our honesty … and therefore the only way to rally public opinion behind us.'

Eglantyne's approach was to organise a new research mission to Vienna under the auspices of a socially well connected but independent medical expert; the society doctor Hector Munro.[2] Munro was a noted left-wing pacifist and supporter of women's rights, but also a well-respected doctor with a flourishing west London practice who had won considerable praise for his war work first with the Belgian Red Cross, and then setting up a private ambulance unit on the Western front. Believing he had now thoroughly fulfilled his moral duty, Munro was rather startled to find Eglantyne, whom he had never met or had any dealings with, pounding on his Seymour Street door in early 1919. Eglantyne was asking a lot of Munro to leave his lucrative London practice for starving Vienna, but her passionate altruism combined with her down-to-earth humour had always made what Ruth Wordsworth called a 'formidable and baffling alliance against all opposition'. 'When she spoke', Munro later wrote, 'everything else seemed to lose its importance and one agreed to do whatever she wished.' He packed that afternoon.

An uncompromising humanitarian, Munro jeopardised his research trip more than once by prioritising the provision of immediate aid above adherence to protocol or even international law. In Austria he helped the wealthy Viennese coffee merchant Julias Meinl to illegally import a large stock of wine from the Romanian occupied part of Hungary so that he could spend the £11,000 commission Meinl gave him on hospital supplies for children. In Romania he effectively closed down a prison for former Hungarian officers whom he found starving in the courtyard, and he later gave his passport and place in a British Military Attaché car to a young man swearing his life depended on crossing the border immediately, thereby stranding himself in Bulgaria. However when it did arrive Munro's Vienna report provided the Famine Council with shocking statistics and anecdotal evidence confirming the extent and impact of the European famine. 'Conditions were indeed terrible,' Munro wrote:

> Children were actually dying in the street. I saw in the Allgemeine Krankenhaus 38 women who were suffering spontaneous fracture of the hips, their bones having lost all solidity. The children's bones were like rubber. Tuberculosis was terribly rife. Clothing was utterly lacking. Children were wrapped in paper, and in the hospitals there was nothing but paper bandages.

'The children were brought in by the score to the denuded hospitals and placed in rows to die,' Eglantyne later took up the narrative. 'Old people killed themselves in order that there might be more food left for the others, mothers murdered their babies sooner than watch the ghastly sufferings.'

Munro was not the only humanitarian observer in Vienna preparing to co-ordinate aid. The Austrian Red Cross had sent out reports of children starving in the city from November 1918, and in response the International Red Cross in Geneva had delegated Dr Frédéric Ferrière to report on conditions. Ferrière was an expert in public health who had worked with the Red Cross for forty years, and had spent most of the war working for civilian relief and protection. He later became one of Eglantyne's great allies at Save the Children, along with his niece Suzanne. Ferrière's report was equally horrific. The blockade had effectively reduced the supply of food and medicine into Vienna to below the level possible for survival, and the children of the city were indeed starving on the streets. Gaunt seven-year-olds still had the physique of three-year-olds, their bodies unable to develop on their diet of cabbages and turnips supplemented only by tiny rations of unwholesome bread. Infant mortality had reached levels unprecedented even during the war, and without wood for coffins, babies were being buried in cardboard boxes or bundles of newspaper. In effect only the rich who could still afford black-market prices were still eating. In spite of overwhelming need, hospitals were closing and those that remained had no medicines. Even basic supplies like soap or coal were lacking. By the end of December 1918 neutral Switzerland, home of the International Red Cross, had sent a convoy of seventy wagons of food to Austria; a fantastic start but far from sufficient to meet the city's needs.[3]

The situation was similar in Germany where huge numbers of children, 'pale and thin as corpses', were dying from the infectious diseases that followed starvation, or were simply no longer able to resist the cold. In a desperate attempt to protect harvests children caught stealing vegetables from the fields were given prison sentences during which prison rations and chronic disease further weakened them. An enquiry about conditions in one German prison infirmary elicited the laconic reply, 'Inmates all dead.' Those children strong enough to keep going were often physically stunted, unable to concentrate, depressed from witnessing the misery and hunger in their homes and driven to theft or prostitution in exchange for meals.

Many killed themselves. Twice as many children died in Berlin during 1919 than in 1913. That April, when the German death toll through starvation and related diseases was estimated at eight hundred people a day, the Famine Council published an inspired leaflet quoting a number of British army officers, returning heroes who opposed the blockade on humanitarian grounds having seen the consequences of the famine in various parts of Germany for themselves. It had little impact. By the following April an estimated one million German children had died through hunger and tuberculosis.

The same picture of ruined nations unable to support their civilian populations was repeated across Central Europe. In 1919 the Hungarian Red Cross stated that of eighteen thousand newborn infants, seven thousand were unlikely to reach their first birthday. There were equally terrifying infant mortality figures in Poland, where new mothers were too undernourished to produce milk, and inquests revealed that many had died of hunger with sand or wood in their stomachs. Adding to the crisis, refugees who had been surviving on grass, bark, berries, wild apples and nettle soup began to flood into the major Polish cities during the winter of 1918/1919. Among them seasonal workers who had been stranded in Germany during the war returned to Warsaw destitute, and in January 1919 thirty-two children were found frozen to death among them. Those refugees who managed to board trains still risked dying from the cold when the trains, fired by wood as there was no coal, broke down and the snow kept falling.[4] Joseph Jakobkiewicz, a Polish Red Cross delegate, described finding small children frozen to death on the naked bodies of their mothers who had wrapped them in their own clothes in an attempt to keep them warm. Some had tears frozen on their cheeks.

In March 1919 Dorothy travelled to Berne in Switzerland to attend a conference on the future League of Nations as a delegate of both the Society of Friends and the Women's League. The Friends had managed to secure a permit to send food and clothing to families

in Austria and Germany early in 1919, and now they authorised
Dorothy and her fellow Quaker delegate, Joan Fry, to spend up to
£1,000 on immediate aid for the children in neighbouring Austria.
In the event Dorothy and Joan spent double the amount – Dorothy
contributing her own funds – to send a railway-truck full of cod-liver
oil, rice, condensed milk, milk-chocolate powder and other essential
foods to Vienna. Ethel Snowden was also at the Berne conference to
represent the Women's Peace Crusade, and recorded her disbelief at
the layers of bureaucracy that hampered the movement of relief
provisions across the Swiss–Austrian border. There were 'endless
delays for no obvious reason', Ethel wrote; 'endless calls on dilatory
officials; endless pleadings with suspicious legations; endless regulations to be subscribed to, and finally the probability that [the train]
would never arrive at its destination'. But with a little manual help
uncoupling and pushing the trucks across the border at blockade
checkpoints, the Friends' provisions including Dorothy's consign-
ment did make it through.

It was the final spur that Dorothy needed. At a Famine Council
meeting on her return that April she proposed that a non-political
relief fund should be established to support the British provision of
immediate aid. One crucial problem remained – how to rouse public concern for the suffering people of Germany and her allies.

It was now that Eglantyne and Barbara Ayrton Gould were
arrested for distributing their leaflets featuring the photographs that
Dorothy had brought back from Switzerland. Their trial took place
a few weeks later, on 15 May 1919.[5] It was a warm day, one of the
first real spring days after a cold and cloudy start to May, and things
quickly heated up inside the busy courtroom at Mansion House, the
city court often used for suffragette trials.[6] The public prosecution's
case hinged on the unauthorised distribution of two leaflets and a
poster with the uncompromising copy: 'What does Britain stand for?
Starving babies, torturing women, killing the old', of which alone
seven thousand copies had somehow been handed out.[7] None of

these papers had been cleared by the government under the 1914 Defence of the Realm Act, and the possible penalty was up to £5 for every copy circulated or a considerable jail sentence. In true suffragette style Barbara demanded 'prison as a protest', but Eglantyne took a different approach, aiming to create a high-profile PR story out of the affair even though the trial – the fourteenth case of the day – was not that intrinsically newsworthy.[8]

Eglantyne conducted her own defence. From the start she took personal responsibility for her actions, testifying that she had prepared the leaflets in a hurry without gaining the sanction of the Famine Council, and resigning immediately as Honorary Secretary. Advised by a lawyer on her technical defence, she then defiantly asserted that she had not broken the law. Her argument was twofold. Firstly she believed that her leaflets fell outside official jurisdiction because they had a humanitarian object rather than being political propaganda, an argument supported by her publisher at the Labour Press. 'It had never occurred to me that a purely humanitarian plea ... had anything to do with the defence of the realm,' she wrote to the papers the following day. As a back-up she also rather cheekily intimated that either the war was officially over, in which case the Defence of the Realm Act should presumably be redundant, or, contrary to the claims of the government, the war was still going on and 'the Blockade is one of our chief war weapons'. She then focused on the moral case behind the leafleting, giving the court reporters, including the journalist and women's rights campaigner Evelyn Sharp, plenty to pad out their stories. 'Without any attempt at eloquence', Sharp wrote, 'she swept aside the technical arguments on which the prosecution had to rely, and spoke only upon the Christian aspect of what she had done ... It left in my mind an unforgettable picture of the woman whose gentleness covered a fire of the Spirit.'

Eglantyne was nevertheless found guilty, and, according to Sharp, Sir Archibald Bodkin, Director of Public Prosecutions and the prosecuting counsel at her trial, did not spare her in his condemnation. But she was only fined £5 without costs or eleven days' imprisonment, 'which, I am told,' she wrote triumphantly to Tye that afternoon, 'is equivalent to victory'. Although technically guilty she had won the moral case, along with the hearts and minds of most of the court. 'The police inspectors had their tea with me,' she continued to Tye, and 'I think that the magistrate was also somewhat sympathetic.' Her greatest coup however, to the amazement and delight of the friends who had come along to provide moral support, was during an interval in proceedings when she won the personal backing of Bodkin. Once the trial was concluded he donated a symbolic £5, the sum of Eglantyne's fine, towards her cause. It was to be one of the first donations put towards a new fund to provide emergency relief for European children: the 'Save the Children Fund'.

Both Eglantyne and Dorothy recognised the PR potential of Eglantyne's trial, but the timing could not have been worse for a 'love thy enemy' press story. The 15 May, the day of the trial, happened to coincide with the state funeral of Edith Cavell, the English nurse who had been executed by German firing squad in Brussels four years earlier, having been found guilty of helping two hundred Allied soldiers escape from occupied territory. Cavell's death had deeply shocked the British public, and had been used by Allied propagandists at the time as evidence of the alleged inhumanity of the enemy, helping both to justify the domestic war policy and precipitate American entry into the war.[9] Her Westminster Abbey funeral, attended by Queen Alexandra and Princess Victoria, was big news, dominating the British papers. With brilliant PR savvy, instead of competing with the story Eglantyne promoted a new angle on the event, writing an open letter to the press which focused not on the atrocities committed by Germany but on the great humanity of Britain's heroine. 'I feel that patriotism is not enough. We must have no hatred or bitterness in our hearts towards anyone,' Eglantyne quoted Cavell's famous last words a year before they were carved on to her London memorial. 'Let us take this message, and live it out in practical action ...' she pressed her case, 'with the saving of the children of Europe, irrespective of their nationality.' Recognising that the plight of children emphasised the essential humanity of her cause, she then deliberately added a maternal–feminist flavour to her appeal:

> I appeal to my fellow country women to help me to lift the whole question of the saving of the child life of Europe out of the political region altogether. Let the women of this country take the lead in a work which the men, in their political groupings, seem powerless to carry forward.

Just four days later, on 19 May 1919, she and Dorothy held a 'Famine Meeting' at the Royal Albert Hall with the aim of capitalising on the trial publicity in *The Times*, *Mail*, *Mirror* and *Guardian* and spread across the cover of the *Daily Herald*, to raise funds for immediate relief.[10] The invitation letter the sisters quickly drafted for their growing contact list is heavy with Eglantyne's unmistakable turn of phrase, torn between blatant flattery: 'I feel sure you are so persuasive you would be able to get people to come,' and the almost painfully personal: 'the question is horribly urgent and I feel convinced that all other questions will be completely thrown into the shade by this one in the course of the next few months ... the whole thing is a nightmare to me from which I can never escape'. Holding the event in such a large and prestigious venue was a huge gamble: 'you can understand how anxious we are to make the Albert Hall meeting a success', the letter ended, adding prophetically if with perhaps more strategy than genuine optimism, 'If it is [a success] it might very well be the start of a real national movement.'

Despite the vast capacity of the Albert Hall, in the event Eglantyne and Dorothy could not supply enough seats to meet demand. Unfortunately though, the crowd that filled the Hall and soon gathered outside on Kensington Gore was not entirely made up of sympathisers – many people were sceptical about the reports of famine and some had arrived with rotten apples to throw at the 'traitors' who wanted to raise money to feed enemy children. Addressing this audience was a daunting prospect even for Dorothy who had had considerable experience of giving political speeches to unsympathetic crowds during Charlie's election campaigns. Eglantyne, who hated public speaking at the best of times, must have been terrified. However, in a well-co-ordinated programme the meeting opened with a shocking eye-witness account of the impact of the blockade on the lives of ordinary citizens in Berlin and Vienna by the journalist Henry Noel Brailsford. Not content with rolling out descriptions of skeleton-thin women and passive, wide-eyed, dying children, Brailsford spoke of seeing unarmed men fighting mounted police in the streets, not in public protest but simply to seize a police-horse which they tore apart there and then for food. It was a shocking picture that brought the desperate realities of starvation home to the audience: England might have plenty of quiet suffering, but no one was driven to butchering trained horses for their meat in the cities' streets.

Brailsford was followed on to the stage not by some well-meaning aristocrat but the controversial and popular miners' leader Robert Smillie. The heavily moustached Smillie was a Scottish socialist and a powerful orator who despite having opposed the war now found his influence as the President of the Miners' Federation was at its height. Already a firm supporter of the Famine Council, he now became one of Save the Children's most powerful champions, publicly aligning himself with the cause for several years, and donating over £30,000 on behalf of the miners' union. 'It is felt that if Mr Smillie believed certain "economies" meant the death of little children he would be quite capable of calling a man who urged them a murderer, but he would know how to do it in parliamentary language,' an American journalist once neatly summed him up. Smillie now moved the resolution that 'this meeting urges the necessity of pressing forward every measure of effective relief to meet the appalling conditions of the famine districts, and especially to stay mortality among the children'.

Eglantyne and Dorothy were next up. Eglantyne kept her contribution short but her message was the more powerful for it. Surely, she asked in a voice at first quiet but gaining force with her conviction, 'it is impossible for us as normal human beings to watch children starve to death without making an effort to save them ... We have only one object, to save as many as possible. We have only one rule, we shall help them whatever their country, whatever their religion.' Dorothy then detailed the case for the Save the Children Fund, opening with the classic line, 'I stand here tonight to appeal to you for the lives of children.' Although she also talked calmly about the political consequences of not providing humanitarian assistance, her immediate appeal – for the children of Poland, Armenia and Vienna – was delivered with compelling emotion:

> Do not let us forget what it means that there are many hundreds of thousands of parents today, whose awful doom it has been and still is to watch their children grow weaker, to see them wither and perish before their eyes, while they are helpless to save them ...

> Every tin of babies' food which private effort can send out comes as a token of sympathy and a message of new hope to some despairing mother.

Looking around at her now-silent audience Dorothy realised that they had carried the moment, and she sealed the success of the meeting with a brilliant piece of ad-libbing. 'There is more practical morality in this tin', she called out, waving a tin of condensed milk above her head to tumultuous applause, 'than in all the creeds.'[11] So the Save the Children Fund was launched as a spontaneous public collection was taken up around the hall.

Eglantyne and Dorothy later credited each other with starting Save the Children.[12] By early 1919 both were convinced that immediate practical measures as well as political campaigning were needed to alleviate the suffering caused by the blockade and the aftermath of the war. But as Eglantyne was serving as Honorary Secretary of the Famine Council it had to be Dorothy, at a Council meeting in April 1919, who raised the idea of organising a distinct relief fund for the starving children of Europe. As a result it was Dorothy who was listed as the Fund's first Honorary Secretary; but in fact the sisters saw the appeal very much as an opportunity to continue working together, their 'hearts and minds', according to Dorothy, 'always working in very close co-operation'. Dividing up the immediate task, Dorothy focused on using her and Charlie's press contacts and political leverage to gain support for the Fund, while continuing to supply information on the famine conditions and existing relief work across Central Europe. This left the actual management of the Fund to Eglantyne, along with heading up the all-important public campaign for donations. 'I do feel it so glorious … that we should have this work *together*; – climbing the same trees like we did so long ago,' Dorothy wrote to Tye that July.

But although she enjoyed working with Eglantyne, Dorothy was a political animal and she soon began to resent the distraction that her commitment to the avowedly non-political Fund required from her advocacy work with the Famine Council and Women's League, and her support for Charlie's parliamentary campaigns. She and Eglantyne would continue to work together for several years, the courage and commitment of each inspiring the other, but Dorothy would focus increasingly on lobbying work until finally extricating herself completely from Save the Children in 1921, when she wrote to a friend that she had 'abandoned politics altogether when I took up the SCF, and now … I think it is time to take up politics again'.[13]

Eglantyne by contrast had never felt more inspired, both by the opportunity to help meet the urgent humanitarian need in Europe, and also by seeing a potential in the Fund beyond immediate relief. This, she believed, was a cause that had the capacity to change the world permanently. It was precisely the non-political profile of the Fund that frustrated Dorothy that Eglantyne found so exciting. Whereas before Eglantyne had supported local philanthropic projects and fleeting party political campaigns, now she hoped to promote a popular and permanent moral revival, breaking down barriers of nationality and shifting international perspectives about people as a whole. Within a few months of Save the Children's launch Eglantyne had replaced Dorothy as Honorary Secretary. She had already become the motive force within the organisation, leading on co-ordinating immediate aid across Europe, and she would soon start to transform it from a one-off British relief 'fund' into a permanent international organisation not only providing emergency relief but promoting sustainable development. Recognising her sister's transforming vision for the organisation as early as July 1919, Dorothy noted that 'Eglantyne is the real soul of our movement. Everybody who comes into contact with her gets inspired and they all worship her.'

It was not just by default to the Fund's first appeal that Eglantyne continued to focus on the needs of children. At first, with her deep commitment to humanitarian work that refused to recognise distinctions of class, gender, nationality, political belief or faith, she had been unsure about the Fund's exclusive focus on the needs of this one social group above all others. Early on she even mooted launching a 'National Relief Fund' along similar lines to Save the Children but to provide emergency aid for adults. Not unreasonably the Save the Children Council quickly squashed the idea, fearing such a fund would damage their own fundraising potential. Eglantyne was not one for giving in to partisan arguments, but she soon saw several other reasons, both strategic and tactical, for sticking with the focus on children.

In the first place Eglantyne and Dorothy were both persuaded that children had a special case for priority relief that was not being met by existing aid organisations. The International Committee of the Red Cross had identified children as the main sufferers in the post-war European famine, but although the Red Cross, along with the American Relief Administration, Friends Relief Society, Salvation Army and others were co-ordinating relief work in Europe, none were specifically focused on the needs of children. Save the Children was the first charity specifically set up for non-domicile children, and coincidentally the first to be founded by women. Dorothy, herself a mother of two, had been moved by the plight of European children for years, writing to Eglantyne from the outset of the war in August 1914 that 'the newspapers are full of headlines about battles, but how many British people know what is happening to children?' Just back from visiting the orphanages and 'soup-kitchens' of conflict-torn Macedonia Eglantyne was also emotionally and intellectually alert to the claims of the child victims of war, but it was not until 1919 that Dr Munro's medical reports from Vienna convinced her that children had a particular case for support because, as she later wrote, both physiologically and psychologically 'grown-ups can adjust themselves, to a certain extent, and recover vitality later on, but children stop developing and it is doubtful whether ground lost can ever be recovered'. This issue of a child's arrested development was reflected in Eglantyne's 'starving baby' leaflets and reiterated in countless articles to the press and letters to potential supporters. 'As a result of prolonged malnutrition, which now amounts to daily increasing starvation, countless children have become almost like living skeletons,' Eglantyne even petitioned the American President Woodrow Wilson for support in early 1919. 'Children of twelve look like children of eight. All are under-developed and reduced to the utmost weakness and apathy.' Her letter ended with the marvellous handwritten PS: 'What we need is an immediate initial credit of not less than 20 million dollars.'

But Eglantyne also subscribed to the popular idea that children represent the future, and therefore an investment in child welfare

was not only an immediate moral obligation but a strategic investment in society.[14] The potential for social change offered by each
generation had always engaged her, drawing her to education theory
while at college, and explored in terms of citizenship in her social
report on Cambridge and through the Boys Employment Register a
few years later. Now she added an international angle to the mix.
'The point is this,' she launched into an earnest explanation to her
sister Em: 'If we want the world to be a better place, obviously the
first necessity is that the children should have what is essential for
their physical, mental and moral wellbeing.' Reflecting the unfortunate influence of contemporary eugenicist ideas she continued:

> The creation of a sub-human race (and at present such a race *is* being
> created through disease) *must* mean a relapse into barbarism: con-
> versely the construction of a better social order demands men and
> women capable of constructing it. The saving of the children who
> are starving now should be the first step towards building up a world
> in which children shall no more starve.

Later Eglantyne would refine this argument into a rather more
appealing sound-bite for public consumption: 'Every generation of
children … offers mankind anew the possibility of rebuilding his ruin
of a world.'

The idea that the inspiration behind Save the Children was the
creation of a 'better social order', as well as individual child welfare,
is compelling. Eglantyne had no great sentiment for children individually, but she had an overwhelming desire to promote a moral
revival based on the essential 'unity' of humankind as revealed to her
through her unconventional faith. Save the Children not only
offered the opportunity to foster better social relations between
Britain and her former enemies in Europe, but also the chance to
reach out to a new generation who, supported rather than abandoned, would be more likely to value and respect the international
community and the common claims of humanity. As Ruth later

wrote, 'to Eglantyne relief work was never more than a clearing away of obstacles so that the real advance of humanity could proceed'.

Promoting an international peace agenda was an incidental benefit of the Fund's work, but also hugely important to both Eglantyne and Dorothy. 'We ... wanted to do our bit if possible, to break down that awful spirit of mistrust and suspicion and hatred which outlived the war...' Dorothy later wrote:

> We thought that one supreme way of doing this would be if we could appeal to men and women of different lands to reach each other through the most intimate source of all feelings, the interests of the child.
>
> We felt that even if some people found it difficult to give up their hatred against their so-called enemies, at least they would not find it difficult to find some pity and love in their hearts for the children of these so-called enemies.

Both sisters intuitively understood that a focus on children would appeal powerfully to the British public. Young children have unique appeal, popularly being seen as innocent as well as vulnerable. Eglantyne may not have shared this view; she was not given over to maternal protectiveness, and did not see innocence as valid criteria for prioritising relief any more than the qualities of respectability and hard work that the Cambridge COS ladies had looked for to demark the 'deserving poor' years before. But she recognised that this perception of children, as somehow innately deserving, could help to overcome the hostility towards aiding the people with whom the country had been so recently at war. In harnessing the image of a suffering child on her leaflets Eglantyne had already brought together two powerful public relations tools – the infant and the photograph – both of which appear to have no language, no involved argument or bias, but simply to present a statement of fact; in this case undeniable need. The emotive use of photographs of children was not entirely unprecedented. Thomas Barnardo had promoted his children's homes with hundreds of photographs of ragged children, some of which were staged, the century before, and other domestic children's charities including the NSPCC were still publishing 'before and after' photographs of the 'rescued' children in their programmes well into the 1930s. Eglantyne's approach was less contrived but in fact more complex: she recognised that the young child's apparent neutrality was actually hugely political in the widest sense, highlighting not only childhood innocence and vulnerability but also shared humanity. Her decision to stick with the focus on children both recognised and exploited this. Furthermore a focus on child relief through the provision of food avoided the politics of economic reconstruction that was indissolubly bound up with the relief of adults.

But if in some ways children were the vehicle for promoting Eglantyne's vision for a just and peaceful society, they were not a tool she was exploiting cynically: children's well-being was the end as well as the means in her vision for the future. Visiting Vienna at the close of 1919 to oversee the allocation of Save the Children's funds to relief operations on the ground, she wrote home to Dorothy:

> To the end of my days, I don't think I shall ever get out of my head the sound of children crying!

> Thank God that our Fund will do something to save them.

Something, however, would never be enough for Eglantyne.

Chapter 13

Hearts and Minds,
1919–1920

The problem is not lack of money, but attitude of mind …

Eglantyne Jebb, 1920

The launch of a campaign to raise money for children in countries that barely six months previously had been at war with
Britain – especially when there was still such obvious need at
home – was courageous. Despite the success of Eglantyne and
Dorothy's public meeting at the Albert Hall, friends like Emmeline
Pethick-Lawrence, who had marched against the blockade in
Trafalgar Square just a few weeks earlier, cautioned that they would
be lucky to raise £100, and many believed any fundraising would be
impossible.

Early attempts to pull together a committee to head the 'Save the
Children Fund' seemed to confirm this. 'I know what some people
mean when then say they won't give English money to help feed
foreign children who will only rise up and kill us again in 25 years,'

Lady Norah Bentinck wrote to excuse herself to Charlie's sister, Victoria, who was co-ordinating approaches. Others, like Violet Hanbury, responded even more emphatically:

> I should not feel inclined to take any part in assisting the enemies of England to recover from the effects of their own lack of honour and humanity. *I do not desire their recovery.* It is well known that in Germany, at all events, there is now no lack of money. Let those in authority commandeer it for the needy in their own country and in those of their allies – Whatever money may be to spare in England had better be spent on those Britishers who have suffered by the War; only half-hearted patriots would wish to relieve enemies whose conduct has disgraced civilisation while one single victim remained in need – or wish to see Germany and her allies strong enough once more to attempt renewing their atrocities.

Lady Norah was of course right that Germany would 'rise up' again, in fact just twenty years later. And no doubt in 1919 when she decided against joining the Save the Children Council her thoughts were with her newborn son, Henry, who would indeed later be wounded during active service in the Second World War.[1] But the return of war was not inevitable in 1919 when the terms of the Treaty of Versailles were being debated and Save the Children established, and it is possible that a more humanitarian approach towards Germany might yet have altered the course of events. Charlie was outraged by these responses to his sister, fuming to Dorothy that there was 'no hope of such people becoming civilised', and another early Fund supporter, Lord Aberdeen, wrote similarly of 'the extraordinary and horrible manifestation of enemy hate which takes the form of objecting to help even the starving infants of the countries with which we were at war … Is this anything less than a genteel form of savagery?'

However even Famine Council members were divided about the advisability of raising funds for relief, because 'at best charity could do

very little to assuage the misery of the famine stricken, and moreover
… the giving of charity would act as a salve to the public conscience
and divert attention away from the necessity of more adequate measures'. Eglantyne felt it was just as plausible that relief might have the
opposite effect on public opinion, by 'arousing the public to the
necessity for economic reconstruction', but she was in any case
determined to stick to purely humanitarian arguments for aid. 'The
sole aim of the Save the Children Fund is to save children,' she wrote.
'It will not diverge one hairbreath into any of those political or economic issues which are the sphere of the Governments.' Later she
would wearily note that 'there are always two classes of people who
are prepared to take sides against the humanitarian view. There are
those who do not believe that the children are worth saving, and
those who do not believe that they can be saved.' It was all about
changing beliefs.

'All your life you will make other people better,' Margaret had
written to comfort Eglantyne nine years earlier when she was forced
to give up her Cambridge social work. 'You will inspire them and
make the impossible seem possible to them.' Now Eglantyne was
doing just that; helping to realise the potential of Save the Children
by communicating her ideas and values to colleagues, volunteers and
supporters in such a way that it seemed to her cousin Gem as if
'people … under the spell of her personality, were for a time lifted
above their normal selves'. Eglantyne inspired others effortlessly
partly because she herself had so much faith in her cause. But part of
her appeal was that despite all her passion she managed to avoid being
overly earnest and putting other people's backs up. The very human
sense of humour that Gwen Darwin had once felt saved Eglantyne
'from the kind of philanthropicalness of most good ladies' now
helped to win over the great and the good, the cold and the cynical.
It was a powerful combination of cause and approach.

Soon a well-connected committee of politicians and journalists
who were also prepared to make the immediate relief of starving

children their priority had been recruited, headed up by Lord Robert Cecil, one of the architects of the League of Nations. The wealthy Liberal politician and philanthropist Lord Weardale, who had married a Russian Countess widowed from the family of Leo Tolstoy, added some glamour to the line up. Weardale was a committed pacifist who had once faced the double indignity of being attacked with a dogwhip by a suffragette for his opposition to the women's vote, but anti-suffrage aside he quickly became a close ally of Eglantyne's and served as an invaluable Chair of the Fund until his death.[2] Eglantyne also wanted to recruit a General Secretary, 'if necessary at a high salary', to complement her own role. 'There must be a clearly recognised differentiation between control of policy and control of the administrative machine', she wrote, continuing with no false modesty, 'inspiration and efficiency are both necessary, and the two are seldom found in the same person'. She appointed Lewis Golden, a well-connected British citizen born in Russia where he had served as the correspondent for the *Daily Mail*. Escaping after the October Revolution of 1917, Golden had just returned from an aid mission to Czechoslovakia when he joined the Fund. He could hardly have been better qualified for the work ahead.

Many of the rest of the team were friends roped in from the *Cambridge Magazine*, Famine Council and Women's League, including Maude Royden, Kate Courtney, Ethel Snowden, Mosa Anderson and the journalist Henrietta Leslie, now at the militant anti-war paper the *Daily Herald*. Inevitably the association with such overtly political organisations caused dismay among some of the Fund's more conservative supporters who feared it would damage the charity's fundraising potential with the upper classes. 'I am horrified … that Miss Royden and Miss Courtenay [sic] are to tour the country for the Fight the Famine Council,' one local fundraiser recorded her indignation in December 1919. 'This means, in many provincial towns, that a fatal spoke will be put in the wheel of this society.'

Less Conservative supporters would be offended in turn, however, as Eglantyne courted support from across the political spectrum, later accepting fundraising help from Lady Cynthia Mosley, the wife of Sir Oswald, future founder of the 'British Union of Fascists'.[3] Within six months Eglantyne had even recruited Margaret Lloyd George, the wife of the Prime Minister, as the Fund's Vice President. In many ways it was a fantastic coup that secured widespread public legitimacy for Save the Children, but it also caused outrage among the Fund's campaigning supporters who objected to the Lloyd George name on its letterhead, 'as if', one wrote bitterly to Dorothy, 'a murderer were to head the public subscription for a coffin for its victim'.[4] As David Lloyd George was directly responsible for continuing the blockade this was not an unreasonable perspective – Eglantyne's move was rather akin to inviting Laura Bush to head up a national relief fund for the children of Iraq. Even the 'Friends Emergency Committee', one of Save the Children's most established partners in the field, was concerned about the Lloyd George association and commented on the importance of the Fund being run 'by persons whose international outlook we trust'. Raising funds for humanitarian relief was proving to be surprisingly political, and Eglantyne's policy of being overtly non-partisan was often diplomatically challenging. 'We collected on our Committee and as officers of the Fund the queerest collection of cranks, fools, and vassals which could well be imagined,' Dorothy summed things up with typical bluntness. Her main concern was focused elsewhere: 'We had neither the office quarters nor the staff competent to deal with the new situation.'

One of Save the Children's first headquarters was a condemned house in London's Soho at 26 Golden Square. Eglantyne had always preferred a modest address and now at last she could justify her economy. The office had no carpet, the trestle-tables and hard wooden chairs were army-surplus, and index-cards were filed in old dress-boxes. Winnie Elkin, the Fund's first temporary secretary in 1919, claimed she was nearly driven mad by the chaos. As no one anticipated that the Fund would develop into a permanent organisation, its first workers were taken on six-week contracts and the office was run by a mix of low-paid staff sustained by their sense of vocation, and volunteer ladies 'easily distinguished … as they always wore hats'. In 1924 when the Fund moved to a Bloomsbury house with more space for its expanding operations, Eglantyne saved money by moving into rooms on the second floor. Save the Children had quickly become the focus of her life, and she worked long hours both in the office and travelling to meetings at home and abroad. A small stash of chocolate helped to sustain her, and she cheerfully advised all her colleagues to keep some in their desks. At weekends she packed her paperwork for visits to Tye at Crowborough where she worked in an unheated glasshouse, nicknamed the 'refrigerator', at the bottom of the garden. The Fund meanwhile was soon chasing more space and cheaper rents around Bloomsbury, finally settling in Gordon Square.

With the exception of the Cambridge society days that Dorothy labelled rather disdainfully as her sister's 'worldly period', Eglantyne had always pursued a romantic bent towards frugal living. Now acutely aware of the human value of every penny, she became obsessive about cutting back her personal expenses. She soon had a seriously austere lifestyle, even taking to constantly wearing practical, brown, rather nun-like clothes. But if simplicity had become a little confused with self-mortification Eglantyne was not entirely unaware of the ridiculousness of her 'uniform' as she called it. 'A great many thanks for all the clothes', she wrote cheerfully to Margaret in 1924, 'the stockings came just in time to prevent … light coloured stockings from introducing a startling inconsequence to my monastic attire'. Although she had not lost her sense of humour this outward sign of austerity was a rather depressing habit that she never kicked; even at her death her clothes included two brown coats, three brown jackets, four pairs of brown trousers, five brown petticoats (two wool, but more pleasingly two satin, one silk), two brown dresses and some brown gloves – although her wardrobe was mildly enlivened by the addition of a mauve dressing-gown and 'a grey knitted dress in a case' among a few other items.

Eglantyne's severe dress advertised her long-standing rejection of spendthrift society and admiration for simplicity of wants; a well-worn theme of earlier English philanthropists neatly captured by Thoreau, who had famously warned in *Walden*, 'beware all enterprises that require new clothes'. Brought up at least with reference to this tradition, Eglantyne and her sisters had always been critical of what they considered the expensive frivolity of fashion. Tye may have regretted this trend among her daughters and their aunt Carrie would certainly have disapproved, but Bun, in many ways their soulmate, would have understood. Bun's own overtly masculine clothes, like those of several of Eglantyne's female Oxford tutors, were an outward indication of her independence of spirit as well as a desire for physical freedom which all the Jebb sisters appreciated. On her return to England from Ottoman Iraq in 1908 Lill had been quite shocked by the complicated and restrictive British fashions, which she compared with the Chinese tradition of foot-binding, enslaving women to 'barbarous custom'. And Dorothy would later admire the utilitarian clothes she saw on a 1928 trip to Russia, commenting that 'dress, in fact, is primarily for use, which brought me to realize how very largely ours is for display, and therefore what a waste of time, of thought and of money it habitually represents'.

But if Eglantyne was seeking both a degree of physical freedom and relief from the time and expense that keeping up a fashionable appearance entailed, she was also not unaware of the importance of clothes for display. 'The ways of women are past understanding,' she had written to her friend Dorothy Kempe as she prepared for her Oxford college leaving ceremony. 'I had fondly believed that I was to be clad in *brown* and *gray*, colours most appropriate to my profession and lot in life. Instead I am sent a robe of purple and gold and a scarlet and bright blue mantle.' Now nearly twenty years later

Eglantyne was finally using her wardrobe to emphasise her professional persona. Victorian and Edwardian women seeking to enter public life had often used voluntary uniforms in this way; from evangelicals in their plain dress to militant suffragettes in purple, green and white. Eglantyne's chosen dress accentuated her age and asexuality, almost certainly giving her greater credibility in her public role and, consciously or not, the habit-like brown emphasised what many saw as her 'spiritual' goodness. According to Ruth 'something in her carriage and the soft brown draperies that matched her hair, but much more in the sense of spiritual force transcending limitations, made one think of a herald angel or of an incandescent flame'. Eglantyne's image was already bordering on the saintly, and now like many who believed they had found inspiration, perhaps even salvation, through dedicating their lives to the needs of others, she could often not understand why everyone else did not share her perspective and priorities.

Top of Eglantyne's list for reform was what she considered the immoral misuse of public funds, both in terms of the central government defence budget – which she left to Dorothy – but also private spending on fashion and small luxuries like cigarettes and cinema tickets. Raising funds was now her first priority and she could not bear the thought of money that could be spent on child relief being frittered away.[5] From now on Eglantyne would be haunted by the knowledge of how many more lives could have been saved had her hands not been tied, as she saw it, by lack of funds. Her poem 'Handcuffed' shows how keenly she felt this awful responsibility:

> I watched them drown, my brothers and my friends,
> There where the cliff descends
> Sheer to the inky waters of the lake.
> With unavailing fury of hate and despair
> They fought for life, and were
> Inch by inch drawn under. I heard them make
> Frenzied appeal to all the powers that be.

Then they appealed to me,
Out of their agony they called, and they,
'Mid the engulfing terrors of their death,
Called still with their last breath.
But on my wrists the heavy handcuffs lay.

Translating this into a moral fervour for fundraising, Eglantyne launched into a very modern dissection of public priorities. 'We must not allow ourselves to imagine that we are without the necessary material resources for putting our ideals into practice,' she argued:

> It is said that in the Unites States of America a million pounds a day is spent on cosmetics and various kinds of beauty treatment. We are willing to spend a million pounds a day on internecine destruction; women are willing to spend a million pounds a day on improving their personal appearance; when shall we be willing to spend a million pounds a day on rescuing the children who are at present left a prey to agony and despair?

Sometimes Eglantyne let her puritanical streak run away with her. In a letter to *The Times* on 21 December 1919 she pleaded, 'Can humane men and women celebrate the birth of Christ in any better way than renouncing self-indulgence and extravagance in order to have something to spend on saving the lives and health of the suffering little ones?' It was not a sentiment that attracted many in the run up to the first real Christmas celebrations after the war, and Eglantyne soon realised that simply hectoring the public through letters to the press was not going to generate much sympathy. What she needed was a much more innovative approach.

Eglantyne and Dorothy's launch appeal for Save the Children went by the very modern-sounding name 'Cows for Vienna', and aimed to provide Austrian children with a regular and cheap supply of fresh milk by bringing over Swiss dairy-cows. Like some of the most successful fundraising today, the idea was to ask people to pay for something specific and appealing that would provide lasting benefit to the recipients. The ambitious target was £1,000, to be raised and spent within ten days.[6] Eglantyne had £5 from the prosecutor at her trial, and half a crown from her housekeeper's apron pocket. Everything else had to be raised from scratch, a fair section of the press and the public were against her, and she had never enjoyed fundraising at the best of times. 'Never were there more hopeless looking beginnings', Ruth commented, 'the first stages of the effort would have deterred any less self-forgetting soul'.

Eglantyne launched the appeal with a familiar campaign of press articles and public speaking. Building on the support of Robert Smillie, the miners' leader, she also established a good relationship with the Labour Party and Trade Union movement, stressing the importance of the 'suffering children, who will be the workers of the future' when she spoke at the Labour Party annual conference in 1920. But even her friends conceded that she was 'not good at collecting money by speeches'. A traditional community-based fundraising campaign quickly followed, but this was not Eglantyne's forte either. Winnie Elkin's patience was now tested again as, she wrote, 'Eglantyne, believing as she did in people ... insisted on trying out the enthusiasts.' It was a policy that added to the number of what Dorothy called 'cranks' in the organisation as Eglantyne gave time to some fantastically hopeless fundraising ideas, and even initially supported a Mr Graham who swore that his 'vita bread', the recipe for which had been revealed to him by heaven, was so nourishing that it would defeat the famine in a few weeks. For an intelligent woman Eglantyne could be surprisingly gullible.

Fortunately the journalist Henrietta Leslie soon took over the local fundraising campaign, pulling together an enthusiastic team who by 1921 were managing over three hundred committees of local volunteers raising money through everything from cake sales to street collections, and from popular dances at the Hammersmith Palais to society events at the Guildhall. Collections were taken up by factory girls and miners barely earning a living wage. An anonymous donation was sent 'from a French governess to a German child'. With her eye firmly on the next generation of citizens Eglantyne was particularly pleased when children sent in contributions, and she often quoted one small boy who wrote to Lord Weardale, 'I have fished 2/6 out of my money box and hope you can now save all the starving children.' 'Life was one long procession of "stunts" …' Henrietta recalled, 'we indulged in every kind of money-making dodge that a highly inventive committee could conceive.' Her team soon became known rather disparagingly as the 'stunts department' by the more conservative Fund volunteers, and there were plenty, like Lewis Golden, who did not approve of her more controversial tactics such as street collections and public debates. 'Such methods – I had inherited them of course from my suffrage days – seemed to him lacking in dignity,' Henrietta realised.

Eglantyne had no such qualms, but she was frustrated by the huge amount of time, effort and diplomacy such fundraising required. Describing the typical fundraising committee to Dorothy's daughter, who was now thirteen and fully caught up in her mother and aunt's work, she wrote cynically that 'there will hardly be a person on it who single-mindedly wants to relieve the famine':

> Some will have joined for snobbish reasons, swayed (unconsciously) by the prospect of working on a committee with people with titles. Others will have some personal axe to grind, or think the work will be to their credit in some way. A bishop may be invited, so as to lend respectability to the work, but he will be full of scruples, over-anxious not to offend the government perhaps.

Henrietta was similarly frustrated by unreliable committee ladies who could often not remember the name of the society they were supposed to be assisting, and once completely failed to turn up for an event because the invites happened to be sent in envelopes the same colour as those used by a society dressmaker, as a result being mistaken for bills and thrown away.[7] 'I never ceased to grudge the overheads and fatigue that had to be expended on such efforts,' Henrietta wrote in a sentiment that many a modern fundraiser might appreciate. 'It made generosity seem a frivolous thing. How much simpler to have given the money outright.'

Eglantyne agreed. 'In this country we have received contributions from a very large number of quite poor people' she wrote to Maynard Keynes in July 1920, and 'it may be said that the money [was] raised "with great labour"'. It had become clear that while many people were very generous and collectively the effort was hugely valuable, such fundraising was also expensive and time consuming. 'The problem is not money, but attitude of mind,' Eglantyne concluded. 'We have to devise a means of making known the facts in such a way as to touch the imagination of the world.'

Eglantyne was always keen on 'introducing business methods into philanthropy', and now she looked to commercial marketing strategies to see what could be adapted for Save the Children. In March 1920 she launched a pioneering campaign that ditched the traditional polite small ads in the personal columns of newspapers for full-page spreads in nationals like *The Times,* similar only to the advertising then given to pills, pens, soap or biscuits. Such ad space was frighteningly expensive and Eglantyne faced considerable opposition from the Fund's Council, many of whom could not believe that their obsessively frugal founder could endorse such a potentially risky investment. Furthermore Eglantyne's copy was certainly far from the conventional polite appeal. 'We have won the war,' screamed one advert:

> We are justly proud. We are spending, on our well-earned amusements and our comfortable meals, **millions of pounds every day!**
>
> And all the time, outside our very doors, a multitude of helpless children and stricken mothers are perishing for want of food and clothes – not One Thousand, Two Thousand, or a Hundred

thousand, but MILLIONS! It is not in China or Tibet. It is in Europe – a mere tourist's trip from where you are reading now. It is not due to natural causes which we might regard as Destiny and for which we might feel inactively sorry. It is part of the price which poor, innocent children are paying for the glorious victory we have won.

Like every good fundraiser she included some emotive statistics: 2/- would provide a child with dinners for a week, £1 would feed and clothe a starving child, £100 would feed a thousand children for a week, if every worker in Britain gave a penny a day for just two months all the children of Europe could be saved, and each donation would be put to use within twenty-four hours. Illustrations of starving mothers and despairing children dominated the copy, and taking the best from the Famine Council leaflets, Eglantyne also quoted British soldiers, heroes, who had shared their own rations with the starving children of their former enemies in Hamburg, Bremen and other cities. Please donate quickly, she invariably ended, 'for every moment you hesitate another innocent life may be forfeit'.

At least one committee lady resigned in protest at the vulgar commercialisation of the approach, and Labour Party friends called the expensive advertising 'repellent'. For Eglantyne, however, it was a simple choice 'between incurring this cost and leaving the children to die'. The public response exceeded all expectations. On average each advert took around ten times its cost. One in the *Daily News* brought in £7,000 over just two days, and another was clipped and returned anonymously with a cheque for £10,000 pinned to it.[8] It was a fundraising phenomenon, and Eglantyne was quick to invent other cost-effective ways in which to build on Save the Children's new profile to capture the public's imagination and support. Soon the Fund was pioneering innovative giving schemes like asking workers for a day's wages, companies for a day's profits, or the public to sponsor a child, all of which have since become well-established fundraising methods.

But in catching the headlines Eglantyne had also exposed the Fund to claims of sensationalism and with it the risk that the organisation would lose credibility. The public was already sceptical about the severity of the situation in Europe and the Secretary of the Charities Organisation Society – focused around British philanthropy – now claimed in the press that 'it is not unreasonable to think that the condition of the children cannot be as desperate as represented in that [Save the Children] appeal'. Determined to secure the public's confidence, Eglantyne and Dorothy approached their list of celebrity contacts. Among others Sigmund Freud, Albert Einstein, the Russian dancer Anna Pavlova, and popular English authors Jerome K. Jerome, A.A. Milne and Thomas Hardy all either wrote movingly about the plight of children for the Fund to quote in their publicity, or signed open letters to the press expressing their support. 'By our pride, by our greed, by our folly, we have brought the children to death's door …' Jerome wrote. 'It is upon the children that we have been making war. Are we not tired of slaying them? It is not time to save those who are left?' The novelist and playwright John Galsworthy, who would be awarded the Nobel Prize for Literature in 1932, even dedicated a poem to the Fund's work:

With doom the children paid the wage
Of war. And now, in trailing peace,
And, ever more, the children die!
Ah, if there's anything we can
You-I-the simple woman-man-
For pity's sake then let us give
That some starved frozen child may live.
… A child's a child!

But in the lingering climate of hostility towards sending aid to Austria and Germany it was George Bernard Shaw that gave Save the Children its greatest PR boost, writing with powerful simplicity, 'I have no enemies under the age of seven.' Dorothy had approached

Shaw some months earlier to write a preface for a disturbing booklet called *Family Life in Germany under the Blockade*, published that July.[9] Although he felt the favour had been extorted from him while he was already 'frantically busy', Shaw quickly knocked off the preface, afterwards fearing that 'it must be rather a scamped job'. In fact it was a perfectly pitched call for some human perspective. 'Are we out, not merely for defeat, but for extermination?' Shaw asked:

> In the early days of voluntary recruiting, we were exhorted from every hoarding to remember that some day our children would ask us what we did in the great war. That question was dropped when compulsory military service was instituted. It might very well be revived in the form, 'Daddy: what did you do when the war was over?' The man who can say 'I shared my ration with the poor starving children in Germany' will have considerable moral advantage over the ardent patriot who has nothing better to say than 'I voted for hanging the Kaiser; and he was not hanged after all.'

Because Shaw was a very public figure, and reputedly the richest writer in the country, he attracted endless charity appeals. Dorothy and Eglantyne had caught him early, but by 1920 he was moaning to the German playwright Julius Bab that it had become 'part of the day's routine to hear that so and so were starving and that there was not a child under seven years of age left alive in Poland'. Soon the constant requests for donations began to irritate him in certain moods, and despite his early support he sent a shocking reply to the Fund's next approach. 'On the whole, the response to my appeals was wonderfully heartening,' Henrietta remembered in her memoirs, 'but Shaw sent me a postcard on which was written: "Better let them die."' 'In the light of subsequent events,' she later commented, 'someone said the other day, he was quite right!' But Shaw, who was prone to a lurking pessimism, was probably simply depressed about the futility of relief and his ability to make a meaningful difference.[10] Henrietta made the best of it, auctioning the card as an autograph so that in effect Shaw unwittingly contributed to Save the Children's funds after all. But his response was a telling precursor of the more widespread charitable exhaustion or 'giving fatigue' that would soon make sustaining Save the Children's early fundraising success difficult. Eglantyne's greatest fundraising coup at the end of 1919 however was securing the active support of the churches. That summer she had approached the Church of England to make an appeal on behalf of the distressed children of Europe but Randall Davidson, the Archbishop of Canterbury, had shown no interest. Undeterred she wrote to Rome to see if the Pope, His Holiness Benedict XV, might be more amenable. Pope Benedict had already tried to promote a negotiated peace settlement during the war and had expressed his support for the Famine Council by extending his blessing to Eglantyne and the other officers. Now he took the unprecedented step of issuing an Encyclical Letter asking Catholic churches around the world to collect for Save the Children on Holy Innocents' Day, 28 December.[11] It was the first time that the Catholic Church had supported a non-denominational cause. 'Our heart bleeds for these suffering little ones,' the Encyclical read:

> Not only are they completely innocent and even ignorant of the san-
> guine struggle which has saddened the whole world, but they are the
> seed of future generations which cannot but suffer from their debil-
> itation … In our grief we have been not a little comforted to learn
> that some humane persons have inaugurated a society to 'Save the
> Children'.

Just before the appeal Eglantyne was granted a Papal audience. Dr Munro, the society doctor who had visited Vienna for Eglantyne, again accompanied her at next to no notice, to provide a first-hand account of the famine conditions. Having been brought up in the Protestant Church Eglantyne was nervous about jeopardising the meeting by some slip in etiquette, but in the event her anxiety was forgotten in the drama of the moment. After a series of audiences the Pope had fallen behind schedule and was trying to make up time as Eglantyne's appointed twenty-minute slot approached. 'As we left the ante-chamber where we had been waiting, we paused at the door to allow some nuns to pass,' Eglantyne later recounted her adventure to Dorothy:

> The man who was showing us the way, turned to us with violent gesticulations, shouting out voluble Italian in which I only distinguished the words 'Come' – Then he turned round again, and to my utter amazement, took to his heels and ran. He was wearing a purple flowing garment like a dressing gown, which blew out all around him as he ran, so that he had the odd appearance of a purple ball bounding along the corridor. There was nothing for it but to run, too. Grasping my mantilla to prevent it falling off, I ran after him, through one gorgeous antechamber after another, where groups of soldiers and gentlemen in-waiting turned to look.
>
> At last, through an open door he turned, apparently too breathless to speak, with a wild wave of his arms. Precipitating myself in his wake, I perceived a small lonely figure like a ghost standing stock still in the vast room, and recollecting that Popes always dressed in white, dropped on one knee. To my relief I found that Dr Munro had run, too and – for he was close behind me – making the poorest attempt at a genuflexion that I ever saw.

Munro was equally unimpressed by what he described as Eglantyne's 'attempt to curtsey', but the Pope simply helped her to a chair and immediately started 'pouring out' questions, keeping the pair of them for over two hours. 'He was obviously attracted to Dr Munro', Eglantyne modestly continued to Dorothy:

> [who] mistrusting his French had got something written down for him on an untidy piece of paper, a statement that it was important to provide for the people's physical necessities, but even more to combat the moral deterioration which was one of the appalling results of

war. This he took out and read in halting fashion. The Pope seized the paper and insisted on keeping it. Then they beamed at each other. It was a strange sight. The Pope beamed with a strained, eager look, Dr Munro with stolid benignity.

Munro's account mentions nothing of his untidy piece of paper, but credits the Pope with making a few notes in 'a rather dirty little note book'. Either which way, the interview was a great success: the Pope contributed £25,000 of his own funds to kick-start the appeal and also promised to repeat the Encyclical for Holy Innocents' Day the following year, 1920.[12]

Eglantyne was impressed by the Pope, thinking him, in an interesting distinction, 'a very sincere man; though not what you would call a great man'. Privately she told a friend 'as I looked at that poor lonely old man in that great apartment, I felt I wanted to do something to make him comfortable'. But the Pope also inspired her by his undiscriminating humanity, asserting that any funds raised by the appeal should not only be allocated for the relief of all children irrespective of their faith, but also that aid should be provided by the most effective agency on the same basis. There were to be no conditions, and no Catholic agenda. The Pope's generosity prompted the Archbishop of Canterbury to reconsider and support the Holy Innocents' Day appeal. Soon the Orthodox churches and many other faith groups from the Jewish community to Theosophists followed suit. After his death in 1922 Eglantyne paid tribute to Benedict XV, calling him the 'Children's Pope' and writing that he died 'before the world recognised the magnitude of the debt which it owes him for his championship of the world's children'. By this time his charitable giving had depleted Vatican funds so much that money had to be borrowed to pay for his own funeral expenses.

While she was still in Rome, in December 1919, Eglantyne attended a Catholic Holy Innocents' Day service in the city. The directness of the appeal amused her: 'Now you mustn't leave the

Church till you have given something for the children,' she para-
phrased for Dorothy:

> No soldi, mind. Why, you spend in going to the café and the cine-
> matograph one lira, two lire, three, four – even ten. Today, *No!* Do
> without your amusements. The Germans inflicted cruel suffering on
> the Belgian children. And they have been terribly punished. DO
> you want the same punishment to fall upon you? It will, if you don't
> help the German children. You just give anything you can. And
> then you'll be rewarded. Your own children will be healthy and
> beautiful and strong. It's a law, you can't escape it. So put your hands
> in your pockets.

Hands around the world delved deep. The combined church appeal
raised an unprecedented sum not just within Europe, but from the
United States, China, India and Samoa. Even the Pitcairn Islands
loaded up 'two boxes and five barrels' of supplies and flagged down a
passing ship to carry them to Europe, care of the Fund. In January the
Vatican wrote to congratulate Eglantyne personally on the 'splendid
success' of her work. At another European conference two months
later Dorothy proudly wrote to Tye, 'I wish you could have heard half
the lovely things about Eglantyne which I did when I was in
Switzerland. It is marvellous all the different types and varieties of
people who adore and profoundly respect her. They all seem to feel
that she is a *very great* person (the Pope included I hear), and it is obvious that she has everywhere made quite an extraordinary impression.'

By now the British reception to Save the Children also seemed to
reflect a growing public mood of reconciliation and sympathy for
those who had like themselves lost so much. Arriving in Oxford for
a conference Eglantyne found the whole city placarded and, she
wrote in delight to Tye – perhaps remembering Trafalgar Square –
'some enthusiast has chalked notices … on the pavements!' Ethel
Snowden also noticed the public mood shifting. Following a publicity tour for the Fund she recalled:

Many times I have had the experience of addressing large public meetings containing men and women who have lost their sons in the war and who have not quite recovered from the pain and the sorrow of their loss, who, after a description of child life in a German city, have come forward and offered to help if they could …

On one occasion, when I spoke of the helpless children I had seen in a slum in Vienna, I remember hearing a voice from the back of the hall shout out, 'Serve them right!' The whole audience turned fiercely on the interrupter who shambled out of the room pursued by hisses and cries of 'shame!'

Looking back, Ruth Wordsworth credited Eglantyne, Dorothy and the Fund with doing much to galvanise this change in the public mood from the 'mass weariness, apathy, disillusion, hatred' of 1918 and 1919 to 'the great wave of directed pity' that replaced it. Eglantyne however cited public generosity and enlightened compassion as driving the Fund. 'I suppose the two sisters' contribution was the focusing of humanity's distracted conscience on what to do first,' Ruth concluded, 'by their singling out of the youngest generation and concentrating on that.'

Certainly under Eglantyne's inspirational direction, and with the support of celebrities and the churches, Save the Children quickly caught the public imagination and donations flooded in. The first grant was allocated for Cows for Vienna at the end of May 1919, less than ten days after the Fund was launched. Two weeks later grants were made to the Friends' relief agency and the International Red Cross for their work with the children of Armenia and Germany, and this all before the Fund had held its first Committee meeting or been registered under the War Charities Act. By the start of July 1919, just six weeks after the launch, the first grant was made for Serbia, and the pace of the work showed no signs of slowing. By the end of the first year a staggering £400,000 had been raised through a wide range of fundraising events and appeals (equivalent to over £13 million today), and the total was up to nearly £1 million (£29 million today) by the end of that year.[13] It was an unprecedented achievement that directly enabled many thousands of lives to be saved, and spared those families that had survived the war the further devastating grief of losing a child in the peace.[14] As Eglantyne had hoped it was also a great assertion of the ability of people to empathise with each other against all the odds; a triumph of the humanitarian spirit that had seemed lost beyond recovery during the Balkans conflict and the First World War. 'I venture to think that when the history of these times comes to be written', Ethel Snowden wrote in her political memoirs, 'the work of the Save the Children Fund will be regarded as one of the redeeming features of a situation otherwise black and well-nigh hopeless.'

By the end of 1920 Eglantyne's combination of passion, compassion and daring publicity had achieved far more than she and Dorothy had believed possible when they launched the Save the Children Fund the previous May. For Eglantyne now the sky was the limit; it was just a question of letting everyone else in the world know what could be done. 'The Save the Children fund is often told that its aims are impossible ... There has always been child suffering; there always will be. It is impossible to remedy it,' she wrote:

> Let us clearly understand that it is not impossible. Three things are required to save children from their misery: Money, Knowledge, Good Will.
>
> We have the money – but we spend it on other things. We have the knowledge – only we do not apply it. Can we not cultivate this good will, which will enable us resolutely to utilise our resources in money and knowledge for the saving of the children of the world and with them the future of the race?

Chapter 14

'Supranationalism', 1920–1923

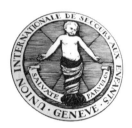

The only international language in the world is a child's cry.

Eglantyne Jebb

E glantyne was never one for boundaries, except in the overstepping of them. Presented with the rulebook on her arrival at college she had sat down on her trunk and considered whether she should leave immediately or 'stay long enough to break all the rules and be sent down'. She cheerfully went on to break plenty of rules, many more social conventions, and even British law when she found it wanting. It was not that she lacked a healthy respect for personal and civic responsibility, quite the contrary, but for Eglantyne human rules, boundaries and codes of behaviour were entirely subordinate to the universal moral laws created by God for all peoples. 'Your cardinal duty to humanity is this,' she wrote in a private note to herself in 1922, 'to realise God's ruling.' In pursuit of this goal, Eglantyne had cheerfully crossed deep-rooted class divides, unstable national borders, and even, she believed, received communications from beyond the ultimate human boundary – the grave. As a result her rather mystical brand of Christianity emphasised not only human equality under God's law,

The Save the Children International Union (UISE) logo, 1920

but the actual spiritual unity of people. Once this 'knowledge of unity' had replaced what she called 'the hallucination of an individual possessing life separate from other lives', it was impossible for her to accept the exclusive self-interest of any person, social group or nation. Co-operation and mutual aid had always appealed to her, and now took on a heightened relevance. Witnessing the power evoked by the suffering of children to rekindle empathy across war-torn Europe, Eglantyne began to see the potential for Save the Children not only to provide famine relief, but to foster reconciliation between nations and promote a new internationalism – 'supranationalism' as she called it – through constructive child welfare.[1] As her niece Eglantyne Buxton later wrote, Eglantyne now saw Save the Children as 'an effective assertion of the oneness of mankind, of the human race being, as it were, one family. [She] wanted the SCF to be a demonstration of that outlook … a common assertion of our common humanity.'

Eglantyne's brand of internationalism was intensely personal, being intimately linked to her faith, but it also responded, and ultimately contributed, to the growth of the new international outlook that began to develop in the 1920s. In Britain this internationalism expressed itself most significantly through the endorsement of the League of Nations by prominent members of the Liberal and Labour Parties, including Ramsay MacDonald, the Labour Prime Minister from 1924, who went on record asserting that 'our true nationality is mankind'. After years of swimming against the tide of public opinion it was hugely encouraging for Eglantyne to begin to hear her own beliefs reiterated in public and political debate. Nonetheless she was aware of the hard political realities of the time; that governments ultimately act from their own national standpoints, and that the movement towards internationalism had a counterpoint in the drive to carve up Europe into smaller nation states. Eglantyne was not opposed to patriotism or nationalism per se; 'national distinctions … can represent an incalculable enrichment to the world, and are to a certain extent the channel through which a nation can make its special contribution to civilisation', she wrote. But in the run up to the war she had developed a deep aversion to what she considered the elevation of the nation state into the 'supreme and ultimate authority' in people's lives. Characteristically she felt that this intense nationalism had become 'almost a religion' for many, albeit one that 'divides the world instead of aiming at uniting it'. The Great War expressed the ultimate consequence of such nationalistic fervour in Eglantyne's eyes, fostering misunderstanding and hatred, and producing only poverty and misery. As a result, despite growing state welfare provision after the war, Eglantyne believed that international responsibilities for children could only be entrusted to voluntary effort, acting both independently from, as well as in conjunction with, governments. Her vision was of a great voluntary movement to be organised and executed along international lines, on the basis of mutual aid between nations as and when the need arose. 'Once … we take the principle of world service as the basis of our policy, it will enable us to build up a civilisation incalculably happier and more secure than that which we see around us today,' she wrote. 'Nobody can indeed be a real patriot at the present day unless his deepest wish for his country is that it should worthily play its part in the wider service of humanity.'

The idea that social responsibility should embrace all humankind was still something new and quite astonishing in 1920 before the League of Nations was well established, and Eglantyne did not have a clear strategy for how to deliver her vision. But things now began to take on a momentum of their own; Eglantyne later wrote that 'the first real prospect of an organised world-effort was opened up by the promise of support from Pope Benedict XV'. The Pope's call for collections to be taken in Catholic churches throughout the world had put Save the Children on the map internationally in a way that neither Eglantyne nor Dorothy had dreamed of when they launched the Fund. Concerned that Catholic churches overseas might not be keen to hand over their collections to a seemingly Protestant organisation sitting in London, Eglantyne proposed an overtly neutral international body, based in the Swiss city of Geneva, to co-ordinate the non-partisan allocation of grants across famine-stricken Europe.[2]

If childhood represented, in Eglantyne's words, a symbolic 'neutral ground ... where all could most easily meet', then Geneva was the geographical equivalent, and the natural home for the new organisation. The International Red Cross had been founded here by Henri Dunant in 1863, followed a year later by the passing of the Geneva Convention to set standards for international humanitarian law inspired by Dunant's work and writing.[3] As the unofficial capital of flourishing internationalism, Geneva was now chosen to host the League of Nations in a new 'Palais de Nations' to be built in a beautiful park overlooking Lake Geneva, then full of busy white steamers, and wooden barges carrying sand and bricks for all the construction work, and with views across to the Alps and, on clear days, Mont Blanc. The Women's International League had also established its head office in the city, at the Maison Internationale, a two-storey house that had previously been the home of another of the city's sons, Lazarus Ludwig Zamenhof, the inventor of Esperanto, which greatly appealed to Eglantyne. She was not only emphasising the neutrality of her umbrella Save the Children organisation when she chose Geneva as its base, but setting it strategically among these well-established and respected bodies as an equal member of the international community. It was a community to which she felt she belonged, 'not so much as a visitor but as a habitant' she wrote to her mother, even as she sat with her back to a radiator in a chilly hotel room early in 1920, 'for I have become so closely connected with international humanitarian work, the interest in which is Geneva's predominant characteristic'.

The Save the Children Fund International Union (Union Internationale de Secours aux Enfants) was formally inaugurated on an overcast day in Geneva on 6 January 1920. It had been a snowy winter and that morning Eglantyne and the new committee members hurried to take shelter out of the raw north-easterly wind in the Salle de l'Athénée, the same hall in which the Red Cross had been founded some fifty years earlier, and where Eglantyne now inspired those present with her own 'burning words'. Romantic as Eglantyne was about historic associations, this choice of venue was not an empty gesture. She saw a strong parallel between the work of the Red Cross, built on a then-new sympathy for the wounded soldier, and that of Save the Children, using the general sympathy towards children, to provide humanitarian aid and to work towards peace. 'War which stops in front of wounded soldiers', she maintained, 'must even more respect the innocent child.' Accordingly she invited Gustave Ador, former President of the Swiss Confederation and President of the International Red Cross, to sit on the new Save the Children International Union board. Ador accepted and the Red Cross accorded its patronage to the new organisation, greatly strengthening its status as the pre-eminent body co-ordinating recip-rocal aid between nations in the field of child welfare.[4]

Eglantyne was now a director of both the British Save the Children Fund and the International Union, and regularly travelling between England and Switzerland. Although she never owned her own home, she kept the keys to Tye and Dorothy's houses in Crowborough and London, and in Geneva she stayed with Suzanne Ferrière, the softly spoken niece of the Swiss Red Cross doctor Frédéric Ferrière, whose reports from Vienna had so affected her and Dorothy the year before. Both Suzanne and her uncle now contributed work for the Save the Children International Union, where Suzanne quickly found her voice to the point of becoming 'quite outspoken on questions of morality'. Even Eglantyne had to exercise considerable tact when challenging Suzanne: it is 'not really a criticism of your leaflet,' she once wrote to her, 'but of the policy it so ably sets forth'. Predictably the two of them were soon firm friends, and the polite formality of their early letters was quickly replaced by an affectionate, even gush-ing, intimacy that was typical of Eglantyne. 'My beloved Suzanne,' she would write, 'I keep looking back with pleasure and joy to the delightful visit I paid you,' and 'How *delightful* to think of seeing my beloved international sister so soon again,' and more tellingly, 'How much I want to see you again. I often feel quite lost without you, especially when Mr Golden and I are taking different points of view and I have uncomfortable feelings that he must be in the right.' Allies in the office, the two women would also occasionally escape from it to eat lunch together and read books in the sunshine beside Lake Geneva, or visit Suzanne's family at their country chalets just beyond the city on Sundays. Suzanne was just what Eglantyne needed: a 'most delightful companion' and vocational soulmate.

Suzanne soon put her small flat in the heart of Geneva's Old Town, at number 14 on the steep Rue Jean Calvin, entirely at Eglantyne's disposal.[5] It was here that Eglantyne came for some quiet during the day, drinking tea on her own in the drawing-room, and where she and Suzanne would sit in the evenings discussing Fund work over Suzanne's thick soups and 'excellent' coffee. Their friend William MacKenzie, artist, journalist, writer of detective stories, and the Pope's representative on the Fund's council, as well as the International Union's Treasurer, had taken the attic flat upstairs, and below them was the meeting hall of a small religious sect whose chants, hymns and psalms could be heard at regular intervals, particularly on Sundays. Suzanne went riding on Sunday mornings, but Eglantyne loved to listen to the 'glorious singing' floating up to their rooms. As a student she had enjoyed tramping around Oxford in the footsteps of 'great men', and now she loved staying on this famous street, surrounded by buildings of religious and historic interest. A small plaque on Suzanne's building informs passers by that Henri Dunant founded the Genevan YMCA there, before moving on to the Red Cross. Higher up the street, number 11 had once been the home of Jean Calvin, the French theologian who put Geneva at the centre of the Protestant Reformation in the first half of the sixteenth century (the commemorative slab was already in the wall in Eglantyne's day). And Pierre Fatio, who in 1707 lent his support to the claims of the people of Geneva for recognition of their rights, in return for which he was tortured and executed, had lived on the other side of them, at number 17. Opposite the lower end of the street is a house where George Eliot once lived. Did Eglantyne enjoy the irony of walking past the former addresses of social novelists at the bottom of the hill, up to those of reformers and human rights advocates at the top, a trajectory that was echoed in her own ambitions? There was certainly plenty here for her to be mulling over as she jangled Suzanne's flat-keys in her pocket.[6]

But Eglantyne was busy. Minutes diligently typed up by Suzanne and bound in fine marble-papered volumes show that Eglantyne managed to attend only two of the first ten committee meetings of the Union in Geneva. The movement was rapidly expanding both in terms of national fundraising offices and programme work in different countries. Independent Save the Children committees had already been formed on the British model across Scandinavia, and now new affiliates were quickly established in Ireland, South Africa, Canada, Australia and New Zealand, all working under the auspices of the Union. Although she never left Europe, Eglantyne was keen to support these organisations, ensuring that learning was shared and that there was a common sense of purpose throughout. 'Members of the movement [must be] prepared to act not as representatives of their own nation', she wrote in an early policy memo, 'but as representatives of mankind.' As a result from 1920 Eglantyne was almost constantly travelling between fundraising offices and field programmes, revelling in the possession of a portable typewriter but losing more than one umbrella as she rushed between the stations of Europe.[7] 'My plan is to go into Macedonia tomorrow', one note to Suzanne ran:

and then return in time to take the Simplon-Orient Express on Sunday evening. This arrives at Milan at 4 o'clock on Sunday and at Lausanne at 11 at night. Miss Young comes with me as far as Paris which we reach at 8.40 on Wednesday in order to see me into the train for Calais. She then returns to Geneva.

When in London Eglantyne stayed at the Fund's offices or with Dorothy, who returned the compliment on her regular trips to Geneva on international work or visiting her two children, Eglantyne and David, now at a Swiss boarding school. Despite their hectic schedules the sisters were intellectually and emotionally closer than ever. However, away from Dorothy and Suzanne, Eglantyne was lonely and when she felt most adrift 'in some foreign hotel' she took to imagining Dorothy walking up from the station, suitcase in hand, to meet her. The punishing schedule, solitude, and often less than comfortable conditions soon took their toll on her; her thyroid trouble was returning and her heart was now also feeling the strain. But Eglantyne seemed almost to enjoy ignoring her own health. 'I once saw her rise from her bed', Henrietta Leslie wrote in her memoirs, 'and packing her rucksack, set off for Bulgaria at an hour's notice, without so much as including a warm coat or a hot-water bottle in her luggage.' It was pure Eglantyne, at once herself inspired and inspiring others by her own almost pointedly disinterested service. She was becoming ever so slightly eccentric.

Eglantyne was now a familiar and instantly recognisable figure rising to her feet to firmly put the case for children on the international conference circuit that was flourishing in the early 1920s. She was just forty-four but, painfully thin with pale, papery skin and rapidly silvering hair, she looked much older. She had recently taken to wearing a heavy silver cross on a dark ribbon from her neck, but otherwise she continued to pay little regard to her appearance, and her brown uniform was, by her own admission, 'dreadfully grubby … and I fear getting ragged as well'. Soon colleagues were affectionately calling her 'the white flame', referring both to the premature white of her hair but more to her saint-like burning passion for her work. 'I am always expected to preach short sermons to these very unsuitable audiences on Christianity and cognate themes,' she laughed to Bun in 1921.

Ironically, Eglantyne had been too ill to attend the International Union's own inaugural conference in Geneva, in March 1920.

Convened to pull together an international relief plan for Europe, the event was nevertheless a great success, and Eglantyne was delighted when her friend Edith Pye reported back that 'the narrow national walls really had fallen at the sound of the trumpet you have blown'.[8] The following year however she sealed her reputation as an inspirational public speaker at the Save the Children International Congress in Sweden. Eglantyne was still uncomfortable appearing on a platform: 'I always dread the atmosphere of a conference,' she wrote to excuse herself from one Paris event, and after the Swedish conference she confessed to Bun, 'I am always too frightened to look back upon such meetings because I know that if I do I shall realise all the blunders I am certain I must have made.' She gave much of the credit for the success of the event to the presence of Prince Carl and Princess Ingeborg of Sweden among the delegates. But although she was delighted to have tea, more than once, at the palace during her visit, to her acute embarrassment she was also cornered by the royal couple in a Stockholm hotel lobby one evening, and forced to make an impromptu speech to their society guests. Having spoken, she believed 'dreadfully badly', she was horrified that people hurried to thank her 'with tears in their eyes'. 'Oh dear, I feel such a charlatan on these occasions', she wrote to Bun, adding she was admired only 'because it is fashionable at the moment to make a fuss over me'.[9]

But Eglantyne clearly did make a profound impression on the many people who heard her speak. The author Anna Lenah Elgström, who had first come to know Eglantyne through the Women's League and met her again at the Swedish Congress in 1921, described her as a born campaigner and great orator, completely absorbed in her work and yet not fanatical. Ruth Wordsworth, invited to a fundraising event in 1922, noticed that 'the speakers all turned towards Eglantyne as if she and the SCF were one'. And after a visit to Geneva Charlie Buxton wrote to his mother that 'there is no doubt that she has raised the conceptions and ideals of all those who have in any way come into contact with her and has in some sense opened a new world to them'. It was quite a turn around for a woman who had always hated public speaking. In 1924 she accepted an invitation to preach from Calvin's famous pulpit in Geneva's St Peter's Cathedral, the roofs of which she could see from Suzanne's flat. 'Which was more astonishing', her great nephew Lionel Jebb later wondered: 'that a protestant and a woman should have been invited to an audience with the Pope which resulted in him asking his church to contribute to her organisation; or that a woman and a confidante of the Roman Pontiff should have been invited to speak from Calvin's pulpit in Geneva?' It was a question that summed up Eglantyne's powerful and pervasive appeal. 'I cannot refrain from sending you a line to tell you of the quite extraordinary effect you have had on all those people from the ends of the earth,' Charlie saluted her on a postcard. 'They speak with bated breath of you. It will be of great use.'

It was. Less than three weeks after the Save the Children International Union was launched it distributed its first grants, totalling £23,000, to Armenia, Germany, Austria, Hungary and Poland, where the famine situation remained desperate throughout 1920. But appalling choices had to be made about the allocation of grants both between different aid agencies, and between different countries. At this point none of the national Save the Children offices had any presence in the famine zones; they were purely soliciting donations within their own countries, with the Union operating as a 'central collecting agency'.[10] The idea was to reduce the expensive competition for public funds, and enable common purchasing for relief supplies and transport. Grants were then allocated to well-established, independent programmes run by agencies like the Red Cross, the Friends' relief society and the Salvation Army, as well as local hospitals, schools and other organisations with which the Fund formed temporary partnerships. However this approach had drawbacks. It soon became clear that if Save the Children discouraged competing appeals their operational partners held them responsible for all their funding needs, something that was not sustainable.

The Fund was receiving constant requests for grants which Eglantyne and the team somehow had to prioritise. Eglantyne was frustrated by well-intentioned but ineffective organisations, and what she called 'benevolent people acting like rogues through sheer muddle-headedness', but at least these were easy to filter out. 'The proposal for the farm colonies is excellent,' she politely but firmly rejected one request for a project endorsed by the Prince of the Netherlands, 'But … it would require a great deal of money … We do not wish to take any responsibility whatsoever for obtaining it, because we should only waste our time in fruitless enterprise.' More difficult was ending existing partnerships when she found the approach or its delivery was failing, such as with international child fostering schemes. At times several city authorities, the Labour Party and the Trade Union movement all supported the evacuation of sick European children to Britain in preference to the export of aid. Through such schemes 'the children of the world might be the means of healing the wounds of war', Eglantyne's ally at the Labour Party, Jim Middleton, wrote optimistically. But Eglantyne withdrew her initial support when she discovered that importing children was neither cost-effective nor 'healing' – especially when the British Secretary of State for Home Affairs specified that no child entering the country could be accompanied by an Austrian or Hungarian adult. When the poorly managed 'Famine Area Hospitality Children's Committee', which brought sick children over to the UK, continued to promote their association with Save the Children, Eglantyne didn't sugar-coat her words. 'I had one of the most painful meetings I ever had in my life', she wrote to Margaret after she 'had to explain' to the agency 'that the only thing for them to do was to give up all their business'.

There was in fact constant rivalry and bickering between different relief agencies. Some, such as the 'Bible Lands Missions Aid Group', did not understand that Save the Children was purely a fundraising body, and objected to Eglantyne quoting from their published articles because, 'from my own personal observations I did not discover one child being supported by your fund'. Others attacked the Fund's claims of impartiality, so that when, in June 1920, the Friends faced criticism for using their charity to promote their religious and political views in cities like Berlin where they had a Quaker Embassy, Eglantyne felt obliged to ensure that future grants were divided between them and other agencies working in the city, even if this was less cost-effective. At least she could enjoy goading Dorothy, who had joined the Quakers not long before, 'if Imperialism is to be avoided, so must Pacifism'.

On top of it all there were often considerable differences of opinion within the International Union, and between them and the national Save the Children organisations, as to which agencies were best placed to administer relief. Eglantyne was a great diplomat in these situations and not above a certain amount of deviousness to get her way while arranging things to appear as if she had not been involved at all. In this way when the British Fund could not agree on a grant to the Quakers, who were seen as pro-Bolshevik, for their Russian programme in 1921, ostensibly because they feared it might prejudice the Fund in the eyes of the British government, Eglantyne quietly suggested to Suzanne that the grant be made by the Union in Geneva. Although she later claimed that 'I am quite unequal to any occasion where a little diplomacy and reserve may be required. Indeed I have invariably made a failure in the past at all such times,' it is clear that Eglantyne was fully qualified in this department. Nonetheless the self-interest of different agencies, including the Save the Children committees, appalled her. 'Everyone wants the Pope's money', she moaned in a letter to Tye as she travelled across Switzerland in November 1920, but '– no one wants very much that anyone else shall have it … Alas for human nature.'

Decisions about prioritising the needs of different countries were even more political than dividing funds between agencies.

Eglantyne's insistence on maintaining absolute neutrality in the distribution of humanitarian aid was well known and respected, and at first the British Save the Children committee attempted to 'reduce to a mathematical calculation by a system of index numbers the proportionate claims of different countries'. Not surprisingly this valiant effort quickly proved to be, in Eglantyne's words, 'so much labour wasted'. But as Eglantyne was increasingly taken away from the British office, concerns grew about the London Committee's political sympathies. Emily Hobhouse, among others, believed that they favoured the relief of Austria above the greater claims of Germany and Russia. 'I can't help thinking that the society has suffered *in spirit* owing to Miss Jebb's continued absences …' she petitioned Dorothy in February 1920. 'I earnestly therefore beg that Miss Jebb take complete control again … of [the] absolute fair allocation of its money – as between nations.'[11]

Eglantyne had first argued the case for Germany in early 1919. The British Fund's Council had agreed in principle, but, according to Henrietta Leslie, 'it also demurred. It was a question of tactics':

'Tactics?' said Eglantyne. 'Right or wrong.'

The Council corrected her. Of benefiting a few children at the expense of the many. She must know that to help German children would be exceedingly unpopular. It might adversely influence the appeal that the Fund had just launched … a German appeal might kill it dead.

'This sort of opposition,' Henrietta commented, 'only stiffened Miss Jebb's resolution.' Of course Eglantyne won the argument and the first grant was given for the children of Germany in June 1919. But German relief always caused the greatest controversy with much of the press critical of the aid operations in practice, if not openly hostile in principle. In a typical article in November 1919 the *Daily Mail* made a damning indictment against the distribution of parcels in Berlin as run by 'four incapable German women', who allowed supplies to be stolen. Less space was given to the need in Germany, which remained acute. In February 1920 the Berlin Children's Aid Society concluded that without immediate relief two and a half million German children were 'doomed to a more or less slow, but certain death' over the next few years, and a further six million were in serious danger. Under Eglantyne's direction, the International Union now allocated grants to children's hospitals and nurseries in key German cities, as well as feeding programmes such as that being run by Emily Hobhouse in Leipzig, the first German town to start feeding schoolchildren. 'For those of your readers who may desire to save a child from the torment of hunger and disease, may I mention that the daily dinner provided under Miss Hobhouse's scheme works out at only 2/- per head per week,' she wrote to the papers, 'and that in this one centre in Leipzig alone 27,000 suffering children are sadly waiting their turn to be fed? Earmarked subscriptions may be sent to the Save the Children Fund.' Both she and Dorothy visited the German programmes over 1920 and 1921, and Dorothy was struck forcibly by 'the hatred felt by people in Germany, who have to look on helplessly at the suffering of their children and the elderly' which, she continued with considerable insight, 'could have disastrous consequences for the future'. Eglantyne was frustrated that the chief representative of the Fund in Germany failed to visit England to put the case personally, making her question whether the German Fund was 'a really competent and active organisation', but for her the issue anyhow was clear. 'We ought not to ask whether they are … enemies or friends' she stormed, adding, 'Personally I find that the people who will not feed German children are generally just as loathe to feed Czecho-Slovak children; and these are the people who in days of shortage will be indifferent to the suffering of the children of the poor in our own country.'

This belief was put to the test in the winter of 1920 when the economic situation in Britain became much worse. Eglantyne had always maintained that the Fund would be happy to assist British children should severe hardship arise, and in early 1921 two national appeals were launched. As the need was still clearly more acute abroad, Eglantyne and Dorothy at first justified the British work by asserting that 'our own children have a closer claim upon us than any others'. It was not a position that sat well with Eglantyne's frequently reiterated belief that aid should be prioritised solely on the basis of greatest need, and suggests that donor interest did hold some influence over funding decisions, as is still the case. She went on to clarify that while Save the Children aimed to give most help where it was most needed, 'it was also its wish to give a little help wherever help was needed, if only as a token of interest and sympathy. For it was clear that to save the children it was not only a Society which was wanted, but a world-wide impulse of pity and compassion …' This might be true, and was certainly Eglantyne's honest opinion, but according to Dorothy's daughter her mother and aunt were in fact 'simply bored' by the English side of the work. For Eglantyne it was even worse; she soon began to see the relative wealth and influence of the British Fund almost as an obstacle to what she was trying to achieve internationally. This could be seen most clearly with the International Union's watershed programme for providing relief in Russia.

Until 1921 Save the Children's stated aim was 'to help children throughout the famine areas' in post-war Europe, and as the European economies gradually recovered there was talk of winding up the Fund. However that summer the devastating famine in Russia became the overriding international emergency, and as a result the Fund's object was changed to 'an international effort to preserve child life wherever it is menaced by conditions of economic hardship and distress'.

Charlie Buxton had visited Russia in his official role of Secretary to the British Labour Delegation in 1920, like many intellectuals enjoying the immense thrill of seeing what was at that time the only socialist country in the world. Once his official business was done he slipped away to stay with a peasant family for a week on a private fact-finding mission, happily debating religion and politics, and on occasion, as there was no soap, washing as the family did in fresh milk. One year later the village where he had stayed was in the centre of a famine zone with no milk, oil, grain or much else. After seven years of revolution, international and civil war, with the loss of twenty-five million lives and the creation of thousands of refugees, Russia had been hit by harvest failure, greatly exacerbated if not directly caused by the new regime's domestic policy. Between fifteen and twenty million people were facing starvation.[12] As flour ran out, people began using acorns, grass and other substitutes to make bread. Livestock was slaughtered or starved. Rural populations fled in their thousands creating a refugee crisis within Russia and across Europe. Eglantyne would soon be writing up eye-witness accounts from the Volga basin of 'heaps of corpses', and survivors trying to live on grass, vermin and refuse, and even turning to cannibalism. The situation was repeated across Russia, in the Ukraine, the trans-Caucasus and Armenia. On 16 July the novelist Maxim Gorky, who sat on the All Russian Famine Relief Committee founded by Lenin, appealed internationally for aid. In response the International Red Cross in Geneva called a meeting of aid agencies including Save the Children, the Society of Friends and Hoover's American Relief Administration (ARA), and established an International Committee for Russian Relief. 'Nobody brought up the point that the measures for relief might simply salve the conscience of those concerned and prevent the necessity of promoting economic measures on a large scale,' Eglantyne wrote to Suzanne, anticipating what would become one of the major contentions around the appeal.

From the start the Russian relief operation could not but be political. Hoover believed that if they were to have any success negotiating access to the famine areas with Lenin then the ARA, which had already unsuccessfully promoted a 'food for peace' plan in Russia, could not be directly involved. They needed a front man from a neutral country, and chose the famous Norwegian Arctic explorer Fridtjof Nansen, who was well respected internationally for having co-ordinated the League of Nations' repatriation programme with Russia for prisoners of war. Nansen agreed both to negotiate the delivery of aid with the Soviet authorities and to head the international fundraising appeal. Eglantyne greatly admired this 'solid Viking', as she called him, pursuing his work regardless of public and press criticism. 'He is absolutely disinterested,' she wrote to Bun, 'working at his own expense, though he is not a rich man, and regretting, I fear, all the time that he is not attending meetings of geographical societies.' She was quite right. Nansen had turned down the League of Nations when they requested he go to Moscow to discuss the refugee situation the previous June because, he apologised, 'it requires a man who would be able to give this great work with his whole soul and give his whole time to it … I am now buried in work here, have three big scientific projects that have been waiting and waiting, and must now be finished, and this is after all my real work.' But just two months later, as Ernest Shackleton set sail on his last expedition to Antarctica, Nansen's 'real work' was again put on hold when he accepted the role of High Commissioner for Refugees.

Nansen's official review of the refugee crisis in various countries showed why he could not in good conscience turn the work down. It also stressed that:

> of all the heartrending problems … that of the children is by far the most distressing … many of them have never known a home in the full sense of the word … they are scattered all over the face of Europe in strange lands, among foreign tongues; they see other children properly fed, clothed and educated when they are starving, ragged, uncared for.

Save the Children first worked with Nansen and several other organisations to feed and educate thousands of Russian refugee children in Turkey and elsewhere. This was fairly uncontroversial and unproblematic work that the Fund was well placed to undertake, earning them the praise of the League of Nations. At the end of August however the International Union agreed to act as agent for the transport and distribution of relief supplies provided by nineteen co-operating nations to one of the worst-hit provinces inside Russia: Saratov on the River Volga. The British Fund was to lead the operation under the direction of their Russian-born General Secretary, Lewis Golden. Adding a new complication to the work, Russia now had no domestic infrastructure for the provision of relief and was virtually a closed country offering no access for independent aid agencies. Previously exclusively a grant-making organisation, Save the Children was now forced to become fully operational, working with Nansen to persuade the Soviet authorities to let them set up their own relief programmes inside the country. This was a significant departure for the Fund, for the first time giving them a presence on the ground.

Nansen negotiated strict terms for the provision of aid with the Soviet authorities in Moscow, hoping to reassure Western donors, who regarded the Communist government with profound distrust, both that relief supplies would reach their intended recipients, and that humanitarian relief would be kept distinct from political endorsement. The terms agreed were quite humiliating for the Soviets, including providing an armed guard and free transport for aid supplies in sealed wagons that could be checked at any time by Nansen's team. Nonetheless back in Geneva Eglantyne still had to counter rumours that Nansen had made an agreement with the Soviet government to supply food for the Red Army. And in Britain too the Fund once again had to win over a hostile press and unsympathetic public who quite reasonably blamed Bolshevik economic mismanagement for the famine, and feared that relief would play into the hands of the government.[13] 'Feelings run very high ...' Eglantyne wrote to Suzanne, 'on our committee I think the majority are anti-Bolshevik':

It cannot be denied that relief given in Soviet Russia tends to the support of the Soviet Government. But in some degree it is true that we support *any* Government anywhere under which we are working, when the government itself takes an interest in child relief. The indirect result of relief is to make people more contented and to stabilise the existing order … But is this sufficient reason for excluding the children from their fair share of our charity? I feel sure it is not.

Even when that principle was accepted, the heated discussions about where to prioritise relief continued, some committee members and supporters objecting to feeding communists in Russia, others protesting that less needy Russian émigré children were being given milk in Europe. At one conference an exasperated Eglantyne reported to Tye that 'there was a great danger that the people who want to do relief in Russia, and the people who only want relief to be given to Russian refugees, would fly at each other's throats, and that I and my colleagues would perish under the attacks from both sides'. Meanwhile the slowing British economy prompted the press to question the prudence of donating funds for Russian children at all when there was growing need at home. It was clear that for a Russian appeal to be successful in Britain the public once again needed to be persuaded that there was a genuine and desperate case for aid. Full-page press advertisements, emphasising that it cost just a shilling (five pence) to feed a child for a week, were losing their impact. Some papers were sympathetic, but several criticised Save the Children and challenged the accuracy of famine reports. 'The magnitude of the famine has been greatly exaggerated', the *Daily Express* reported in November 1921, and when Randall Davidson defended the relief programme the paper responded with surprise that 'the Archbishop of Canterbury sees fit to accept the word of Dr Nansen, who is a foreigner, against that of a British journalist'. The dispute rumbled on with the paper questioning Save the Children's motives, finances and efficiency, while running headlines emphasising domestic need, such as 'Folly of Feeding Russia', 'Huge Sums for a Dubious Famine: What of England?' and 'Moment Ill-Chosen to Appeal for Funds: Needs at Home'. As tensions grew Save the Children flag-sellers were threatened with a dip in the Thames, and groups of unemployed men demonstrated in the street outside the Fund's office.

Eglantyne's brilliant response was to send a well-known press photographer, George Mewes from the *Daily Mirror*, to film first the famine conditions, and later the Fund's feeding centres in operation. 'Often I saw children who had gone far beyond the stage where English food and medicine would help,' Mewes reported, 'children in such a condition, that had they been animals, one would have destroyed them where they lay.' His films, shown privately as well as in cinemas up and down the country, were unlike anything seen before or much since, including heart-rending images of starving and dead children huddled together, and bodies being buried, as well as soup and milk kitchens in operation and children recovering their strength and health. It was the first time that film had been used in this way, and the shocked public responded generously; collections at film showings alone raising over £6,000. More importantly, the films provided evidence not just of desperate need, but of the real possibility of saving lives. 'No advertisements, articles, verbal or printed appeals', the *Daily News* reported in 1922, 'could have produced such an overwhelming impression upon the audience as did the staggering realism of these pictures.'[14]

That year Nansen was awarded the Nobel Peace Prize in recognition for his his work as a League of Nations High Commissioner, and the following February he visited Britain to give a lecture on the famine at the Albert Hall and to speak at a number of private dinners and fundraising events organised by Eglantyne. 'His name worked magic,' she wrote to a friend after several successful evenings. Nansen's appeals were remarkably similar in approach to Eglantyne's. 'Never in the world's history has help been more desperately needed,' he reportedly pleaded. 'Only one thing is required, and that is for one part of the human race to help another suffering part.' Although opposites in many ways, both he and Eglantyne were loners, almost reluctantly driven to social work by their deep moral conscience, and they saw eye-to-eye on a range of issues from the absolute importance of international co-operation and non-discrimination to the value of every penny that could be spent on relief. Having worked out that just £1 could save a Russian from starvation, Nansen's wife Sigrun bitterly recorded that he would travel 'second class … thus saving £5 = five human lives!' It was very like Eglantyne, and she quickly became quite a fan of the great man, even agreeing to support his appeals to South American States 'in my personal capacity' over and above her existing Fund commitments.[15]

The combined effort brought results. Amid a blaze of publicity, on 7 September 1921 the SS *Torcello* chartered by Save the Children set off for Russia with a cargo of six hundred tons of aid. Lord Weardale came down to the Millwall docks to see the ship off under a large banner reading 'Food for Russian children'. The *Torcello* reached Riga, in Latvia, by the end of September, and the food was quickly unloaded. At once rumours circulated in London that ships in the port had been looted, but Save the Children's supplies in this and future consignments were dispatched safely for Saratov. It was now a race against time before the Volga and the port at Riga froze over for the winter, making transport virtually impossible, but less than two months after Russia's request for aid the first feeding centre was opened. The so-called children's 'menus' are still filed in Save the Children's archive; essentially three variations of rice, beans, milk, flour, sugar, salt, fat and bread, each in carefully controlled measures. In all over 157 million rations were issued, occasionally cheered up by over a thousand tons of herrings and nearly three hundred tons of cocoa. In total the supplies would have filled a train eleven miles long. Over the winter of 1921 and most of 1922 these daily meals kept over 300,000 children alive, as well as 375,000 adults fed on behalf of the Russian Famine Relief Fund and Nansen's organisation.[16]

Save the Children closed its Russian feeding programme in the summer of 1923. The work had been difficult and sometimes dangerous: one staff member had died of typhus, another committed suicide. But, unlike the American Relief Association, several of whose staff were arrested and accused of being spies, the Fund had maintained good relations with the Soviet authorities, and as a result gained an international reputation for providing effective emergency relief in the most challenging diplomatic and geographical circumstances.[17] Above all Eglantyne was inspired by the unprecedented level of international co-operation achieved, with nineteen nations and many different relief agencies eventually supporting the Saratov feeding programme. It was an example that would inform all of the Fund's future work. 'We set out to save the lives of children', Eglantyne wrote of the Russian relief effort, 'but if we remain true to this ideal [of international co-operation] … we may make a worthy contribution to the task of saving the soul of the world.'

By the time the worst of the Russian famine was over, it was clear that there was an ongoing need for Save the Children. Many of the Fund's programme managers transferred directly from Russia to Greece to set up emergency feeding centres for the million refugees expelled from Asia Minor at the close of the Greco-Turkish war, others began co-ordinating aid both for Armenian orphans and the children of the Turks. That same year the Fund for the first time also supplied aid outside Europe and the Near East, providing grants to Egypt and Chile, and emergency relief to Japan following earthquakes that had left over 200,000 dead.

But Eglantyne was no longer satisfied with responding to emergencies. She had always found the limitations of relief work frustrating. In July 1920, when after a year of aid Vienna was still dependent on continued relief, she had written to Maynard Keynes that despite raising and spending over a million pounds, she deeply regretted that the Union 'has had so little result'. 'We cannot possibly go on maintaining children by charity for ever and ever,' she continued: 'our funds are certain to become exhausted, and it will be heartbreaking indeed if it comes about that we have only saved them from starvation one year in order to leave them to starve the next.' It was unusual for Eglantyne to venture into politics, and it shows how at a loss she felt that she now rather patronisingly suggested Maynard pull together a programme for economic reconstruction to be carried out by the governments of Europe.[18] Whether he found the time to politely thank his sister's dear friend for her suggestion is not recorded, but in any case Eglantyne soon wisely turned her attention back to what could be achieved through the International Union. 'The great point to realise is that relief alone cannot save the children,' she wrote. 'If we really want to save them we must add to our work of relief other activities.'

Eglantyne had always insisted that wherever possible aid should be delivered in partnership with local child welfare organisations, strengthening existing provision to avoid creating dependency; policy that is still respected today. Now she went a step further, promoting a range of constructive child welfare programmes looking at education and housing as well as health and nutrition. Soon Save the Children was supporting projects ranging from anti-tuberculosis campaigns to model orphanages and training in trades for girls – including most famously that run in Budapest by Eglantyne's good friend Julie Eve Vajkai. In 1925 Eglantyne returned to the Balkans to witness a regional 'population exchange'. It was clear that running a feeding programme would not provide a long-term solution to the refugee situation, so the Fund bought some marsh land with part funding from the Bulgarian government, drained it, and worked with some landless families to build houses and farms on the site. The result was a model co-operative farming village which was called Atlovo, in honour of the Duke of Atholl, then President of the Fund. Eglantyne returned to Atlovo the following year accompanied by King Boris of Bulgaria, on the way back relishing the adventure of dodging express trains on the railway line after the breakdown of their car in the snow forced them to travel some way by trolley. She was in her element. 'Relief work', she wrote:

> does not consist entirely – whatever one is sometimes tempted to think – in wearisome meetings, wearisome appeals, wearisome statistics, and a yet more wearisome struggle against uninteresting misery. It has its moments of enchantment, its adventures, its unexpected vistas into new worlds.

The Union was soon acting as a centre for international research and a forum for developing and sharing best-practice, like the Atlovo refugee settlement, that pioneered innovative and sustainable solutions to child poverty and distress through constructive development. Eglantyne opened a research library for anyone interested in child welfare at the office in Geneva, and the Fund regularly published its work in its journal, *The World's Children*, as well as producing the first world survey of child welfare.[19] They also ran a series of international conferences from 1925, at the first of which Eglantyne seemingly anticipated citizenship classes, albeit with an international flavour, when she spoke on 'the education of children in international goodwill'. The following year, having rejected the idea of establishing an International Institute of Social Service in Geneva after consultation with William Beveridge, Eglantyne fostered links with existing research institutes and welfare organisations, and in 1925 she was appointed an advisor to the League of Nations Committee for Protection of Children.

Eglantyne now turned her attention to the welfare of children in Persia, India and Africa, giving the Fund a truly global remit. Her idea was to establish a world-wide system of mutual aid, rather than a one-way flow of charity, based on the principle that all countries were expected to give, for domestic as well as international programmes, but that all also had a right to receive in times of need. This reciprocity was neatly demonstrated when the city of Vienna, remembering their debt from 1919, sent £1,000 for milk for the children of Welsh miners during the general strike in 1926. Eglantyne was delighted, but her ambition was for more than a tit-for-tat exchange of aid between nations, however generous. The 'supranationalism' she envisaged was a global sense of community whereby all nations recognised that their best interests were aligned. 'Our economic interests are so intertwined', she argued, 'that the prosperity of one nation makes for the prosperity of all, while the poverty of one impoverishes the others.' But for Eglantyne the giving of aid also worked at a higher level. 'It is a fact', she wrote, 'that a country loses nothing by financial contribution to international social work. The ledger account between any two countries balances perfectly. Receipts and expenditure tally. There are no debits and no credits. On the one hand there is a technical, on the other a spiritual gain.'

Eglantyne's faith had remained her constant support and inspiration. 'As time goes on the essentially *spiritual* character of the work for the children impresses me more and more,' she had written to one of the British Fund's council members, Lady Sara Blomfield, in October 1920. Lady Blomfield was a prominent member of the British Baha'i movement, which emphasises the spiritual unity of all humankind, a belief that chimed closely with Eglantyne. 'It would be an incalculable help to us', Eglantyne continued, 'if we had friends all over the world who … prayed with a true understanding of the great issues involved.' At the back of her mind Eglantyne might have wondered whether a request for prayers might translate into vital donations from members of this growing international movement, but if so it was not her primary concern. She was absolutely committed to the power of prayer. 'Words quite fail me …' she wrote on receipt of messages of support from 'Abdu'l Bahá, the head of the Baha'i movement. 'How grateful I am for the encouragement – and oh! much more than encouragement – real direct help, the incalculable spiritual help we so much need.' However although Eglantyne was completely in tune with the basic Baha'i principle of the 'oneness of humankind', she never joined the movement. Her own faith was enough to sustain and, she believed, guide her. 'In these tragic days, so full of darkness and terror', she wrote, '– what happiness and peace can nevertheless be ours if we can realise Christ in our midst. He, here with us now … giving us directions day by day as to the ways in which we are to undertake practical service for His Kingdom.'

Eglantyne had had grand ambitions when she launched the Save the Children International Union in 1920. 'It is essential that we put the world in order, and put it in order without delay,' she had written. 'To this end we must develop a powerful international organisation for child saving which would extend its ramifications to the remotest corner of the globe.' Within a remarkably short time she turned a national famine relief fund into a successful international society devoted to the welfare of the world's children. At times, she confessed to Margaret, she felt overwhelmed by the great momentum that the organisation had achieved. It has 'grown much too large for me', she worried, 'the only thing to be done is to let the movement go on by itself, and try and not hinder it by dropping out of it ourselves if we possibly can'. Within five years of its launch there were forty national committees affiliated to the International Union, £4 million had been raised internationally, help had been given to children in thirty different countries, and systems were in place to ensure that child welfare could in future be undertaken collaboratively by different agencies and the state sector, working both within and across national borders. Today the International Save the Children Alliance is the world's largest independent organisation for children, with twenty-seven member societies collectively working to improve the lives and life chances of children in over 110 countries around the world, including within each member country. All of this work is still informed by Eglantyne's commitment to long-term, sustainable, constructive work delivered in partnership both with specialist agencies and local communities. Eglantyne would have been delighted, though not perhaps surprised by this lasting legacy. However while she always regarded setting up the

International Union as both much more difficult and much more significant than establishing the Fund in Britain, her ambitions went even further.

Eglantyne had identified what she called 'a new feeling of international responsibility', and in 1928 she sketched out her hopes for developing this in an article in *The World's Children* she called 'The Dawn of a New Era'. With typical drama, and enthusiastically mixed metaphor, she wrote of the great sense of liberation that 'the people who have been accustomed to have their outlook limited by a high wall' will find when 'the fetters of narrow provincialism suddenly drop from their wrists'. Perhaps this described her own moment of inspiration when she realised the potential for Save the Children to act as a transnational organisation, not only representing the interests of different nations, but the common concerns of humanity. She now hoped that the International Union would make a contribution towards an eventual world community where mutual help between nations would be seen as a normal social obligation. But Eglantyne had one more idea to release on the world before she considered her own contribution done, and, she wrote confidently from her new internationalist perspective, 'it should be plain to us that we cannot close our frontiers against ideas'.

Chapter 15

The Rights of the Child, 1922–1925

I believe we should claim certain rights for the children and labour for their universal recognition.

Eglantyne Jebb, 1924

When, as a new mum, I stuck a bright yellow 'baby-on-board' sign in my car rear-window I quickly became the butt of friends' jokes. 'Be careful!' they sniggered. 'There is a child in this car, so you definitely don't want to hit it. Go hit the car of someone without a baby on board, like that old lady's over there – because, you know, old people are comparatively devoid of any social value!' It turns out that baby-on-board signs were first designed to alert the emergency services to check for a baby on the floor of a car in the event of an accident, before the legal requirement for child car-seats made this unnecessary. Now technically redundant, they can be pressed into another service, as a metaphor for the encoding of children's human rights. Why do children need specific rights over and above existing human rights legislation that serves well enough for the driver behind and the old lady over there? Eglantyne's immediate answer would have been that children are particularly vulnerable, both physically and psychologically, to abuse and neglect. Rights provide grounds for respect, protection and redress. Without a specific statement of their rights children might continue to fall off the adult agenda.[1] Only when car-seats have been designed with children in mind do the signs to remind adults to check for children on the floor become unnecessary.

Legend has it that one cloudless summer Sunday in 1922, Eglantyne climbed to the summit of Mont Salève, the great rocky plateau on the edge of Geneva. From the top she had a fine view of the city sprawling out from around the curve of the lake, and, on the far bank, the League of Nations' offices. Here she settled down on the crisp turf, her hair flying in the breeze and, in the silence and calm above it all, she took out pencil and paper and drafted a five-point 'Charter for Children'. It was the first major statement of children's universal human rights, and the forerunner of all subsequent international children's rights treaties including one of the world's most influential pieces of international legislation: the United Nations Convention on the Rights of the Child.

Romantic though it sounds, there is almost certainly some truth in this story. Eglantyne had always loved climbing in the Tyrol and the Dolomites, and one of her special reasons for liking Geneva was that the mountains surrounding the city were visible from so many of the streets. 'Such a heavenly vision of Mont Blanc up in the skies,' she would typically interrupt her letters. Occasionally when Dorothy visited, the two of them would escape to the mountains together; Henrietta Leslie reported the sisters discussing current affairs on the Salève in 1920. More often though Eglantyne climbed alone to find some solitude in which do her thinking. Her friend William MacKenzie, the Save the Children International Union's Treasurer, remembered that when in Geneva she would frequently ignore doctors' orders to rest, instead fleeing for the mountains 'almost surreptitiously, and with all the suppressed excitement of an elopement', having quite reasonably excused herself, ' "But I am always so much better there." ' 'The spirit free,' MacKenzie commented, 'how should the body not fare well?'

Nearly ninety years later, on a cold November morning, I took a break from the Geneva archives to go up Mont Salève myself, albeit travelling most of the way in the cable-car that was strung up the cliff face in 1932, four years after Eglantyne died. Mont Salève has no foothills, just the towering presence of almost vertical rock for over a thousand meters. Eglantyne's Tyrol training must have served her well, and presumably she would take some bread and cheese, a thermos of Suzanne's fine coffee and a few squares of chocolate to sustain her; all the same not bad going for a woman with recurring thyroid problems and a developing heart condition. Over six months pregnant on my visit, it felt achievement enough to clamber the last few hundred meters from the cable-car station though scrubby beech woods to the windswept summit, where it drifted snow on me and across the huge view down to Geneva. 'The first great thing is to find yourself, and for that you need solitude and contemplation: at least sometimes,' Eglantyne's 'solid Viking', Fridtjof Nansen, wrote. 'I tell you, deliverance will not come from the rushing, noisy centres of civilisation. It will come from the lonely places.' It is easy to understand why Eglantyne might have found this lonely mountain summit inspiring; perhaps less easy to see why instead of sticking with constructive welfare solutions she made the leap to asserting that children had certain unique rights that ought to be stated and defended.

Rights themselves may be considered in abstract terms, as universal and exempted from history, having been endowed somehow metaphysically by God or nature. But statements of rights at least are constructed within specific cultural and historical contexts. Eglantyne's declaration of children's rights has now been slotted into its appropriate place in the history of human and civil rights: 125 years after Thomas Paine asserted the Rights of Man, but jostling along with international campaigns for women's rights and suffrage. Retrospectively Eglantyne recognised the power of this heritage, and firmly aligned her statement of children's rights with the historic rights movement by comparing it to the 'inalienable rights of man proclaimed by the National Assembly of France in the famous Declaration of the Rights of Man'. Also with hindsight, early Save the Children staff would refer to Eglantyne's work as her 'suffragette movement for children'. However neither the historical development of human rights nor contemporary civil rights campaigns had greatly inspired Eglantyne. Universal male suffrage had left her pretty cold in 1900: '"one man one vote" is a horrible idea' she had commented, although she later relaxed her attitude. If she was aware of the child rights activism that was going on in British schools between 1889 and 1911 while she was toying with teaching, she passed no comment on it. Even the campaigns for women's franchise, which she agreed with in principle and her uncle Richard promoted in parliament, had failed to draw much active support from her.[2] This lukewarm interest in rights, taken in conjunction with her lack of particular affection for children, seems to make Eglantyne an unlikely champion of children's rights. But her ideas were firmly of their time – indeed she was usually just one step ahead of the zeitgeist, which is partly what made her so effective – and her conceptualisation of children's rights was heavily informed by both the Victorian development of protective child welfare and later New Liberal ideas surrounding citizenship and social responsibility.

In the nineteenth century social reformers began advocating protection for children in the workplace, along with educational reform and the development of a distinct juvenile justice system. Arguably the resulting policies, which aimed to turn working-class children into model future citizens, were as much about controlling the development of society as they were about children's immediate welfare. Eglantyne later had no problem with this sub-agenda: 'there is a wonderful Catholic association which takes the boys and turns them into excellent citizens', she enthused to Tye in one 1924 letter. However, interventionist legislation also contributed to the idea that children inhabited a distinct social space, and so required specific legal protections to safeguard their right to develop through play, rest and schooling – although there was as yet no idea of specifying children's rights as a general principle.

By the turn of the century children were receiving more concerted attention. In 1900 the educationalist Ellen Key proposed that the new century be devoted to the welfare of children. Eight years later the Liberal Party passed the first British 'Children Act', informally known as the 'Children's Charter', which established juvenile courts, introduced the registration of foster parents, prevented children from working in dangerous trades, and raised the minimum age for execution to sixteen. Local authorities were also granted powers to keep poor children out of the workhouse and protect them from abuse, which eventually led to many councils setting up social services and orphanages. As a Cambridge social worker Eglantyne had been greatly inspired both by such welfare policies, and the developing New Liberal ideas around participative citizenship. She had already begun to extend the idea of citizenship to children when, with the first rumblings of the Great War, a new international focus overtook her domestic agenda.[3] The war and its aftermath not only raised public awareness of the universal vulnerability of children in the face of disaster, but also invested children with a new symbolic potential, not just as the next generation of citizens, but as ambassadors for future peaceful international relations.[4] It was between 1919 and 1922 that the first international child protection treaties were developed, by the International Labour Organisation, an offspring of the League of Nations that Eglantyne greatly admired.[5]

This was the climate in which Eglantyne framed her own charter for children on the heights of Mont Salève. 'The moment appears to have come when we can no longer expect to conduct large relief actions,' she wrote to Suzanne. 'If we wish nevertheless to go on working for the children … the only way to do it seems to be to evoke a co-operative effort of the nations to safeguard their own children on constructive rather than on charitable lines. I believe that we should claim certain rights for the children and labour for their universal recognition.' It was March 1922 when Eglantyne first proposed that Save the Children adopt a document 'defining the duties of adults towards children, which each country should recognise either by means of State intervention or by private action'. A few months later she circulated a draft of her 'Children's Charter' to the British Save the Children for comments, and that autumn she started work on three separate papers: a declaration of rights, a legislative code to be embodied in a future Convention of Geneva, and an outline of work to be done by both the State and private organisations. The actual declaration of rights was to be 'general and fundamental and such as to command universal assent', Eglantyne wrote. 'They are in the nature of principles. They should be sound, indisputable and universally valid.'

But Eglantyne's was not the only children's charter under discussion in 1922. The International Council for Women was developing a detailed document with seven categories marshalling fifty-one clauses into order, 'based on the principle that every child is born with the inalienable right to have the opportunity of full physical, mental and spiritual development ...' Lady Aberdeen, the President of the International Council for Women, was also a member of the British Save the Children Fund, and it was soon suggested that this charter should inform, or even replace, the briefer Save the Children document of which Lady Aberdeen disapproved. By January 1923 Eglantyne's proposed 'Children's Charter: A Declaration of the Rights of Childhood' had been fundamentally compromised. The 'Declaration of Rights' subtitle had been dropped, the fifteen clauses extended to twenty-eight and tangled up in welfare details, and the opening phrase of each clause: 'It is the right of every child ...' had been changed to 'Every child should ...' as in 'should be brought up, as much as possible, in the open air and sunshine'. In effect it was no longer a bold statement of children's rights, but a rather woolly list of the responsibilities of governments towards children; a not-so-subtle shift that made the child the recipient of state protection rather than the bearer of rights and responsibilities appropriate to his or her age.

Eglantyne was hugely critical of the Women's Council charter for 'summing up the duties of the state towards children', while at the same time being 'to my mind too socialistic'. 'At present however', she now furiously told Suzanne in a series of letters written in both pen and pencil, whichever came to hand first, 'I prefer Lady Aberdeen's charter to ours, for the SCF council has cut out all its more important provisions, retaining the questions of detail which are puerile without the others.' 'The Charter I drafted originally has been entirely spoilt,' she was still going two days later, 'the result is ludicrous.'

Somewhat tactlessly, and naively, in January 1923 the British Save the Children council proposed that Eglantyne take the revised Children's Charter to the February meeting of the Save the Children International Union in Geneva for approval. Eglantyne had other ideas: 'I am hoping the Union will turn it down!!' she confessed to Suzanne. With the support of Étienne Clouzot, the Union's General Secretary who had been her close ally since the days in 1920 when they were both involved in setting up the international organisation, she quickly revised her own brief statement, translated it into what she called her 'execrable French', and pressed for it to be adopted. Months of painful consultation and revisions followed, with more than one vote for a clause to cover the child before birth which was ultimately rejected on the grounds that it would reduce the unity and simplicity of the document. Finally the 'Declaration of the Rights of the Child' was adopted by the International Union on 17 May 1923. Eglantyne had always valued Clouzot's tact and clear thinking and now she also praised his ability to 'mould a great world policy on broad and general lines'. While not quite as strident as Eglantyne had first intended, the final draft was at least clearly descended from her uncluttered statement of principle:

THE DECLARATION OF THE RIGHTS OF THE CHILD (1923)

By the present Declaration of the Rights of the Child, commonly known as the 'Declaration of Geneva', men and women of all nations, recognising that Mankind owes to the Child the best it has to give, declare and accept it as their duty that, beyond and above all considerations of race, nationality, or creed:

I. THE CHILD must be given the means requisite for its normal development, both materially and spiritually.

II. THE CHILD that is hungry must be fed; the child that is sick must be nursed; the child that is backward must be helped; the delinquent child must be reclaimed; and the orphan and waif must be sheltered and succoured.

III. THE CHILD must be the first to receive relief in times of distress.

IV. THE CHILD must be in a position to earn a livelihood and must be protected against every form of exploitation.

V. THE CHILD must be brought up in the consciousness that its talents must be devoted to the service of its fellow-men.

Four of these five points focus on the child's rights to protection and provision, based on Save the Children's experience in international relief and development. Eglantyne had no concept that children's rights might later be discussed in terms of empowerment or the right to degrees of self-determination, but protection has remained the enduring basis of children's legal rights. However she was very aware of the problems involved in trying to reconcile individual and cultural differences in a statement of the universal. 'Everything should be done to avoid imposing a uniform type of culture …' she wrote with impressive vision; 'the methods of child nurture must necessarily vary greatly according to differences of climate, race, traditions, beliefs, etc. But nevertheless there are certain fundamental principles which should be respected, however much the means of their practical application may differ in different localities.'

Eglantyne's last, rather innovative interpretation of what a right entails, that the child 'be brought up in the consciousness that its talents must be devoted to the service of its fellowmen', was clearly the product of her own climate, reflecting the importance she attached to New Liberal ideas around citizenship, and the twinning of rights with responsibilities. Eglantyne's focus here was not with the immediate needs and rights of children as children, but with the child as future citizen; the symbolic child that represented the next generation. 'The future of the world is with the child,' she scribbled on the top of an early draft.

Despite the fierce anti-German sentiment, the post-war period was also a time of great public idealism. There was an overwhelming feeling that lasting peace *must* be secured, and that the opportunity to make the world a better place in which international relations should be based on new ideals of justice and conciliation should be seized. For many this translated into support for the League of Nations with its declared object of ending war, as proposed in the famous 'Fourteen Points' brought to the Paris Peace Talks by the American President, Woodrow Wilson.[6] In April 1919 the Allies adopted a watered-down version of the plan, and the League office was founded in Geneva on 10 January 1920, four days after the Save the Children International Union was inaugurated in the same city. Charlie Buxton would become Britain's Chief Delegate to the League in 1924, but although he and Dorothy initially had high hopes for what they believed promised to be 'a genuine form of supernational Government, representing the interests of all states, and capable of being called into account by the humblest of them', they, like many, would become bitterly disappointed with the reality of the League. Nonetheless it remained the main channel for developing a new basis for international relations in 1920.

At the First Assembly of the League, Gustave Ador of the Swiss delegation, the International Red Cross and the Save the Children International Union brought a resolution in support of agencies working 'on behalf of children affected by war', and proposing a High Commissioner for Children be appointed to co-ordinate the relief work already being undertaken. Although the General Assembly got excited about the role, optimistically recording that 'these millions of children rescued from death and deprivation will remember, when they become men, the debt they have contracted towards the League of Nations when it [was] just beginning', in fact the idea of a Children's Commissioner soon fell off the agenda.[7] It was not until June 1921 when a joint letter from the Red Cross and Save the Children asking the Council of the League for a section dedicated to the protection of children led to the formation of an independent bureau, reflecting the growing sympathy towards the child as an instrument of peace. 'Henceforth the children of the world will be under the protection of the League of Nations,' the English press reported. After several different incarnations this bureau became the League of Nations Child Welfare Committee in 1924. Eglantyne was appointed an assessor.[8]

Eglantyne had never been a fan of 'dull committee meetings', and it took her a couple of sessions to find her feet. One of her first contributions was to propose that 'the League of Nations should recognise the question of the protection of children as one of its fundamental duties …' on the rather Victorian premise that 'every child whose normal physical, intellectual or moral development is hindered is a potential source of disorder and a danger to the community'. After a silence so tangible it can almost be heard in the minutes, the next point raised proposed that 'the Committee should confine itself to resolutions dealing with definite points to be discussed'. Even so, being composed of an eclectic collection of 'experts' commenting on a shared agenda, it inevitably took the Committee a while to become effective: 'this is a not a subject in which I personally take much interest', the Girl Guides Association representative reported on the subject of Family Allowances. Eglantyne could be even blunter, submitting notes like 'I … regret that we can give you no useful information,' and the files are full of handwritten PS's asking, 'Do we really have to respond??'

Before long however Eglantyne was making valuable and some-times quite uncomfortable contributions, such as pointing out that of the twenty-two members of the committee, which was meant to offer global representation, eighteen were European, and of those six were English. Only two members represented the Americas, and one Asia. Africa had no representation. As a result many of the issues under discussion, such as family allowances or 'the effect of cinema on the mental and moral wellbeing of children', were of little or no relevance to children in the majority of the world. Eglantyne herself only submitted reports when she felt the subject was of international relevance, such as a sixty-four-page memo on 'the assistance or repa-triation of foreign children who are abandoned, neglected or delin-quent', which stressed that children should be considered within the context of their families and communities, and given assistance within their own country wherever possible; policy that was later reflected in the relevant convention and is still considered best prac-tice today. After thanking the committee for their positive response to her report, she commented rather dryly that 'judging by the num-ber of conventions in existence, it might be imagined that the prob-lem had been solved; but this was not the case'. It was later agreed to limit the field of investigation to such international issues to avoid invading the domestic policy of member states, as well as over-whelming the committee. On this basis Eglantyne and Suzanne pre-sented a report on the constructive work of the Union around the protection and welfare of children, which was well received, and Eglantyne supported a range of proposals from the central collection of reliable information for use by voluntary associations, to the ban-ning of children under fourteen from employment. Often the work led to new conventions, not all of which were well received. 'We would not sign your resolution because child refugees are not a prob-lem here,' the British government responded with ill-concealed irritation to one proposal, 'it would therefore only create unnecessary admin …'[9]

Eglantyne's main agenda while at the League, however, was to promote the Declaration of the Rights of the Child. It now became evident she had been wise to keep the document short: 'the more deeply a convention goes into a question', one footnote to discussions ran, 'the less likely it is to be concluded.' Even so at first there was some ambivalence towards the declaration and its authors within the League; once the emergency work of the famine became less pressing there was a feeling that the Save the Children International Union had lost its focus. But with the support of Charlie and the British delegation, the declaration was finally brought before the Assembly on a wet September day in 1924.

Eglantyne did not have the authority to address the Assembly herself, but on 26 September Giuseppe Motta, President of the Assembly of the League and a former Swiss President, supported by the Labour Prime Minister Ramsay MacDonald, brought the declaration before the League's Fifth Commission, dealing with child welfare. A motion of approval, chaired by Valdes Mendeville, the candidate from Chile, was carried unanimously. 'The Assembly endorses the declaration of the rights of the child, commonly known as the Declaration of Geneva', the minutes record, 'and invites the State Members of the League to be guided by its principles in the work of child welfare.' In an idiosyncratic act of thanksgiving Eglantyne arranged for a service of dedication at St Martin-in-the-Fields in Trafalgar Square, at which representatives of the Church of England, Free Churches, Orthodox and Armenian Churches all took part.

The next job was advocacy. At a conference called by the Save the Children International Union in both Vienna and Budapest, a month after the declaration had been endorsed by the League, Eglantyne called on participating nations to adopt their own children's charters against which to regularly assess the situation of their country's children. Information cards given out had the Declaration printed in full on the reverse, and it was quickly reproduced in national papers across Europe. Germany, Belgium, Sweden and Canada all used it as the basis to form national laws for child welfare. Eglantyne then set off on a promotional tour to get the leaders of Europe to sign the Declaration. Sometimes she hovered anxiously in government rooms, uncertain as to what reception she might expect. Occasionally the ceremony of the meetings surprised her. In Hungary the great parliament staircase was lined by children in national dress, boy scouts and, to her amazement, young criminals in prison uniform, many holding flags. 'I knew it couldn't be an ordinary meeting at all which was going to be held somewhere at the top,' she wrote home to amuse Tye. She was right. Several hundred people filled the hall where the young Archduke Albrecht presided over the meeting. Encouraged by his ambitious mother, the 'fair and fat' Archduchess Isabella, the Archduke had taken the charitable movement in Hungary under his wing. 'You know I have always felt that unemployed royals might find useful scope in this direction!' Eglantyne continued mischievously to Tye. But she was also affected by the significance of the occasion. 'We had come, English and French, as well as neutrals like the Swiss …' she wrote 'to ask the help of our former enemies in working for a better world for the children.' A week later Eglantyne finalised arrangements at a meeting with the Archduchess in the palace. In a fluster to please, she darted where directed 'like an arrow from a bow', and dropped into her allocated chair 'like a billiard ball into a socket [sic]', and yet after ten minutes' conversation she found her host's attention beginning to wander. 'Distracted and irritable', the Archduchess reminded Eglantyne of the Duchess in Alice in Wonderland, and when no cakes arrived with their tea Eglantyne 'felt sure it would end in someone being beheaded'. Nonetheless the declaration gained one more signature.

Other signatories over the next year included King Boris of Bulgaria, Frau Marianne Hainisch, mother of the first President of

Austria, and the Prime Ministers of Britain, Australia, South Africa, New Zealand, Canada and Newfoundland, then a separate territory. In the Republic of Ireland the declaration was the only document to be signed by both the President of the Irish Free State and the Republican leader, Eamon de Valera. In France the Minister for Public Instruction ordered a copy to be hung in every school. Eglantyne, who had always wanted the declaration to be actively supported by everyone in contact with children, not just government departments making policy, was delighted by this last idea. She quickly organised a children's drawing competition among schools in fourteen countries to illustrate the declaration's clauses. Two thousand entries were exhibited internationally, generating huge press coverage and public interest.

The following year, 1925, the Union organised the first 'General Congress on Child Welfare'. Seven hundred delegates attended this seminal event in Geneva, including the representatives of thirty-eight governments and fifty-four nations. If their diverse interests presented certain problems, from Eglantyne's perspective it meant that the event was 'rich also in possibilities of which you had scarcely dreamed'. Above all, she felt that the discussions, structured around the clauses of the declaration, highlighted the need to 'universalise the work which is being done in small patches here and there', and set the scene for a new 'concerted effort'. 'Sometimes you feel you turn a corner and pass through a door,' she concluded: 'Is it too much to hope that it may mark our entrance into a new era when the Declaration will be made the charter of a new civilisation?'

A new civilisation is ambitious, but this is a new era for children's rights. Eglantyne's simple declaration has now evolved into the 'United Nations Convention on the Rights of the Child', which, ratified by all but two countries around the world, is the most universally accepted human rights instrument in history, making children a central concern of the global community. In encoding children's rights into international law the Convention provides agreed standards against which a country's progress can be both organised and independently assessed, and makes governments legally accountable for failing to meet the needs of children.[10]

Many valid criticisms can be made of the modern convention. The UN did not consult children and young people about their rights before drafting their document any more than Eglantyne did up her mountain; however, under-eighteens were represented by non-governmental organisations like Save the Children who do themselves actively consult children and young people, and the drafting process was unique in being approved by consensus. Nonetheless in aiming to both protect children and give them a voice, the fifty-four clauses are inevitably open to criticism as both too disciplining and too liberal.[11] And in seeking to be at once universally relevant and culturally inclusive, they can be seen as both culturally imperialistic and as making too great a compromise towards diversity. The difficulty is finding the balance between the simplicity Eglantyne advocated to ensure universal relevance and appeal and, now that the principle has been established, sufficient detail for the convention to have applied value as a set of enforceable standards.

However, the most serious criticism is that if children's rights are now recognised, arguably they remain on the international agenda because of the world's failure to meet its obligations under the convention. Somalia, which does not have a fully recognised government, and the USA, which wants to retain its legal rights both to execute children under eighteen and put them in the front line of battle, are both yet to ratify the convention. And, perhaps worse, many ratifying governments have failed to develop a coherent strategy or allocate sufficient resources to implement the convention. All over the world children are neglected and abused, forced to become soldiers or work long hours, detained in immigration centres, denied healthcare, education and even the playtime simply to be children. 'The principle of "all children, all rights" is still much too far from being a reality,' the former UN Secretary General Kofi Annan has admitted, and Save the Children has reported that 'millions of lives … have been barely touched by the UNCRC'.

But if not the complete solution, the convention *has* had powerful impact for many millions of children around the world. Eglantyne's declaration for the first time enshrined the moral equality of children with adults, and its endorsement by the League of Nations put children's rights, as distinct within broader human rights discourse, firmly on the international legal map. The convention now provides the impetus for governments to make a reality of children's rights through consultation, legal protection and the provision of welfare services, with independent agencies like Save the Children, UNICEF and national children's ombudsmen able to hold those governments to account. And there is currently an international campaign underway to secure a complaints mechanism for breaches under the convention, which if successful would serve to augment the current reporting process, and really put ratifying governments under the spotlight with regard to their human rights obligations to children.

It is perhaps too hopeful to imagine a world with no neglect or abuse of children, the utopian 'new civilisation' that Eglantyne had hoped for. But the promotion of children's rights has structured the work not only of governments and development organisations, but all the social institutions that impact on children's lives, from schools and medical practices to courts and detention centres, around the world. The modern perception of child welfare being a right rather than a privilege, and the increasingly active climate of consideration of children, would have pleased Eglantyne, who recognised that any declaration or convention only becomes valuable when applied, and that real progress in making a reality of children's rights lies in a new respect between children and adults being reflected not only in conventions and laws but also in social institutions, practices and attitudes. 'It is not much use in passing laws unless the whole community are endeavouring to carry out the principle underlying them,' she wrote to Suzanne in 1923. 'Everybody ... everyone who in any [way] comes into contact with children – that is to say the vast majority of mankind – may be in a position to help.' Eglantyne put children's rights on the world's agenda; the responsibility for upholding them now lies with us.

Chapter 16

Blue Plaques, 1920–2009

Thou canst not touch me, death,
Thou canst not dim
The brightness of my spark of life divine.

Eglantyne Jebb, 1929

Despite her penchant for climbing mountains Eglantyne was, in the words of one of her colleagues, 'far from being an athletic type'. In fact she had always loved horse-riding, walking and swimming in the sea as well as climbing; the problem was that she was seriously ill and photographs show a rapid transformation from the elegant social worker of 1920 to a hollow-faced old lady just eight years later. Eglantyne's illness had quickly returned after her goitre operation in 1916, and was now complicated by a heart condition. In February 1920 she discovered she needed two new operations: surgery to remove another lump from her thyroid – this one the size of a 'small marble', which she referred to ominously as her 'growth'– and an unrelated operation to remove a toe, which was just as depressing if less serious. The toe went, but she was not deemed strong enough for the thyroid operation, so the marble stayed. Her London doctor advised her to stop working completely, but it was not a good moment to cut back on commitments: she had launched the Save the Children International Union in Geneva just the month before. Recognising her predicament her doctor capitulated, but insisted on continuing to treat her without charge out of sympathy for Save the Children. 'It seems important for me to go on for the sake of the Fund. In a few years' time the famine might have righted itself, and then I shall have time to be ill!!' Eglantyne wrote to Margaret that August, adding bluntly, 'My life can't be weighed against those of the children, and if I can help to save a few at the cost of shattering my own health, it's cheap at the price!'

Now animated by an almost frantic energy, according to Dorothy's teenage son, his aunt Eglantyne was 'most vivid' and full of 'sparkle and originality …' and his elder sister described her as 'an exhilarating personality'. But this verve was increasingly interrupted by bouts of debilitating exhaustion. Eglantyne frequently worked from bed, her brown petticoat hidden beneath a 'beautiful white coat', a gift she rather guiltily accepted from Margaret as it enabled committee meetings to be held in her room with participants sitting on her bed when there were not enough chairs.[1] When brighter she would plant herself on a makeshift couch in the Fund's London office, often working there through the night until colleagues got used to seeing her rush through the corridors in the morning, her white hair still down on her shoulders, en route to grab a cup of tea, or lying on the long chair in the committee-room, 'frail and white', making decisions and giving orders in her 'low voice'. Henrietta Leslie remembered her fainting three times on the journey to Brighton before making an eloquent and moving speech at a crowded meeting, and a relief-worker in Salonika reported watching her being carried ashore by her friends, utterly exhausted from her journey, only to respond to his report by starting for Macedonia early the next morning. When she could not do everything herself Eglantyne's guilt and frustration overflowed into her letters. 'I want you to explain to Mr Clouzot that I cannot come to Geneva and that truly it is not my fault,' she wrote in a typical letter to Suzanne in 1920. 'I would have come if I could …' Soon the letters were going back the other way as colleagues urged her to cut back on commitments. 'I am quite conscious that your vibrant spirit cannot brook easily inactivity …' Lord Weardale, Chair of the British Fund, wrote to her, but 'complete recovery requires absolute rest'. Eglantyne was in an impossible position; her work both exhausted and, perversely, sustained her. Enforced idleness, otherwise known as rest, sent her stress levels soaring, counteracting any benefit to her heart.

Eglantyne's thyroid problems may have both responded and contributed to her ongoing depressions. Her suicidal thoughts certainly continued and she later recalled that after 1920 'whenever I went across a bridge or a high landing on a staircase, I heard a voice saying to me, "Throw yourself down, throw yourself down" … Once we had realised the suffering caused to the innocent children by the ghastly, unthinking cruelty of men, life was too miserable to be endured.' But, she continued, 'I had no intention … of obeying the suggestion: it simply made me react, brace myself, and go straight on.' Her agonies were exacerbated, however, when after the spectacular launch appeals the Fund's income inevitably steadily declined through the 1920s. 'The thought that we might after all have to abandon the work has never seemed far distant,' she poured it all out to Dorothy in 1926. 'It has weighed on me, gradually crushing out my strength … I often said to myself that if only we had money enough, I should be quite well.' Now she tore round the country on fundraising tours, always travelling economy, and sometimes wondering whether she would still be alive when she reached her destination.[2] Disappointed with the results she confessed, 'it was strange that I knew perfectly well that I was killing myself, and that I was killing myself for nothing'.

When Tye, now in her late seventies, began her final decline in 1923, Eglantyne started to feel she was facing 'a bottomless abyss of despair'. Tye was already emotionally dependent on Eglantyne. 'She craves for E's frequent letters … and she exists largely in her pride of her,' Em wrote to Bun. 'She lives E's life vicariously, there on her bed.' Hardly able to look after herself, Eglantyne now cared for her mother until she died two years later, followed the next month by her dearly loved and 'incalculably aged' aunt Bun. Eglantyne had dreaded losing Tye for years, and occasionally dreamed of them both, and Bun, 'all crossing the border together'. Her death must have reminded her of her own mortality, but her vivid belief in the afterlife, which had been affirmed by her mother's last vision of peace, happiness and reunion with her loved ones, gave her consolation. Now 'that that apparent separation has come …' she typed rather unevenly to Suzanne from Crowborough, 'I do not feel separated at all. She always used to say that her physical limitations constituted a barrier – a kind of separation – which death would sweep away, and now I feel her influence so strongly …' Nonetheless Eglantyne's own health was causing increasing concern.

According to her surgeon's notes, by the June of 1924 the lump on Eglantyne's remaining thyroid gland had grown from the size of a 'marble' to that of a 'small egg'. It seems she had a multi-nodular goitre, not uncommon for women of her age, but there is no note that the lumps were toxic or hyperactive. Eglantyne found it comforting to attribute her long history of mood swings to her thyroid, but in fact her depressions pre-dated her illness and continued after her 1916 operation, so her goitre might have been coincidental to her hypomanic personality. In any case it is unlikely that James Berry would have wanted to operate a second time on a gland already scarred by an operation, and Eglantyne now underwent some unsuccessful X-ray treatment instead. At the same time her heart specialist prescribed rest, slow walking, and a contradictory diet avoiding 'everything cooked in fat' but with plenty of butter, cream and milk to fatten up his 'terribly thin and frail' patient. There was no improvement. Eglantyne reassured her sisters 'you must not imagine me crawling miserably about with bent shoulders and a white face', but the truth was that for six months of 1927 she hardly got out of bed. She was finally carried into a Geneva nursing-home for a series of operations in the summer of 1928.

Eglantyne knew that her situation was critical. Secretly she had already written her will, arranged for her debts to be recovered, a few mementoes, mostly books, to go to friends, and asked William MacKenzie to act as her executor, trying to keep the tone light by apologising that this meant 'if I should by chance die under the operation, your holiday would be made shorter'. She also asked, repeatedly, to be buried under a plain Latin cross on Mont Salève, although she recognised that logistics meant 'it might be a question of transferring the coffin later'. At the same time her letters are full of apologies in case it was all so much fuss for nothing. 'I have taken an unexpected turn and am much better,' she told MacKenzie in July, and to Lill, 'with my usual inconsequence, I now seem to be recovering as rapidly as I fell ill'. She was indeed deemed much better – better enough to have her operations, but not to no longer need them.

Eglantyne greatly respected her doctors, but she dreaded the surgery, particularly the morphine, which made her feel like she was losing her mind, although she laughed to friends, 'if they go on operating on me every other day, I suppose I will get used to it'. There are 'two kinds of doctor' she now wrote conspiratorially to Charlie: 'the wicked scientific materialists and the good man dealing in spiritual influences, I prefer myself the former'. If true this was by a narrow margin. With typical enthusiasm for anything alternative she had already tried treatment by the 'vibratory radio-waves' of the American quack doctor Albert Abrams' 'oscilloclast machine', which seemed to Eglantyne just as logical as X-ray treatment.[3] She was soon advising Dorothy, who suffered from epilepsy, to try a 'nature cure', and after hearing of 'well over a million attested cases of Christian Science cures', she wrote to Lill, who had been diagnosed with cancer: 'here is hope for us all'. In between her own surgery Eglantyne saw a range of 'healers of other schools of thought', to whom, along with the love of her friends, she gave much of the credit for her post-op recoveries. 'The prayer of my friends and the spiritual power which seemed to pour through them, was like a light, defending me on every side,' she wrote after the final surgery. The next few months were spent recuperating with Dorothy and a succession of visitors on her clinic balcony looking across to the Salève. Here she discussed an invitation from the Persian government to research a national child welfare movement, planned an international African conference which took place in 1931, talked of visiting India and Russia in February, and began studying Mandarin in anticipation of setting up projects in China.[4] 'I think that a voyage to the East … would be no more tiring than office work,' she told Dorothy cheerfully. She still had an irregular heartbeat and the clinic tried to get her to rest more, but rest had never appealed to her.[5] 'You are the "sister" of the whole world, Miss Jebb,' her exasperated doctor sighed when she tried to wheedle him into letting her have extra visitors.

When unable to work Eglantyne seized the opportunity to write. In April she had had a collection of verses published under the title *The Real Enemy*, aimed at fighting public apathy towards humanitarian causes. 'One or two of them are very disagreeable', she wrote in delight to Dorothy, to whom she had dedicated the book, begging her not to look at them until they were together because 'the disagreeableness will come out much more forcibly when I read them aloud!' Now, having received some good reviews, she was working on a second collection with the working title *Poems of Old Age*, allowing her to explore death through the fictional perspective of an elderly man. Some of the verses hinted at loss and regret; 'the ghosts of the dead, come now and walk in the garden with me', one read, another; 'I hear their call at last, but oh! the bitterer woe; to hear it and to know my chance to help is past.' But many more spoke of the reassurance found in faith:

Singing bird, I am lying
In my darkened room dying,
Dying alone,

Like to a light on the darkness
Flashed on my trouble your song,
And I turned on my weary pillows,
Glad for a moment to be strong,
Like a breeze from the mountains
Wafted your melody to me,
And an answering beat to its rapture
Pulsed for a moment through me.
Surely your song to companion me
To the unknown shores is sent,
God! Give me birds in heaven – birds, and I am content!

She also wrote notes for a play, and a short story to amuse Dorothy's daughter who was now twenty-two and planning on joining her favourite aunt on a trip to Persia for the Fund the following year. Written from the perspective of her niece as an old lady, the story looks back on their travels together, sending up Eglantyne mercilessly as a 'poor old thing' who was 'half crazy … but very plausible, as crazy people often are'. But soon a cable announces:

'Aunt Eglantyne severe heart attack from seeing children making carpets contravention of B.I.T. regulations STOP dies while speaking on the subject in market place STOP had expressed wish to be buried summit Mount X with Geneva Declaration in Ashanti on tombstone'

Why Ashanti?

I don't know, I'm sure. Probably she thought it was the language spoken in the neighbourhood. Geography was never her strong point.[6]

Death might not have been far from her thoughts but Eglantyne was clearly enjoying herself. 'I cannot tell you what pleasant days I have here,' she wrote to Lill, and when Dorothy was with her, it felt 'like a holiday'. 'The brilliant autumn sunshine was not more brilliant than her smile,' Ruth wrote with her normal purple prose when she visited the clinic that October: 'she was full of fun and interest in everything; sixteenth-century Geneva, old Oxford friends ... The old passion for solitude, the craving for physical freedom, the super-sensitiveness, had been transcended by a gracious power of loving, a spiritual freedom, a calm that was reflected in her face.'

It was typical of Eglantyne's contradictory nature that her darkest times were often partnered by moments of great spiritual calm and optimism. 'It is a strange circumstance that amidst all this over-whelming tragedy of the suffering of the famine areas, one cannot help feeling at times the happiness of a great hope,' she had written to MacKenzie in April 1920. Four years later, when forced to dismiss staff to cut Save the Children's costs, she again found comfort in her faith: 'My distress is not about the movement ...' she wrote, 'because we are standing for the truth – the truth which always triumphs even across the dead bodies of its disciples! I have a profound conviction that our cause will succeed beyond our hopes.' Eglantyne had four more years torn between anxieties about the Fund and the belief that she could 'rely on a guidance which can never fail' before she was checked into her Geneva clinic. Once there, Ruth testified, 'she fought – oh how she fought! – to live, in order to go on fighting. It was as if her eyes were on a clock, wondering: "Can I live long enough to get this over to the world? Can I? Can I? I must!" ' But finally Eglantyne seemed to feel a release. 'I haven't the slightest wish to do anything which can be called "work"!!' she wrote in November 1928, and the following month she told Dorothy that 'a deepening conviction comes to me that all is well, I can trust God with the future of the SCF. How very odd, how ridiculous it would be, if I could not.'

A few days later Eglantyne was deemed ready to convalescence in Sierre, deep in the Alps. She spent the day laughing and joking with friends, and accepting some farewell chocolates from her doctor. At supper that evening she suffered a major stroke. Em, at that moment the healthiest of the sisters, quickly travelled over from Ireland, providing comfort with a series of thin jokes and the more sustaining fact of her presence. Later she wrote a distressing account of her sister's last days of semi-consciousness, 'moaning like some animal caught in a steel trap' and holding on to her hand 'like a drowning sailor to a rope'. On 17 December 1928, the weather turned colder, snow filled the air, and Eglantyne died following an emergency operation on her stomach. Her last words, dictated to her nurse in a moment of lucidity that morning, began, 'I have been weighing lately the thought that life is happier than we know ...'

Eglantyne had apparently kept going by sheer force of will for so long that many of her friends were deeply shocked when death finally came, including Margaret, who later bitterly regretted not having visited her. As Henrietta put it, 'one had the feeling that it was ... essential for millions of innocent and afflicted children and for millions more, as yet unborn, that she should live, that she simply could not die'. But those closest to Eglantyne found comfort in their faith that her passionate and mischievous spirit, always the strongest part of her, lived on. 'Long before death came to break the last fragile bond one felt ... that with her the spirit had already found a very unusual measure of release,' Dorothy wrote in 1929, and her cousin Gem wrote that 'Eglantyne was so much more spirit than flesh that one can't exactly feel sorrow: death doesn't remove her as it removes other people.' MacKenzie felt similarly. 'Not many memories are easy to bear,' he commented; 'hers is easy, for it is a presence,' and Eglantyne's Baha'i friend, Lady Blomfield, even wrote on the card with her funeral flowers, 'with loving devotion, to the inspiring, beloved spirit, who *is* a Member of our Committee'.

The funeral was held at the English Church in Geneva, after which Eglantyne's mortal remains at least were buried in St George's cemetery, two miles south of the city and in full view of the Salève. Her coffin was draped with the silk banner of the International Union embroidered – by nuns – in blue, white and gold, and completely covered in flowers which were quickly blown with snow. On the same day a memorial service was held for many more friends and dignitaries at St Martin-in-the-Fields in Trafalgar Square with singing led by the Save the Children carol choir. Condolences flooded in from around the world, and obituaries were printed from Paris to Perth. 'I think she would have been glad to know, for the sake of the movement for which she was always willing to be exploited, how good a "press" her passing produced,' Edward Fuller, the editor of the Fund's journal, wrote to Dorothy.

While in Geneva I visited Eglantyne's grave. Buying flowers, fresh cut roses in full bloom, I suddenly found I was crying. It was ridiculous; I had never known Eglantyne – she had died eighty years before. Finding myself somehow embroiled in a story about a deceased aunt with the flower-seller, I mentally blamed the pregnancy hormones, made my excuses, and moved on. Eglantyne's is a remarkably unromantic grave. Zone 25, plot 1,443, she is on the end of a sparsely occupied row, beside a gravel path. To her left, presuming she is facing up, are Mr and Mrs Mehling in a double plot. No one currently opposite. Her slab of marble could do with a bit of a scrub, but then it is not a kitchen worktop. A simple brass cross is slightly inset, followed by her dates, including the foundation of the International Save the Children Union in English and French, and a quote from Matthew XXV.[7] I was just six feet, and eighty years, away from her, but having got all emotional buying flowers I could not now find the connection I had somehow hoped for at the cemetery. It was mid-afternoon on a clear day. Some undistinguished birdsong failed to hide the traffic hum. People wandered about with pots of flowers and the occasional watering can. I sat on her gravestone and tried harder to emote but now another side-effect of my pregnancy, apart from the easy tears, became evident: I inadvertently farted on Eglantyne's grave. Disaster. I have the deepest respect for Eglantyne and have spent much of the last six years in her company; this was not the moment I had had in mind. But perhaps Eglantyne would have preferred this ridiculous incident to my foolish wished-for sentiment.

The next day I found her will at the city archives, along with a pathetic list of possessions at death; mostly brown clothes plus among other bits forty-two handkerchiefs, two tea-towels, a small black cloth bag containing rubber bands, and some medical accessories in a tin. Her books were similarly representative: mainly religious and spiritual, some poetry including her mother's verse, the lives of Calvin, William Penn and Pestalozzi among others, More's *Utopia* and some maps of the Tyrol. The few personal items included her gold cross on its brown ribbon, various diaries and notebooks with titles like 'Combating Sin', some watercolour sketches, and a bundle of valentines made by Eglantyne and her siblings when children for Tye. Unlike her mother, Eglantyne was not a hoarder and it was easy to see how she once fitted everything she needed for a journey into one of the two leather pistol holsters that Lill had taken on her adventure to Baghdad. Now these last possessions were sorted out by Em, ever the practical eldest sister, to be sent home, given or thrown away.

It was MacKenzie who arranged Eglantyne's funeral, sent the 1,946 francs to cover the cost of her grave, and specified the simple gravestone with, intriguingly, 'no fibs', and a cheap wooden coffin with 'inexpensive fittings. And *no* name-plate.' It is 'a barbarous habit to label a coffin as tho' you were inside it!!!' he wrote, and in the end Eglantyne's coffin just bore her initials. Perhaps MacKenzie was thinking of her poem 'A Last Message':

> If I be dead, yet still I am not there,
> For what you love is not my mortal frame;
> I would not be confused with a corpse;
> O! let not, then, a corpse assume my name!

Certainly as a devout Catholic he agreed with the sentiment that once the spirit has flown, the rest is dust, and for him Eglantyne was probably already back on her mountain. Nonetheless with Dorothy's support over the next few months MacKenzie began to organise a

memorial to Eglantyne high on the Salève in deference to her wish
to be buried there, and perhaps he even intended to transfer her coffin there later. The memorial blue-prints show a large stone cross set
on a curving base designed as somewhere for people to sit while
admiring the view over Geneva. But it proved too expensive: 'what
would my poor sister have thought', Dorothy exclaimed, 'had she
known that the sum put down for the *architect alone* would be £170!'
From Dorothy's perspective the 'only possible worthy memorial' to
Eglantyne was a fund to endow specific Save the Children project
work. To kick-start an appeal in 1929 she collected and published
Eglantyne's last poems under the title *Post Tenebras Lux* (After the
Darkness, Light), both in her sister's memory, and as a fundraiser.
Seven years later the money raised went to fund work in Ethiopia. As
a footnote, ironically in 1990 some oversight meant that the lease on
Eglantyne's Geneva grave was not renewed, and somebody else was
nearly allocated her plot. Eglantyne might have been amused by her
various close encounters with disinterment, both proposed and acci-
dental. 'Thou canst not touch me,' she had written in 1928, 'Death,
thou canst not dim, The brightness of my spark of life divine.'

Eighty years after her death there is still no memorial, not even a
park bench, to Eglantyne on Mont Salève. There is a community
sports-hall in her name in Ellesmere where she grew up; a glass chandelier, each drop the shape of a white flame in testament to her burning spirit, in her Oxford college chapel; a portrait in St Peter's
Church in Marlborough close to where she once taught schoolgirls
their letters; and the thriving village of *Xheba* in Albania, built on the
Atlovo model in the 1920s and named in honour of Eglantyne *Jebb*.
An English rose has been named after her and a blue plaque has been
proposed for the Cambridge site where she once had her charities
office, but is yet to go up. Less materially, Eglantyne has a day of
remembrance marked on the Anglican calendar and, perhaps most
pleasing of all, since she 'delighted in the incongruous', Princess
Anne called her famously vicious English bull terriers Eglantyne and

Dottie, no doubt after the founders of one of her favourite charities.[8] Altogether though it is not a lot to remember a woman who in her fifty-two years launched an international aid operation, saved the lives of millions of children, redefined how child welfare operates, and wrote social policy of permanent world significance, all in an era when women did not even have the vote.

Eglantyne was a forceful, eccentric and contradictory woman. Nicknamed the 'White Flame' towards the end of her life, afterwards she was celebrated as 'more flame than woman', an 'apostolic spirit', and a 'saint' who 'lived on a different plane from ordinary mortals'.[9] But Eglantyne was not all spirit; her physique was weak but significant *for* that, for it was partly fear of this crippling frailty that drove her. And although she personally rejected the material and physical in favour of the spiritual, becoming ever more ascetic in her own life, she was saved from over-bearing intensity by her keen sense of humour and her readiness to laugh at herself. She was, in the words of her cousin Gem, always 'alive to the ridiculous as well as the transcendental'. Above all she never limited the scope of her concerns for children to their spiritual well-being: however much she aspired to what she called the 'higher plane of living', she knew that bodies and minds came first in the material world.

Dorothy's homage to her sister was, typically, more grounded. Quoting Étienne Clouzot, who had called Eglantyne 'humanity's conscience', she commented that this must have been the type of conscience of which Coleridge sang, 'which is the pulse of reason'. Eglantyne's idealism and determination to keep an open mind sometimes made her seem naive, but she never lost sight of what was truly important and later she burnished her half-formed thoughts into better policy. She and Dorothy were among the first to call people back to sanity during the First World War and Eglantyne was among the few who continued to champion common, human sense and moral reasoning at an international level in the post-war years that were full of fear and jingoistic hatred. An idealist determined to be practical, she was 'not fond' of children individually but dedicated her life to child welfare because she had the sensitivity to prioritise the immediate needs of children, and the sense to see that children held both universal appeal in the present, and collective responsibility for the future. It was an insight that caught the mood of a generation.

A year after she died, at the tenth anniversary of Save the Children's launch, Ramsay MacDonald eulogised about how Eglantyne had 'offered herself up as a sacrifice for her ideals'. But although she probably did hasten her death by not accepting her physical limitations, Eglantyne also refused to be constrained by social expectations about her role in life. She had not so much sacrificed herself as sought and found fulfilment in dedicating herself to her work. It was deeply sad that Eglantyne relegated the personal to the humorous and inconsequential, but she found lasting emotional and intellectual satisfaction through focusing on the broader human picture. On this scale her credo was essentially one of inclusion and endeavour, not sacrifice and denial. These were the principles that drove the international Save the Children movement. They also inspired the concept of universal children's rights, which, through the hard work, support and co-operation of so many, continues to save, protect and enhance the lives of many millions of children around the world. For Eglantyne above all the universal was personal. 'A leading characteristic of modern thought is its insistence upon the unity of mankind. And at long last this truth begins to find a more ready echo in the heart of the individual,' she wrote with some relief the year she died, concluding: 'now at last, we have an opportunity such as we have never had before, a real working possibility of bringing a decent human life with its normal responsibilities and joys within the reach of all mankind'.

Epilogue:
Truths and Lives

A friend of mine once said to me that our minds, contemplating the truth, were like so many cameras turned towards the same building; no two cameras can be in exactly the same position, even when they are not turned towards it from opposite directions, so that no two precisely similar photographs can be taken; hence also, though some may be better than others, no single photograph, always supposing that it had not been faked, will be without its value.

Frieda Jones, *Eglantyne's fictional alter ego*
The Ring Fence, c.*1908*

What constitutes the truth is the central dilemma in biography. The 'facts' of a life may present one picture, but more often several, and the human truths behind them require some further degree of interpretation. It is a funny thing to search for the truths of someone in the archives of public libraries and between the lines of private letters. Sometimes Eglantyne would remain obscure, more often she'd emerge in fits and starts, her character developing through half-finished poetry and better-considered policy, her heart consistent but her approach at times contrary, and occasionally she would surprise me by her sudden vivid presence. Her irreverent pen portraits and ink sketches are startlingly immediate, and even her handwriting is very expressive, sometimes in pencil, occasionally the propelling kind, but usually a fast untidy scrawl in black ink. Anything she had touched soon held a particular fascination for me; a fact in its existence, a fiction in its romance. Eating from the plates – rather fine, gold trim – from which Eglantyne and Margaret would once have dined, while I was visiting Margaret's granddaughter Susannah Burn, caused me to pause. And Eglantyne's great nephew, Ben Buxton, a former archaeology lecturer with an intuitive understanding of my need to grapple with evidence from the past, once even produced a curl of her baby-hair, still radiant red, from an aging manila envelope. Clearly it is ludicrous to obsess about relics: Richard Dawkins claims that every time you drink a glass of water the likelihood is that you will imbibe at least one molecule that passed through the bladder of Oliver Cromwell, so no doubt we have all shared a few atoms with Eglantyne as well. Pleasingly I think this molecular trivia would have appealed to Eglantyne, given her fascination with the shared nature of life, and the direct relationship between the individual and the universal.

Although typically Eglantyne believed 'it was an illusion to think any great cause ever really depended upon certain individuals', she was a keen reader of biography throughout her life.[1] 'History seems to be written for the sole purpose of conveying information, and that in the most disagreeable way,' she once complained from college. On the other hand, she continued pithily, 'if a book appeals to one's emotions one may take it for granted that it may be untruthful'. Biographies navigate these problems by offering person-shaped insights into social history, while examining the relationship of the individual to the whole. 'The experience of the human race is something that should be available for all,' Eglantyne later pronounced, 'the true heroes and saints of mankind have left a message which was not for one nation only, or for one generation.' Although she never attempted a biography herself, as a young woman she tried to convey individual human experience and universal moral truths through endless dramatic poems and novels.[2] Later she gave talks, wrote articles and harnessed press advertising, photographs and film-footage to open the public's eyes to the desperate truths of post-war starvation across Europe. 'In the first place, we have to devise a means of making known the facts in such a way as to touch the imagination of the world,' she wrote.

The 'facts' that Eglantyne had in mind were not just the harrowing statistics on material need and the provision of relief that Dorothy so competently compiled, but also wider 'truths' about human interdependence, and social and moral responsibilities. She had spent a lot of time contemplating these 'truths'. Eglantyne was born imaginative, had a powerful sense of social responsibility instilled in her as a child, and illness, unrequited and impossible love affairs, and a regular need for solitude later gave her plenty of time to think. In her late thirties, unmarried, lonely and surrounded by the division and conflict that marked the descent towards war, she began to construct the personal philosophy that would help her make sense of the world, and her place within it. Slowly she found her own 'truth' in what she believed to be the artificial tension between the individual and the universal. Eglantyne was not a sentimental woman, but she was a great humanitarian; as friends testified, 'her interest in children had always tended to be rather theoretical than individual'. So the idea that there was a very direct relationship between humankind in general, and the particular person, appealed to her deeply. From this perspective individuals could have no exclusive self-interest; all were unknowingly stranded parts of the same whole. Once, as she explained it, 'knowledge of unity' had replaced 'the hallucination of an individual possessing life separate from other lives', Eglantyne had the formula to make sense of life at both personal and political levels. Soon her aim was not only to save individual lives immediately, but also to foster a new international respect for the common claims of humanity. Her greatest and most creative assertion of this association between the personal and the political came with her promotion of the universal rights and responsibilities of each individual child.

'A leading characteristic of modern thought is its insistence upon the unity of mankind. At long last this truth begins to find a more ready echo in the heart of the individual' Eglantyne wrote with some relief the year before she died. The bearing that our lives have upon each other is reflected in biography as well as human rights. It is a truism that we are known by our deeds. But it is a person's being, not just his or her doing, that is endlessly fascinating; a being that must be at once reassuringly familiar and curiously unique. Eglantyne was at once ordinary, a recognisable product of her time; and extraordinary, pushing the boundaries of accepted ideas in all sorts of directions. If the facts of her story continue to touch the imagination, it is not only because of the importance of her legacy in the international Save the Children movement and the UN Convention on the Rights of the Child, but also by some of the truths she illuminated about human community that underpin these. 'We want men and women everywhere', Eglantyne wrote, 'to take up their stand on the common, simple things of every day life which should unite us all.'

The International Save the Children Alliance

Britain and other nations who were once enemies are pledged in their souls never to forget the Unknown Soldier, who represents all that young manhood that died in the war: but I think we ought also to adopt in our hearts the Unknown Child, who is still alive and who needs our help and our charity, the Unknown Child in all the countries of the world.

Philip Gibbs, British war correspondent, 1931,
inspired by meeting Eglantyne in Vienna

I want to have a long life. Even if you are poor it is nice to live.

Ciano, age 10, The Philippines

People paint young people as being a bad lot, but we've got so much to give … After all we are the next generation.

Joanne, age 14, Newcastle, Britain

The International Save the Children Alliance is now the world's largest independent international children's development agency, fighting for children's rights and delivering immediate aid and lasting improvements to children's lives in over 120 countries around the world through twenty-seven Save the Children member organisations.

This global work still relies on the support of individuals who have adopted unknown children in their hearts.

www.savethechildren.net/alliance
www.savethechildren.org.uk

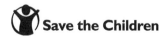 Save the Children

Endnotes

Cast of Principal Characters

1 Carole Angier, *Margaret Hill* (unpublished, 1978)

Chapter 1

1 Mrs Charles Roden Buxton (Dorothy Jebb) and Edward Fuller, *The White Flame: The Story of the Save the Children Fund* (London: Weardale Press, 1931)

2 Francesca Wilson, *Rebel Daughter of a Country House: The Life of Eglantyne Jebb* (London: George Allen & Unwin, 1967)

Chapter 2

1 A family of Jebbs, almost certainly related, had been tenant farmers on the land since at least the eighteenth century.

2 Arthur was the sole surviving son of R.G. Jebb. His elder brother, Richard, had died in 1845 aged eight. Arthur may have been cossetted as a result.

3 John Ayscough (Drew Bickerstaffe-Drew), *Gracechurch* (London: Longmans Green, 1913)

4 Arthur did produce one book, a metrical version of the Psalms, which was much loved by his family and well reviewed when published after his death, but little read more widely.

5 'The prickles and aloofness, grace and delicate, bewitching beauty of an eglantyne rose were all there.' Ruth Wordsworth, *Recollections of Eglantyne Jebb*, II, Oxford, p. 15

6 Eglantyne Jebb, 'A Youngest Sister', undated (Jebb archive)
7 Eglantyne Jebb 'The Land of a Hundred Flags' in *The Real Enemy* (Weardale Press, 1928)
8 Lill eventually went on to serve on the council of the national 'Home Arts' organisation that evolved from this work.
9 He later carved a lectern in the small Welsh church of Isycoed to Tye's memory.

Chapter 3

1 Gertrude Bell, later famous for her role in creating the modern state of Iraq, was among the first students at LMH to study Modern History and left with first-class honours five years before Eglantyne arrived. It was almost certainly about Bell that a male Oxford undergraduate wrote with some begrudging admiration:

I go every day to my crammer,
And he marks all my verses with 'gamma';
While that girl over there
With the flaming red hair,
Gets 'alpha plus' easily, d★★★ her.

Despite the red hair, the girl could not have been Eglantyne, as distracted by extra-curricular activities she could not compete with Bell's grades, and would eventually leave with a second.
2 Titular degrees would not be granted to women until 1923.
3 Eglantyne Jebb, 'Ode to Euclid', undated, *c.*1896 (Jebb archive). Euclid was a Greek mathematician of the Hellenistic period, known as 'the father of geometry'.
4 Eglantyne Jebb, 'To My History Lecturer', undated, *c.*1896 (Jebb archive)
5 Margery Fry became a prison reformer and the first female magistrate; Eleanor Rathbone became most famous for successfully campaigning for Family Allowances; Maude Royden became a leading suffragist and peace campaigner, and an early supporter of Eglantyne's own later campaigns with the Fight the Famine Council.

Chapter 4

1 In her influential book *The Century of the Child*, published in 1900, the Swedish educationalist Ellen Key argued that children's education needed to be transformed so that it focused on the nurturing of children's personality and the cultivation of their potential to do good.

2 On 15 May 1901 Sir John Gorst, Vice-President of the Board of Education, announced a bill to extend the scope of secondary education and reform the administration of elementary education. Not everyone agreed that free secondary education should be available to all.

3 Eglantyne's influence over the two girls was enormous: both went on to university and became pioneering educationalists, Gem as the Principal of Bedford College and Eglantyne as the Principal of the Froebel Institute.

Chapter 5

1 As early as 1861 Carrie, then Mrs Caroline Slemmer, had travelled to Washington with her brother-in-law Charles du Puy, and successfully requested an interview with President Lincoln. Lincoln later jotted down a 'list of officers I wish to remember when I make appointments for Officers of the Regular Army: Major Doubleday, Major Anderson ... Lt Slemmer – his pretty wife says a Major or First Captain'. Mary Reed Bobbitt, *With Dearest Love to All* (London: Faber, 1960) p. 46

2 Among other events Eglantyne looked forward to what she called 'a *reformed* dinner party', the first of an intended series at which social issues of the day were to be discussed under the leadership of George Trevelyan, whom she described as a 'fiery youth'. 'Three courses and Truth!' Eglantyne wrote to a friend enthusiastically. 'This is too terrifying for words!!!'

3 Eglantyne was tutoring her two Irish cousins, Gem and Eglantyne Jebb, in history and literature through a combination of correspondence and study tours. 'I have tours in my head from Stonehenge down to the field of Waterloo' she wrote, and, adopting the Victorian view of history as

one of linear social progress, she planned visits to institutions ranging from the Post Office to the Blackwall Tunnel.

4 Eglantyne put her whole heart into the love letters that Hugh wrote to Frieda, letters which she herself had perhaps only received in imagination.

5 Elsie's brothers were (John Wynford) Lord St Davids, (Owen Cosby) Lord Kyslant, (Laurence Richard) Lord Milford, Sir Ivor Phillips, MP who restored Pembroke Castle, and Bertram Phillips, who is alleged to have once cried when bitten by a parrot.

6 Marcus Dimsdale, *Happy Days & Other Essays* (Cambridge: W. Heffer, 1921)

7 Marcus was not always laid low by depression. During the war he became a Classics master at Winchester to substitute for younger teachers called up for military service, and he was also a leader of the Cambridge Corps of Guides.

8 'To live ahead of one's generation must be to live dangerously, catching glimpses of larger ideas that are just coming into view,' Francis Cornford, who was in the same Cambridge circle, once observed of Jane Harrison. See Anne Hamlin, *Pioneers of the Past* (Cambridge: Newnham College, 2001)

9 Em's son Percy became the respected author and critic Arland Ussher whose publications included collections of Celtic legends and pen-portraits of George Bernard Shaw, W.B. Yeats and James Joyce, as well as a curious 'alphabet of aphorisms' which included the pronouncement that 'great writers are failed talkers. There is nothing so tragic as a bad writer – except a good one.' It was an idea that his aunt Eglantyne, who would exchange her own novel writing for humanitarian lobbying, might have enjoyed. See Arland Ussher, *An Alphabet of Aphorisms* (Dublin: The Dolmen Press, 1953)

10 Mrs Roland Wilkins (Lill Jebb), *By Desert Ways to Baghdad* (Thomas Nelson, 1908). Lill referred to Victoria as 'X' throughout the book. I have amended this here for ease of understanding. The book caused a sensation on publication, and was later widely read again by British troops serving in Mesopotamia during the First World War.

Chapter 6

1 It has been argued that the 'language of self-sacrifice' adopted by the idealist Hegelian Oxford philosopher T.H. Green, which inspired Arnold Toynbee and a generation of male graduates to work in the slums in the 1880s, and then in local and municipal authorities, had appropriated this traditionally female form of social action. See Anne Summers, *Female Lives, Moral States: Women, Religion and Public Life in Britain 1800–1930* (Newbury: Threshold Press, 2000) p. 133

2 In 1893 an estimated 20,000 women were paid charity officials and 500,000 worked semi-professionally.

3 Alfred Marshall and Mary Paley Marshall, *The Economics of Industry* (London: Macmillan, 1879)

4 For a while Charlie edited the *Albany Review*, and wrote articles for the progressive *Independent Review*. See Charles Roden Buxton, 'A Vision for England', *Independent Review*, 1905, volume 7, pp. 146–157

5 Like Booth, Eglantyne included a rent map, hers beautifully drafted by Gwen Darwin, betraying the skill and attention to detail that would later make her famous as the artist Gwen Raverat. 'I am *so* busy now,' Gwen wrote to her sister Margaret. 'Every afternoon I can I go to help Eglantyne. She is making a Booth map of Cambridge ... It's very interesting – and I do like Eglantyne so very much – more and more. For she's got a sense of humour, which saves her from the kind of philanthropicalness of most good ladies.'

6 Mary Carpenter's 'Ragged School Movement' was founded in the 1840s. Barnardo's was founded as the 'Infant Life Protection Society' in 1876. The Children's Society was founded as The Church of England Waifs and Strays in 1881. The NSPCC was founded as the London SPCC in 1884.

7 Margaret Keynes, *The Problem of Boy Labour in Cambridge* (Cambridge: Bowes and Bowes, 1911)

8 *The Cambridge Register of Social and Philanthropic Agencies* (Cambridge: Bowes and Bowes, 1911) reprinted in *Tracts on Social and Industrial Questions, 1860–1911*

9 Eglantyne was devoted to her baby niece, writing to Charlie that one-month-old Eglantyne was 'the first baby to have found its way into my heart', and asking Dorothy 'can I come and rock the cradle?'

Chapter 7

1 When Margaret ultimately gave up book-binding Lytton Strachey bought all her equipment.

2 Maynard would also have known Charlie Buxton independently as both had been members of the Eton Literary Society, meeting regularly to read papers on literary topics.

3 Eglantyne almost certainly went to Mrs Humphrey Ward's Boys' Settlement in Bloomsbury to gain some experience, and where she was later followed by Florence and Margaret Keynes.

4 'My thoughts of you are like a talisman, always there and it gives me strength. I try to think what you would do, what you would like me to do when things are difficult ...' Margaret wrote to Eglantyne in September 1910.

5 David Hill later wrote of Margaret, his mother, that 'she was basically serious-minded, but had a streak of comic, slightly mischievous whimsicality'.

6 After several sittings Duncan Grant abandoned his portrait of Margaret and no record of it remains. Margaret described Duncan to Eglantyne in September 1910 as 'an artist with most of the usual traits – very absent minded, very impecunious, rather nervous in manner but entirely free from affectation. He has black hair which stands on end when he is excited and a very nice face.'

7 At the time it was a common superstition that the first to rise from dinner for thirteen would have misfortune. Agatha Christie wrote a thriller called *Lord Edgware Dies* (London: Collins Crime Club, 1933) reprinted in the USA as *Thirteen for Dinner*, which uses this superstition as its central motif.

8 Margaret was succeeded by Margaret Darwin, who would not long later marry Geoffrey Keynes, so replacing her friend as Margaret Keynes in name as well as in occupation.

9 'Polly' was Margaret's chosen nickname for her baby while still in

utero, and unknown to her daughter had of course also been her own pseudonym in her letters to Eglantyne.

Chapter 8

1 Victoria de Bunsen, *Macedonian Massacres: Photos from Macedonia* (London: The Balkans Committee, n.d., *c.*1907)
2 Austria did indeed attack Serbia after Sarajevo, provoking the First World War.
3 The bullet, which could not be removed from Charlie's lung, probably exacerbated the lung cancer that finally killed him in 1942, aged 67.

Chapter 9

1 Richard Holmes, 'Author's Statement', British Council: Contemporary Writers website, www.contemporarywriters.com/ authors, accessed October 2007. Richard Holmes is the author of *Footsteps: Adventures of a Romantic Biographer* (1985) and *Sidetracks: Explorations of a Romantic Biographer* (2000) among many other books.
2 Nora Sidgwick's analysis of 17,000 questionnaires, excluding any ambiguous results, found 'death-day apparitions' occurring at 442 times the rate predicted by chance.
3 Eglantyne may well have been familiar with Freud. A.V. Hill, Margaret Keynes's husband, was well versed in his theories and later in touch with him for some years, and Freud later lent his name to Save the Children's early appeals.
4 Evelyn Underhill, *The House of the Soul* (London: Methuen, 1929). *Prayer* by Evelyn Underhill was listed amongst the books and articles in travelling case 'B', among Eglantyne's effects on her death in 1928.

Chapter 10

1 Eglantyne's brother, Richard Jebb, being forty and married with three children in 1914, was not expected to volunteer for service, and did not qualify for health reasons when conscription was brought in two years later. At first only single men and childless widowers aged 18 to 41 were called up, but by 1918 compulsory service had been extended to all

men aged 18 to 51. More than 2.3 million conscripts were enlisted before the end of the war in November 1918.

2 Tennyson's 'The Charge of the Light Brigade' was one of the first poems the Jebb children had to learn by heart in The Lyth schoolroom.

3 Statistics vary, so I have consulted a range of sources including:

> Colin Nicolson, *The Longman Companion to the First World War* (Essex: Longman, 2001) p. 248;
>
> Parliament publications and records online; www.parliament.uk/parliamentary_publications_and_archives/parliamentary_archives/archives____ww1_conscription.cfm;
>
> Encyclopaedia Britannica online, http://info.britannica.co.uk

4 A 1921 census revealed there were 1.75 million more women in the population than men.

5 The AOS supported the introduction of Women's Institutes to Britain, where they operated under the guardianship of the Board of Agriculture. It was in no small part through Lill's advocacy that the WI became an independent, self-governing organisation in October 1917. There would be over 1,400 local Women's Institute groups by 1919.

6 Mrs Roland Wilkins, ' "To the Land!" Britain's Battle-Cry to the Women To-day!' *The Times*, *c*.1915. There were of course always women, mainly the wives and daughters of farm labourers, who worked on the land, though their jobs were limited in range.

7 The Hurler on the Ditch (Emily Ussher), *The Trail of the Black and Tans* (Dublin: The Talbot Press Ltd, 1921)

8 Charles Roden Buxton, 'Lost Opportunities', Women's Peace Crusade leaflet no. 9 (London: Ethel Snowden, 1918)

9 Hansard records several occasions when Charlie's publications were referred to in parliamentary debate. A typical response was: 'This leaflet has been considered but the government do not propose to make expressions of opinion such as those contained in it, unfounded though they are, the subject of legal proceedings.' 'Expressions of Opinion', Hansard, November 1916.

10 'Thomas Atkins' had been used as a term for the common British

soldier from the eighteenth century, and was allegedly the name used generically on specimen army forms from 1815. The term 'Tommy' gained wider usage after Rudyard Kipling took the name for his 1892 poem about the lot of the anonymous soldier, part of his *Barrack-Room Ballads* themselves dedicated to T.A., and the name was particularly associated with soldiers during the First World War.

11 An estimated 100,000 soldiers died at the Second Battle of Ypres, which saw the first use of poison gas on the battlefield.

12 Eglantyne Jebb, 'Who Makes War?' undated, unpublished manuscript. The primary goal of the League of Nations, founded in 1920, was to prevent war through collective security, and the Kellogg-Briand Pact of 1928 solemnly renounced war as an instrument of national policy. Among many other cultural contributions to the debate, between 1918 and 1919 the French film director Abel Gance made the first version of his visionary anti-war film *J'accuse* – remade in 1938; in 1932 Sigmund Freud and Albert Einstein contributed a public exchange of letters titled simply 'Why War?'; and in 1938 Virginia Woolf published reflections on the roots of war in her essay 'Three Guineas'.

13 Of all her siblings only Dick was as quiet as Eglantyne during the war-years, most of which he spent on home soil serving modestly as a musketry instructor in his position as a Captain in the King's Shropshire Light Infantry on the Isle of Man. Originally Dick had intended to enter the Indian Civil Service, but the deaths of his father and brother left him financially independent, and he spent the years between 1897 and 1901 travelling overseas, accompanied by Eglantyne in Egypt. Inspired by visiting the colonies, Dick became a progressive authority on Empire and Colonial Nationalism, with several books and a column in the *Morning Post*. However his humiliating defeat as a Tariff Reform candidate in the January 1910 General Election led him to withdraw from politics, and his public career effectively came to a close with the outbreak of war in 1914.

14 If Eglantyne had developed thyrotoxicosis or Graves' disease it would only have been in recent years, so she was wrong to attribute 'the fits of depression which have been such a tiresome trouble to me all my life' to this condition. After 1916, when the goitre was removed, her

symptoms including depressions and weight fluctuations continued, so it is possible that the tumour had been benign, and she simply had a hypomanic personality.

15 In her social novel *The Ring Fence* Eglantyne made the materialistic Hugh criticise Frieda for wanting to invest her inheritance in the social good, describing her as being 'possessed of a mania the opposite of kleptomania'. It was a tendency all the more serious in his eyes as to him 'it was just her possessions which made her what she was'.

16 It would be interesting to know what Charlotte Toynbee made of Eglantyne's experiment of living on a working–class wage. Her own great-great niece, the journalist Polly Toynbee, published a book about a much more sustained experiment in living on the minimum wage in 2003: Polly Toynbee, *Hard Work: Life in Low-Pay Britain* (London: Bloomsbury, 2003)

17 Sir James Berry, FRCS, FSA, later President of the Royal Society of Medicine, established much of the solid foundation for thyroid surgery through his book *Diseases of the Thyroid Gland and Their Surgical Treatment*, for many years the standard authority in the field.

Chapter 11

1 British press censorship would not be so tight again until the start of the British campaign in the Falklands in 1982 when Margaret Thatcher banned direct television transmission and restricted access to only two photojournalists.

2 After writing to her last known address, Eglantyne received a postcard telling her that her governess, Heddie Kastler, had died during the war. In fact Kastler survived both the war and subsequent famine in Germany, and wrote to Eglantyne in June 1920 asking for help to find a position in England. 'After all the tears I shed for her!' Eglantyne wrote to Dorothy in June 1920.

3 Not everyone was charmed by Ogden's eccentricities. Marcus Dimsdale's college friend Arthur Benson referred to him as 'that ass Ogden'.

4 Often Ogden also printed humorous articles such as 'Suggestions for the Council of Trinity College' by the philosopher G.E. Moore, which

proposed the prohibition of 'dangerous meetings' such as attendance at College Chapel. 'The maxim *"Love your enemies; do good to them that hate you"* actually occurs in one of the books habitually read in Churches,' Moore wrote, continuing, 'Here, again, it may, of course, be argued that nobody ever takes seriously what they hear in Church. But I can again assure the Council, from personal knowledge, that this is not absolutely *always* so.'

5 The then German Chancellor, Bethmann Hollweg, who put out the feelers for peace, later had to resign.

6 Marian Ellis and Lord Parmoor made a good team. They had already worked together to organise an international Christian conference during the war, and when the Fight the Famine Council brought them together again in 1918 love blossomed. Not always so slow to act, Parmoor proposed in May 1919 and they were married that July. 'I could not try to express all that this marriage brought in strength and encouragement to my life,' he wrote in a romantic interlude in his mainly political memoirs. 'The greatest gift which heaven sends us is the companionship of a perfect marriage.' See Charles Alfred Cripps, Lord Parmoor, *A Retrospect: Looking Back Over a Life of More Than Eighty Years* (London: William Heinemann, 1936)

Chapter 12

1 The 'Women's International League for Peace and Freedom', also known as the Women's League or WILPF, was the organisation that grew from the women's international peace congress in The Hague in April 1915. It is the oldest women's peace organisation in the world, and now has member organisations in thirty-seven countries.

2 In 1919 Austria had a population of six and a half million, of whom two million lived in Vienna.

3 A year later, in December 1919, Sir William Goode, KBE, British Director of Relief, finally arrived in Vienna, reporting back that 'It is not unusual to see the traffic in one of the main streets which leads to the cemetery held up by hearses – nine tenths carry the bodies of children.' Earlier British aid might have reduced these statistics.

4 Dr Hector Munro described travelling on his research mission through Europe by a train running on, and then running out of, wood, and having to wait for horse-loads of wood to arrive to replenish stocks.

5 The trial prevented Eglantyne from attending the Second Women's International Peace Congress in Zurich that May, where Emmeline Pethick-Lawrence moved the motion that the Allies raise the blockade and provide immediate relief to Europe. The Congress cabled their proposals to President Wilson at the peace talks in Paris who responded with sympathy but pessimism: 'Your message appeals to both my head and my heart, and I hope most sincerely that ways may be found, though the present outlook is extremely unpromising, because of the infinite practical difficulties.' Eglantyne's replacement, Helena Swanick, noted, 'I have never witnessed or imagined so remarkable an affirmation [of humanitarian spirit].'

6 Mansion House is the only British home with its own court of law and holding cells since the Lord Mayor of London, whose official residence it is, serves as the chief magistrate of the City. Unlike the suffragette Emmeline Pankhurst, neither Eglantyne nor Barbara was held in the cells. More recently Mansion House has been used as a venue for SCF fundraising events.

7 The second leaflet, entitled 'Our Blockade has caused this', was officially published by the Women's International League and featured a distressing photograph of two starving Austrian children, aged seven and ten.

8 The court case was covered in at least five national papers, in several with more than one article, and in one it was claimed that Eglantyne had also declared her intention of refusing to pay the fine imposed and of going to prison in default. The Police Authorities frustrated any such plan. See 'Those Wicked Leaflets', *The Daily Herald,* Friday, 23 May 1919, p. 2

9 Edith Cavell was executed by German firing squad at noon on 12 October 1915. Tradition has it that many of the firing squad deliberately missed, and one Private Rimmel was himself executed for refusing to fire on Cavell, and was buried beside her. Her London memorial adjacent to Trafalgar Square was unveiled by Queen Alexandra on 17 March 1920.

10 'Raise the Blockade Leaflets', *The Times*, 16 May 1919, p. 9; 'Blockade Poster Fines', *The Daily Mail*, 16 May 1919, p. 3; 'Raise the Blockade', *The Daily Mirror*, 19 May 1919, p. 5; 'Raise the Blockade Leaflets', *Guardian*, 17 May 1919, p. 12; 'Those Wicked Leaflets', *The Daily Herald*, 23 May 1919, p. 2, and earlier cover spread.

11 Dorothy must have ad-libbed this powerful line as it is quoted word for word in several different sources but a different version appears in her speech notes in the Buxton archive: 'I hold in my hand a tin of condensed milk. It may avail to save the life of some starving baby. All the statesmanship there is left in the world, all the true religion there is left in the world – is symbolised in this.'

12 'If it had not been for her persistent work the SCF would never have been started, although she always tries to give me the credit which belongs to her,' Eglantyne wrote to Suzanne Ferrière in April 1920.

13 After the Albert Hall meeting the Famine Council lobbied Lloyd George and President Wilson at the Paris peace talks, urging them to consider German appeals for a modification of the peace terms impartially and sympathetically. 'We believe that a peace willingly signed by the German government as a representative of the German people is of infinitely greater value than one forced on them by threats of famine, and a far better foundation for the new world order to which we are looking forward,' the letter signed by various Lords, Bishops, Sidney and Beatrice Webb, and C.P. Scott among others read. Dorothy, Lord Parmoor and others continued campaigning, and the Famine Council was reconstituted for a while in the spring of 1921, but it had already done the best of its work. The Women's League also lobbied the Big Four in Paris, mainly through President Wilson, but with similarly little success.

14 The concept that children represent the future of a new nation did not start with the war, but in 1918 the greatly declining British birth rates and high infant mortality during a period of international instability heightened concern about child welfare. Thus the CMO report for 1917–1918 argued that 'the European war has now given new emphasis to the importance of the child as a primary national asset'.

Chapter 13

1 Norah Bentinck continued to support the Fund however, and in 1929 she was invited to join the Save the Children International Union Council. Her son, Henry Noel Bentinck, was wounded twice in the Second World War before being taken prisoner, having felt unable to continue his initial position as a conscientious objector after the death of a close friend.

2 In 1910 Lord Weardale served as President of the 'National Peace Conference'. Ten years later he was still leading the British group in the 'Inter-Parliamentary Union': the first permanent forum for political multilateral negotiations set up to promote the peaceful arbitration of conflicts. In 1912 he and Lord Curzon became joint Presidents of the National League for Opposing Woman's Suffrage. He was attacked with a dogwhip at Euston Station two years later, by a suffragette who had in fact mistaken him for the Prime Minister, Herbert Asquith.

3 Lady Cynthia Mosley was Chair of the Save the Children appeal for German children in 1923.

4 Florence Haughton's October 1919 letter to Dorothy continued to condemn not only working with 'these individuals whose inhumane and cold-blooded actions have caused the Fund to be formed, but actually thus exalt them as saviours of the children' and enable them to 'advertise their humanity (!!)'.

   According to Sir William Goode, British Director of Relief, by the end of December 1919 the British government had allotted £12,500,000 towards relief in Europe, providing railway material for Poland and Romania, and food for Serbia, Poland, Czecho-Slovakia, Austria and other countries. US relief directed by Herbert Hoover meanwhile delivered nearly $500 million worth of foodstuffs between the signing of the Armistice and December 1919. 'Plight of Central Europe', *The Times*, 6 December 1919

5 Eglantyne often focused her appeals on this theme. 'Much of this suffering is unnecessary. We excuse ourselves by saying we have not enough money to save the children. But so long as the world has money

enough for cigarettes and cinemas and numbers of little pleasures and comforts, it has money enough for the saving of child life,' she argued from Calvin's Pulpit in St Peter's Cathedral, Geneva, August 1924.

6 In the end nearly £10,000 bought nearly 1,500 cows for Austrian farmers who paid for them by donating milk to welfare centres. Some 3,000 tons of cattle fodder was also distributed to maintain the yield.

7 Celebrities also sometimes required the most complicated conditions for their support, like the aging star of the musicals Marie Tempest who agreed to a stage performance on the proviso that she would not have to sing or even speak a word.

8 £10,000 in 1919 is worth over £300,000 in today's money.

9 Lina Richter, *Family Life in Germany under the Blockade* (London: National Labour Press, 1919)

10 George Bernard Shaw would later regain his sympathy, and contributed to numerous charitable appeals until his death, including drawing a pig while blindfolded for the book *Famous People's Pigs*, published as a fundraiser for the Famine Relief Fund in 1943.

11 Holy Innocents' Day is the day on which Christians remember the children of Bethlehem put to death by King Herod after he heard of the birth of Jesus. Archbishop Randall Davidson suggested this date for the appeal.

12 The second encyclical, given at St Peter's, Rome, on 1 December 1920, included the line 'We cannot desist from offering a public tribute of praise to the society entitled "Save the Children".' 'The Encyclical Letter of His Holiness Pope Benedict XV on behalf of Suffering and Starving Children, MCMXX'.

13 In fact the funds raised were much greater as these totals do not reflect the funds collected by the churches for Save the Children's appeal, which were sent directly to relief agencies in the field, and from 1920 the government's matching grants were also collected directly by the societies supported by the Fund. Funds raised by churches in the USA and administered through the American Relief Administration were also accounted for separately.

14 By comparison, in purely fundraising terms, subscriptions to the Children's Society, established in 1881, had just reached £200,000 in 1918.

Chapter 14

1 ' "Supranational" was one of her favourite terms' Edward Fuller wrote in his obituary of Eglantyne, December 1928.

2 Quite reasonably Hoover wanted to administer American funds through the American Relief Administration, rather than through Save the Children. This caused a flurry of letters as Eglantyne quickly agreed so as not to jeopardise church collections in the USA, and with them the whole idea of a global appeal.

3 In 1872 Henri Dunant wrote that 'although I am known as the Founder of the Red Cross and the originator of the Convention of Geneva, it is to an Englishwoman that all the honour of that Convention is due. What inspired me … was the work of Miss Florence Nightingale in the Crimea.'

4 The links between the International Red Cross and the International Save the Children organisations were strengthened by the officials they held in common, including Gustave Ador on the Honorary Committee, and Étienne Clouzot serving as the Save the Children International Union's first General Secretary.

5 'It is very kind of you to say I may come to the Rue Calvin whether you are there or not; that is indeed to make it my home; and I so deeply appreciate it; it is a wonderful home to have,' Eglantyne wrote to Suzanne in August 1922.

6 'You feel that the place is full of the ghosts of the grave Genevese who burnt each other so solemnly for their religious convictions,' Eglantyne wrote to Tye, 6 August 1922.

7 'She delighted to turn a railway carriage into an office: I recall a journey from Budapest to Ostend, when most of our waking hours were occupied by her dictating while I typed, much to her joy, on a portable tripod stand,' Edward Fuller paid tribute to Eglantyne in February 1929.

   'I've just left your umbrella at Geneva,' Eglantyne wrote in one of several references to lost umbrellas, in November *c*.1920/1921.

8 Apparently ignoring the Women's International League European peace conferences, the campaigning journalist Henry Wood Nevinson

reported in *The Nation* in March 1920 that this was the first event at which belligerent nations on both sides met on common ground.

9 Prince Carl and Princess Ingeborg of Sweden had also met, and been impressed by, Dorothy the year before.

10 Eglantyne's concept of a 'Central Collecting Agency' anticipated the approach taken by the 'Disasters Emergency Committee' today, co-ordinating the fundraising appeals of relief agencies and the British media in the first days of any major humanitarian emergency.

In March 1920 Eglantyne was horrified when the idea of a second central collecting agency was mooted, to co-ordinate fundraising for adult relief. 'It is no use ignoring this difficulty,' she upbraided Lewis Golden, the British Fund's Chairman, 'nobody gains by its being hushed up and shoved away in a corner. It should be boldly faced and dealt with.'

11 Emily Hobhouse later resigned from the Council of the British Save the Children Fund, outraged by what she considered the continued injustice to German children. However, by March 1924 The British Fund had established kitchens for 1,250 children and the International Union was feeding 4,000 children in Berlin, as well as making regular grants to 70 other children's institutes in the country.

12 *The Chicago Daily News* journalist F.A. McKenzie reported that the famine area embraced fifteen million people, of which 'six million are on the edge of absolute destitution, and the remainder possess the barest minimum for maintaining life'. Fridtjof Nansen estimated twenty to thirty million faced famine conditions of whom at least ten million were threatened by death. Both quoted in *The Daily Express*, 23 November 1921.

13 The Fund's team in Russia were contractually committed 'not to take any active part in political or other movements connected with Russia or Russian affairs and ... not to make any statement public, or which may be likely to become public, with regard to relief questions'.

14 In his play *Fram* about Fridtjof Nansen, the poet–playwright Tony Harrison captures Eglantyne's visionary gift for fundraising in verse she might have enjoyed herself:

> What could happen to the world if lantern slides could be projected in people's homes while they were having tea?

If these actualities could be seen by the whole nation
Surely it would mean an end to the horrors of starvation.

15 Tye was impressed by Eglantyne's enthusiastic reports of Nansen in February 1922, and the description of him always closely hugging his box of irreplaceable slides prompted her to comment he was obviously a wise as well as a great man.

16 The collective effort saved the lives of more than seven million people, of whom six million were children. However millions who either lived outside the main relief zones or were too old to qualify for Save the Children, or the ARA's rations, died. In February 1922 Suzanne Ferrière reported from Saratov: 'In another hut I found four persons: two were young men aged 18 and 21, i.e. too old to benefit from our meagre rations, and two younger boys who were going to the SCIU kitchen every day. The father had died of hunger a week earlier, the mother the preceding day. The two eldest boys knew that their turn was not far off.'

17 Nonetheless the ARA alone fed three million children across Russia.

18 Eglantyne's suggestion in July 1920 was that Keynes pull together an economic programme for reconstruction to be supported by the fledgling League of Nations, the 'Common Sense' group led by Francis Hirst (who led the Liberal opposition to Keynes), and The Labour Party, collectively to bring pressure to bear on the British government, and the governments of Europe to carry the programme out.

19 This survey became a regular publication: Edward Fuller (ed.), *The International Handbook of Child Care and Protection*

Chapter 15

1 In 2006, for example, Victim Support expressed concerns that the *British Crime Survey* did not measure offences committed against children, although children are twice as likely as adults to be victims of crime. And Michael Freeman has highlighted that UK Education Acts in the 1980s and 1990s purported to extend parents' rights while ignoring the rights of the primary education consumers. See Michael Freeman, 'Laws, Conventions Rights' in *The Moral Status*

of Children: Essays on the Rights of the Child (The Hague: Martinus Nijkoff, 1997)

2 Children's civil rights activism mainly took the form of a series of school strikes against corporal punishment, and disorganised action against unpopular teachers. Eglantyne presented a sympathetic account of poor teaching and the ill treatment of children in schools in her novel *The Ring Fence*. As MP for the University of Cambridge Eglantyne's uncle, Richard Claverhouse Jebb, spoke at length in favour of the Women's Suffrage Bill in 1896.

3 The idea of an international office linking the efforts of states to ensure that 'the idea of child protection triumphed more and more in the civilised world, to help defend abroad the rights of children against parents who forgot their duties' was already being raised in Switzerland in 1912. And while the British Foreign Office at this time refused to include child welfare in its concerns, the Swiss were keen to promote child protection in their international discussion, arguing that 'in many … states the powerful idea of protecting children and youth is becoming more and more the dominant preoccupation, not only of official spheres, but also of all classes of the population'.

4 Children were increasingly being valued as the future power of a nation, whether as peace-keepers or soldiers, an idea most dramatically developed with the rise of the Hitler Youth.

5 Ruth Wordsworth wrote that the ILO was 'very dear to Eglantyne's heart, as she had a firm belief in the practical possibilities of its usefulness to the whole world'.

6 Eglantyne's Aunt Carrie, now an old lady back living in the USA, was not such an idealist. 'You know I think the League the craziest proposition man ever made, human nature being such as it is, even divine nature, for the matter of that,' she wrote to her niece, Lady Darwin, in January 1921. 'Wasn't there war among the Angels, and didn't Lucifer, son of the morning, fall almost as badly as our Wilson did?'

7 It was another eighty-five years, in March 2005, before the British government appointed Professor Al Aynsley-Green as England's first Children's Commissioner.

8　League of Nations' specialist committees were composed of state representatives with voting rights, and voluntary representatives appointed
   as advisers and assessors. The League asked the Save the Children
   International Union to nominate a representative for the Advisory
   Committee, 'really as a compliment' to Switzerland who did not have
   state representation. 'We had understood that a Swiss would be
   appointed,' Dame Rachel Crowdy wrote in a memo in February 1925,
   'although in fact they have now nominated an Englishwoman, Miss
   Jebb, to represent them.' Eglantyne served as an Advisor to the
   Committee until May 1927.

9　Reply from the British government to the questionnaire regarding the
   'Draft International Convention on the Relief and Repatriation of
   Minors of Foreign Nationality', 17 March 1927 (UNOG archive).
   Britain is still yet to respect the rights of children who have emigrated
   illegally to the UK, many of whom are placed in detention centres,
   contravening several of their human rights under the UNCRC,
   including access to suitable housing and education.

10　The UNCRC is the only international human rights treaty that
    expressly gives non-governmental organisations a role in monitoring its
    implementation. The Committee of the Rights of the Child acts as a
    monitoring body, systematically gathering and responding to reports
    from UN member states regarding their progress towards meeting the
    standards set forth in the convention.

11　The preamble to the 1989 UNCRC highlights that 'the child, by
    reason of his physical and mental immaturity, needs special safeguards
    and care, including appropriate legal protection'. Article 12.1 makes
    explicit provision for the child's voice to be heard, but Article 3.1
    stresses that it is 'the best interests of the child' rather than his or her own
    views that 'shall be a primary consideration'.

Chapter 16

1　'I ought to send [the coat] to the famine areas, but it will be such a saving to me for years to come that I think it would be more economical
   to keep it. It will be lovely for wearing over my uniform, or in bed. I

intend to wear it a good deal in bed,' Eglantyne wrote to Margaret in 1920.

2 'Sometimes I wondered whether I should still be alive when I reached my journey's end,' Eglantyne later wrote. 'At the mtgs I hardly knew whether I was standing on my head or my heels. And those efforts were useless.'

3 In 1923 Dr Albert Abrams developed a treatment called the 'Electronic Reactions of Abrams', or ERA, which held that all diseases have their own electronic vibratory rate, which could be measured and treated by his electronic boxes. Dr Abrams was dead by 1928, but although his work was exposed as fraudulent in the US *Scientific Monthly* in 1925, his 'magic boxes' enjoyed a revival in 1928 after a Dr H.H. Wilkinson reported advances in the technique.

4 The conference on the children of Africa took place in 1931, largely organised by Charlie's sister, Victoria. Over two hundred delegates attended although only seven were black and only five from Africa. Nonetheless the conference represented a major shift away from the self-regarding focus of Europe, and the International Union was further distinguished when it became one of the first international humanitarian organisations working in Africa.

5 Mme Manoukian, Eglantyne's nurse, mentioned her patient's heart tremors in a series of letters to Dorothy between October and December 1928. A hyperactive thyroid can cause an overactive heart and actial fibrillation (irregular heartbeat), and high blood pressure, but Eglantyne's weak heart could also have been caused by other factors including catching rheumatic fever as a child, leading to rheumatic heart disease; ischemic heart disease, which would make her prone to heart attacks by reducing the supply of blood to the heart; or valvular heart disease.

Mme Manoukian had not known Eglantyne before November 1928. After her death she wrote, 'I feel an immense gratitude for having known her … I have got from this a new and better conception of life, for life sometimes seemed to me very ugly during these last years. Through Miss Jebb and her family and friends, confidence and faith in humanity have returned to me.'

6 The 'B.I.T.' was the regulatory Bureau Internationale de Travail.

7 The stone reads:

> Eglantyne Jebb, born Ellesmere, Shropshire 1876, died Geneva 1928
>
> Fondatrice de l'Union Internationale de Secours aux Enfants 1920
>
> Verily I say unto you in as much as ye have done it unto one of the least of these my brethren, ye have done it to me. Matt. XXV

8 HRH, The Princess Royal, Princess Anne is the President of Save the Children. Her two bull terrier bitches, Eglantyne and Dottie, both attacked members of the public on different occasions, leading Princess Anne to plead guilty under the Dangerous Dogs Act, having become the first member of the royal family to be summoned to court on criminal charges.

9 'Her greatness was the greatness of the spirit – the White Flame, as we used to call her' and 'Apostolic spirit', Julia Eva Vajkai
'Plus flamme que femme' (More flame than woman), Count Carton de Wiart, Belgian delegate to the 10th Assembly of the League of Nations
'Saint', Viscount Cecil of Chelwood
'Different plane', Winifred Elkin

Epilogue

1 Eglantyne's listed possessions at death included about sixty books, almost all poetry, religious books, reference and biography. Among the latter were the lives of 'the Mystics', St Francis of Assisi, Joseph Vance, William Penn, Ludvic Zamenhof, Martin Planta, Johann Pestalozzi and Calvin.

2 Her most polished social novel, *The Ring Fence*, was rejected for publication after Eglantyne refused to edit it. 'Mother likes it', she wrote to Dorothy Kempe, but 'unfortunately publishers have not got the same standards as mothers, and the general public will never have a chance of judging'. She finally published a book of poems, *The Real Enemy,* in 1925, and four years later Dorothy published a second collection, *Post Tenebras Lux*, after her sister's death.

Bibliography

Manuscripts, Primary Leaflets, Press and Journal Articles

The British Library Manuscripts and Newspaper Archive, London

'Raise the Blockade Leaflets', *The Times* (16 May 1919), p.9
'Blockade Poster Fines', *Daily Mail* (16 May 1919), p.3
'Raise the Blockade Leaflets', *Guardian* (17 May 1919), p.12
'Raise the Blockade', *Daily Mirror* (19 May 1919), p.5
'Those Wicked Leaflets', *Daily Herald* (23 May 1919), p.2

Letters

Maynard Keynes to Duncan Grant (1913) (MSS 39 and 44)

Burn family archive, Cambridgeshire

The GEM, Keynes and Glazebrook families' newspaper (1898)
A.V. Hill, 'Memoirs and Reflections' (1973)
Margaret Keynes, diary (1907–1908)
John Maynard Keynes, 'Remarks made by John Maynard Keynes at a
  Luncheon in King's College Cambridge for his father's ninetieth birth-
  day and diamond wedding' (August 1942)

Letters

Margaret Keynes / Eglantyne Jebb (1910–11)
John Neville Keynes / Florence Keynes (1907–1912)

Buxton family archive, Dorset

Eglantyne Jebb's passport (issued 18 February 1913)

Fight the Famine Council minutes (1918–1919)

Mosa Anderson, 'The Cambridge Magazine: 1915–1920' (1920)

Dorothy Buxton, table of journals used in compiling 'Notes from the Foreign Press' (*c.*1916)

Dorothy Buxton, list of postal subscribers to the *Cambridge Magazine* (n.d.)

Dorothy Buxton, 'Hunger Politics', *Union of Democratic Control*, 4(7): 323 (1919)

Dorothy Buxton, 'Psychic Experiences' (1962)

Eglantyne Roden Buxton, 'Notes on Eglantyne Jebb and Dorothy F. Buxton' (n.d.)

Eglantyne Roden Buxton, 'Note on Eglantyne Jebb's "Princess Peg" story' (n.d.)

Eglantyne Jebb, 'The Claims of the Children', address, St Peter's Church, Geneva (1924)

Glen Storhaug (translator), article in *Stockholms-Tidningen*, Sweden (1920)

Letters

Charlie Buxton to Dorothy Buxton (1917) and Eglantyne Jebb (1920)

Dorothy Buxton to Tye (1919) and David Buxton (1929)

Bonaventura Cerretti, Archbishop of Corinth, to Eglantyne Jebb (1920)

Polly Hill to David Buxton (1974)

Eglantyne Jebb to Miss Sidgwick (1915), Tye (1918), and Miss Fraser Smith (n.d.)

Gilbert Murray to C.K. Ogden (1917)

Philip Snowden to Charlie Buxton (1918)

Churchill Archive Centre, Churchill College, Cambridge (A.V. Hill papers)

Margaret Keynes, notebook of wedding gifts (1913)

Margaret Keynes, 'Notes and Memoirs for an Autobiography' (n.d.)

Letters

Margaret Keynes / Eglantyne Jebb (1913)

Corporation of London Records Office, London

Mansion House Justice Room Register, vol. 1 (1918–1919)

Dimsdale family archive, Hertfordshire

Essendon 'Visitors' book'
Anon press cutting, 'Wife's Tragic Find: Shot Gun Suicide of Fellow of Cambridge' (1919)

Humphrey family archives, Cambridge and London

Letters

Eglantyne Jebb / Margaret Keynes/Hill (1907–1924)
Eglantyne Jebb to Florence Keynes (1913)
A.V. Hill / Margaret Keynes (1913)

Jebb family archive, Shropshire

The Briarland Recorder, Jebb family journal (1891)
'The Homes Arts and Industries Association', Royal Albert Hall flier (c.1894)
'In Memoriam. Died at Littlefield, Wednesday, March 11, Arthur Gamul Jebb, Aged 16 Years', *Marlburian* (25 March 1896)
'Farmers and Co-operatives: Successful Working of Manchester Society', *Preston Guardian* (7 February 1914)
'MP Who Was Shot At', *Daily News* (c.1914)
'Expressions of Opinion', *Hansard* (November 1916)
Lord Bledisloe, 'Mrs Roland Wilkins', *The Times* (29 January 1919)
'What Does Britain Stand For', *Daily Herald* (16 May 1919)
'Report on the Work of the Fight the Famine Council 1919–1920'
Letter to the Editor, *Manchester Guardian* (15 March 1920)
'The Encyclical Letter of His Holiness Pope Benedict XV on behalf of Suffering and Starving Children, MCMXX' (c.December 1920)

'The Compassion of Benedict XV for the Children of Central Europe' (1924)

'Report of the Heart Specialist on E.J.' (June 1924)

'Death of Mrs E.H. Ussher, Cappagh House' (1935)

Miss Burns, 'The True and Authentic History of the Six Young Jebbs' (1878)

Charles Roden Buxton, 'A Vision for England', *Independent Review*, 7 (1905)

Dorothy Buxton, 'Our Second Mother' (n.d.)

Dorothy Buxton, 'Comment on Eglantyne's Balkans report' (*c*.1913)

Dorothy Buxton, 'Saving the Children of Europe', *Manchester Guardian* (31 May 1919)

Dorothy Buxton, 'Typical hostility to SCF – What the great world thinks!' (n.d.)

Anne Clough, 'Particulars about Eglantyne Jebb' (n.d.)

Emily Hobhouse, 'The Worst Phase of the Famine', *Manchester Guardian* (31 May 1919)

Eglantyne Jebb, childhoood writing: 'History of Ellesmere' (1884); 'The Mischief Pot' (*c*.1886); 'A Youngest Sister' (*c*.1886)

Eglantyne Jebb, diary (1885–1886, 1898, 1900)

Eglantyne Jebb, unpublished poems including: 'Ode to Euclid' (1896); 'To My History Lecturer' (1896); 'Consultations' (1919); 'To my old German Governess, Dying in Consequence of the Blockade' (1919); 'Poems of Old Age' (1928)

Eglantyne Jebb, 'My Standard Three' (25 December 1900)

Eglantyne Jebb, 'A Liberal Portrait Gallery', *Cambridge Independent Press* (n.d.)

Eglantyne Jebb, *The Ring Fence* (*c*.1908–1912)

Eglantyne Jebb, Oetz journal (*c*.1911)

Eglantyne Jebb, 'Notes on the Psychic Life' (*c*.1911), 'The Soul's Roadbook' (*c*.1913), 'Conversations with the Dead' (1914), 'Book of Dreams' (1918), 'Experimenting with Dreams' (1918), 'Dreams and Psychical Experiences of Eglantyne Jebb' (1918)

Eglantyne Jebb, 'Letters From the Balkans: The Next War' (1913)

Eglantyne Jebb, 'Where War Has Been Lady's Work in Macedonia', unknown publication (30 May 1913)

Eglantyne Jebb, 'The Price of Power', *Glasgow Herald* (26 August 1913)

Eglantyne Jebb, 'The Barbarous Balkans' (1914)

Eglantyne Jebb, 'Who Makes War?' (*c*.1915)

Eglantyne Jebb, 'How to live on 6/- per day' (1915)

Eglantyne Jebb, draft letter for Mrs Lloyd-George (1919)

Eglantyne Jebb, 'Conclusion' (*c*.1919)

Eglantyne Jebb, 'Account of Last Meeting with Mr Graham' (1923)

Eglantyne Jebb, 'The Claims of the Child', address, St Peter's Cathedral, Geneva (1924)

Eglantyne Jebb, 'An Account of Our Visit to the Archduchess Isabella' (1924)

Eglantyne Jebb, 'The Education of Children in International Goodwill', *Premier Congrès Général de l'Enfant* (1925)

Eglantyne Jebb, 'International Social Service', report of the First International Congress on Social Welfare (1928)

Eglantyne Jebb, 'Autobiographical' (1928)

Eglantyne Jebb, 'A Foolish Story: to Amuse ERB' (1928)

Eglantyne Louisa Jebb (Tye), 'Rights of Women', *Temperance Visitor, Ireland* (n.d.)

Eglantyne Louisa Jebb (Tye), 'The Home Arts and Industries Association', *Magazine of Art* (1885)

Eglantyne Louisa Jebb (Tye), 'Recreative Learning and Voluntary Teaching', *Contemporary Review*, 48 (July–December 1885)

Eglantyne Louisa Jebb (Tye), diary (1885)

Eglantyne Louisa Jebb (Tye), 'Mysticism' (*c*.1907–1912)

Lionel Jebb, address, St Mary's Church, Ellesmere, Shropshire (1994)

Jerome K. Jerome, 'Our Children' (*c*.1920)

E. Lawrence, 'Random Memories of the SCF from 1921' (1921)

Hector Munro, 'Memories of the Time After the War' (n.d.)

Anna Pavlova, 'Hunger' (*c*.1920)

James Ramsay MacDonald, Save the Children tenth anniversary speech (1929)

Canon Reginald Smith, Sermon, Marlborough School (1896)

Emily Ussher, 'Notes on Our Home and Childhood' (n.d.)

Emily Ussher, 'Personal Memoir of EJ' (n.d.)

G.F. Watts, 'The Homes Arts and Industries Association', *The Times* (26 November 1894)

Mrs Roland Wilkins (Lill Jebb), '"To the Land!" Britain's Battle-Cry to the Women To-day!', *The Times* (1915)

Henry Wood Nevinson, *Nation* (6 March 1920)

Letters

Charlie Buxton to Eglantyne Louisa Jebb (Tye) (1920)

Dorothy Buxton regarding her biography of Eglantyne Jebb: Edward Fuller (1928); Gem Jebb (1928); Maud Holgate (1933–1934); Miss Pullen (1935)

Eglantyne Jebb to Dorothy Kempe/Gardiner (1899–1914), Dorothy Jebb/Buxton (1908–1928), Board of Trade, Labour Exchanges and Unemployment Insurance (1913), Florence Keynes (1914), Margaret Keynes/Hill (n.d.), Tye, Bun and Em (1919–1924), Lewis Golden (1920), Lord Weardale (1920), Lady Blomfield (1920), John Maynard Keynes (1920), Maud Holgate (1928), Lill Wilkins, née Jebb (1928), and Charlie Buxton (1928)

Jebb family correspondence (1871–1903, 1919–1922, 1928)

Margaret Keynes/Hill to Eglantyne Jebb (1908–1928)

Mme Manoukian to Dorothy Buxton (1928) and Victoria de Bunsen (1928)

Save the Children correspondence: Douglas J.F. Parsons, Friends Emergency Committee (1919); Violet Hanbury / Mr M. Sheepshanks (1919); Florence Haughton to Dorothy Buxton (1919); Lady Norah Bentinck to Victoria de Bunsen (1919); M.P. Willcocks, SCF Exeter and District Branch to Dorothy Buxton (1919); Dora Sanger to Lord Weardale (n.d.); Lord Aberdeen to Lord Weardale (1920); Emily Hobhouse to Dorothy Buxton (1920); Dorothy Buxton / Marian Ellis (1918); Miss Durham / Mr Christian (1913); Rev. Samuel W Gentle-Cackett to Eglantyne Jebb (1919); The Official Committee for Relief in Europe to Dorothy Buxton (1920)

Labour History Archive, People's History Museum, Manchester

Jim Middleton, Assistant Secretary, the Labour Party, internal appeal (18 February 1920)

Vienna Emergency Relief Fund, appeal advertisement, *Nation* (10 January 1920)

Letters

Dorothy Buxton / Jim Middleton (1920)
Eglantyne Jebb / Jim Middleton (1920)
Arthur Jenkins / Jim Middleton (1941)

Lady Margaret Hall archive, Oxford

Dorothy Gardiner, née Kempe, 'Eglantyne Jebb, 1876–1929' [*sic*], *Lady Margaret Hall's Little Brown Book* (1929)
Eglantyne Jebb, assorted sketches and illustrated programmes (1895–1898)
Geraldine Jebb (Gem), 'Recollections of Eglantyne Senior' (n.d.)
Lilias Milroy, 'Memoirs of Eglantyne Jebb' (n.d.)
Lilias Milroy, 'The Crickets' (n.d.)
Hector Munro, 'Visit to the Pope in 1920 by Dr Hector Munro' (n.d.)
Mildred Preston, 'Memoirs of EJ for Mrs Buxton' (1934)
Ruth Wordsworth, 'Recollections of Eglantyne Jebb' (n.d.)

Letters

Maud Holgate to Dorothy Buxton (1929)
Ruth Wordsworth to her mother (1902)

League of Nations Archives Collections, the United Nations Office at Geneva (UNOG), Switzerland

High Commissariat for Russian Refugees, memo (March 1922)
'League of Nations: Protection of Children, Report of the Fifth Committee to the Fifth Assembly', Geneva (September 1924)
'Programme of the Fourth International Congress of Childhood', Vienna and Budapest (October 1924)
League of Nations Advisory Committee on the Traffic in Women and the Protection of Children, minutes (May 1925)
'Draft International Convention on the Relief and Repatriation of Minors of Foreign Nationality', footnote (June 1926)

League of Nations Child Welfare Committee, minutes (March–April 1926, May 1927)

British Government reply to 'Draft International Convention on the Relief and Repatriation of Minors of Foreign Nationality' questionnaire (March 1927)

League of Nations Advisory Commission for the Protection and Welfare of Children and Young People: Child Welfare Committee; Legal Sub-Committee: Draft Convention for the Assistance and Repatriation of Minors (February 1928)

Sir Austen Chamberlain, report on the 'League of Nation's Advisory Commission for the Protection and Welfare of Children and Young People: Child Welfare Committee' (June 1926)

Dame Rachel Crowdy, memo (February 1925)

Eglantyne Jebb, 'Memorandum Concerning the Assistance or Repatriation of Foreign Children Who Are Abandoned, Neglected or Delinquent' (March 1926)

Eglantyne Jebb, 'Reply Received by the Social Section of the League of Nations from the Save the Children Fund (International Union)' (November 1926)

Letters

Katharine Furse to Dame Rachel Crowdy (1926)
Fridtjof Nansen to Frick (1921)

National Meteorological Archive, the Met Office, Exeter

Weather records

Shropshire: 24 August 1876; winter 1894
Marlborough, Wiltshire: 11 March 1896
Cambridge: 28 August 1902; 26 December 1913; 28 July 1919
London: 1904; winter 1914; 11 November 1918; early May 1919; 15 and 19 May 1919
Geneva: 6 January 1920; 4 March 1923; 26–27 September 1924; 13 December 1928; 17 December 1928

Newnham College Archive, Cambridge

The Newnham Register

'Obituary of Miss Louisa Wilkins', Newnham College Roll Letter, pp.44–48 (1930)

'Obituary of Mrs M. Dimsdale (E. Philipps, 1898–1900)', Newnham College Roll Letter, pp.47–49 (1950)

Royal College of Surgeons of England Archive, London

Medical Records of Dr James Berry, 'Operations for Goitre' (1916–1928)

The Save the Children Fund Archive, London

'Extracts from *The Cambridge Magazine*', section on Famine and War (29 December 1917)

Fight the Famine Council leaflet, 'Economic Notes: No. 1' (London: December 1919)

Fight the Famine Council leaflet, 'Starving Baby' (London: National Labour Press, 1919)

Save the Children Fund accounts (1919)

The Save the Children Fund, 'The Most Awful Spectacle in History: Millions of Children Naked and Starving in Europe', advertisement, *The Times* (4 March 1920)

'News Sheets and Notes for Speakers', no. 32 (Save the Children Fund, 25 March 1920)

Press coverage of the Russian famine 1921–1922 including *Daily Express* (November 1921), Save the Children archive papers (December 2001)

Untitled clipping, *Daily News* (26 January 1922)

Edward Clively's employment contract as Assistant in Russia (*c.*1922)

'Total Supplies Administered by the Save the Children Fund Organisation in Russia' (*c.*1923)

Mosa Anderson, 'New Educational Ideals: Recollections of Talks with Miss Eglantyne Jebb', *World's Children* (September 1929)

Rodney Breen, Save the Children archive papers (1995)

Rodney Breen, 'Thirty-Four Things You Didn't Know About Eglantyne Jebb' (*c.*1998)

Anthony Brett Young, 'Fifty Years On! An interview with Kathleen Clark', *World's Children* (1975)

Corder Catchpool, 'Charles Roden Buxton', tribute offered at his funeral (1942)

Eglantyne Jebb, 'A Journey to the Balkans on Behalf of the Macedonian Relief Fund' (February/March 1913)

Eglantyne Jebb, 'Notes for English Delegates to the Council Meetings of the Save the Children Fund (Central Union) Geneva' (1920)

Eglantyne Jebb, various articles, *World's Children* (1921–1929), including: 'Building a Village: Some thoughts on Atlovo' (1926); 'The World Policy of the Save the Children Fund: an Essay' (1928); 'The Dawn of a New Era' (January 1929)

Eglantyne Jebb, 'The World's Children', *Contemporary Review,* 128 (July/December 1925)

Eglantyne Jebb, 'Memo on the Policy of the Save the Children Fund' (1928)

E. Lawrence, 'Time Past', *World's Children* (1959)

George Mewes, 'Filming the Famine', *Record of the Save the Children Fund* (1922)

Letters

Eglantyne Jebb to: Dorothy Kempe/Gardiner (1895–1903, 1920); Margaret Keynes (*c.*1911); Suzanne Ferrière (1919–1926); President Wilson 'Memorandum from the Comité International de secours pour les enfants to President Wilson' (1919)

Margaret Keynes/Hill to Eglantyne Jebb (1906–1911, 1921–1924)

H.L. Woolcombe to the *Westminster Gazette* (15 January 1921)

The State Archives of Geneva, Switzerland (UISE – International Union of Save the Children – papers)

Official Reports of the Executive Committee, UISE (1920–1928)

Executive Council of UISE, minutes (1923)

Last Will and Testament of Eglantyne Jebb (1928)

List of personal articles belonging to Eglantyne Jebb (1928)

Lady Blomfield, card from funeral flowers for Eglantyne Jebb (1928)

Dorothy Buxton, draft leaflet for a memorial appeal in Eglantyne's name (1929)

Suzanne Ferrière, 'Report from Saratov' (1922)

Edward Fuller, 'Miss Eglantyne Jebb', obituary press release (1928)

Edward Fuller and William MacKenzie, untitled tributes to Eglantyne Jebb, *En Mémoire d'Eglantyne Jebb: Extrait de la Revue Internationale de l'Enfant*, VII.38–39 (February–March 1929)

Eglantyne Jebb, 'Miscellaneous Thoughts about My SCF Work', Chamonix (1922)

Eglantyne Jebb, untitled typed manuscript re situation in Russia (1922)

Eglantyne Jebb, 'The Geneva Congress on Child Welfare: an impression' (1924)

Eglantyne Jebb, 'An Interview between Miss Jebb and Sir William Beveridge, Director of the London School of Economics' (1926)

Eglantyne Jebb, untitled manuscript, Vevey (1928)

Eglantyne Jebb, 'Notes on Life', Geneva (1928)

Evelyn Sharp, 'The Common Home: Some Spiritual Aspects of Child Welfare Work', *New Chronicle* (31 January 1929)

UISE Honorary President, 'Eglantyne Jebb', *International Union for Child Welfare: 50 Years* (June 1970)

Letters

Eglantyne Jebb to: Dorothy Buxton (1919); Étienne Clouzot (1920–1924); Suzanne Ferrière (1920–1926); William MacKenzie (1920–1928); Charlie Buxton (1928)

Dorothy Buxton to William MacKenzie (1931)

The Times Archives, London

Obituary, Colonel H.L. Pilkington, C.B. *The Times* (6 March 1914), p.9

'Memorial Service, Mr. M.S. Dimsdale', *The Times* (31 July 1919), p.15, Issue 42166, Col.B, Deaths

'Funerals, Mr. M. Southwell Dimsdale', *The Times* (4 August 1919), p.11, Issue 42169, Col.B, Deaths

'Plight of Central Europe', *The Times* (6 December 1919)
Obituary, 'Mrs Roland Wilkins: Work for Women on the Land', *The Times* (25 January 1929)
Obituary, Margaret Hill, *The Times* (22 June 1970)

William Ready Division of Archives and Research Collections, McMaster University Library, Ontario, Canada (C.K. Ogden papers)

Dorothy Buxton, 'Notes from the Foreign Press', a guide for translators (*c.*1915)
'Congratulations on Mrs Buxton's Notes', *Cambridge Magazine* (27 November 1915)
G.E. Moore, 'Suggestions for the Council of Trinity College', *Cambridge Magazine* (27 November 1915)
Philip Snowden and Charles Trevelyan, 'Quotations Showing the Effect in Germany and Austria of the Extreme Proposals in this Country as to the Objects of the War' (March 1916). A selection of translations from the *Cambridge Magazine* including: *Berliner Tagblatt* (November 1915); *Vorwärts* (24 November 1915); *Tägliche Rundschau* (24 February 1916); *Dresdener Neueste Nachrichten* (23 November 1915); *Kölnische Volkszeitung* (10 December 1915); *Vossische Zeitung* (8 December 1915)

Letters

Charlie Buxton / C.K. Ogden (1915–1919)
Dorothy Buxton / C.K. Ogden (1916–1919)

The Women's Library, London

Charles Roden Buxton, 'Lost Opportunities', Women's Peace Crusade, Leaflet 9 (London: Ethel Snowden, 1918) (vault C, Bentick collection)

Primary Source Books

Anon, *The Cambridge Register of Social and Philanthropic Agencies* (Cambridge: Bowes & Bowes, 1911), reprinted in *Tracts on Social and Industrial Questions (1860–1911)*

Jane Addams, Emily Green Balch, Alice Hamilton, *Women at The Hague* (1915, reprinted NY: Garland, 1972)

John Ayscough (Drew Bickerstaffe-Drew), *Gracechurch* (London: Longmans Green, 1913)

Gemma Bailey, *A Short History of LMH 1879–1923* (1923)

A.C. Benson, *From a College Window* (London: Smith & Elder, 1906)

Helen Bosanquet (ed.), *Social Conditions in Provincial Towns* (London: Macmillan, 1912)

Helen Bosanquet, *Social Work in London 1869–1912: A History of the COS* (London: John Murray, 1914)

Vera Brittain, *The Women at Oxford: A Fragment of History* (Oxford: George G. Harrap, 1960)

Victoria de Bunsen, *Macedonian Massacres: Photos from Macedonia* (London: The Balkans Committee, *c*.1907)

Victoria de Bunsen, *Charles Roden Buxton: A Memoir* (London: George Allen & Unwin, 1948)

Josephine Butler, *A Letter to the Mothers of England* (1881)

Charles Roden Buxton, *Memoirs of Sir Thomas Fowell Buxton* (London: John Murray, 1855)

Charles Roden Buxton (ed.), *Towards a Lasting Settlement* (London: George Allen & Unwin, 1915)

Charles Roden Buxton and Noel Buxton, *The War and The Balkans* (London: George Allen & Unwin, 1915)

Charles Roden Buxton and Dorothy Buxton, *The World After the War* (London: George Allen & Unwin, 1920)

Charles Roden Buxton, *In A Russian Village* (London: The Labour Publishing Company, 1922)

Charles Roden Buxton, *The Alternative to War: A Programme for Statesmen* (London: George Allen & Unwin, 1936)

Dorothy Buxton, *The Challenge of Bolshevism* (London: George Allen & Unwin, 1928)

Mrs Charles Roden Buxton (Dorothy Buxton) and Edward Fuller, *The White Flame: The Story of the Save the Children Fund* (London: Longmans, Green, 1931)

Noel Buxton, *Travels and Reflections* (London: Allen & Unwin, 1929)

Charles Alfred Cripps, Lord Parmoor, *The Policy and Work of the Fight the Famine Council* (London: Hodgson, n.d.)

Charles Alfred Cripps, Lord Parmoor, *A Retrospect: Looking Back Over a Life of More than Eighty Years* (London: William Heinemann, 1936)

Marcus Dimsdale, *Happy Days and Other Essays* (Cambridge: W. Heffer, 1921)

Anne Lenah Elgström, *Tidens Kvinner* (Women of the Time) (Stockholm: Albert Bonniers, 1948)

Edward Fuller (ed.), *The International Handbook of Child Care and Protection* (London: Save the Children/Longmans, 1924)

Caroline Jebb (ed.), *Life and Letters of Sir Richard Claverhouse Jebb* (Cambridge: Cambridge University Press, 1907)

Eglantyne Jebb, *Cambridge: A Brief Study in Social Questions* (Cambridge: Macmillan & Bowes, 1906)

Eglantyne Jebb, *Manual of Prayers for Private Use in the General Election* (London: GJ Palmer, January 1910)

Eglantyne Jebb, 'A History of the Save the Children Fund', *Record of the Save the Children Fund*, III. I (1922)

Eglantyne Jebb, *International Responsibilities in Child Welfare* (Geneva: UISE, 1927)

Eglantyne Jebb, *The Real Enemy* (London: Weardale Press, 1928)

Eglantyne Jebb, *Save the Child! A Posthumous Essay* (London: Weardale Press, 1929)

Eglantyne Jebb (ed. Dorothy Buxton), *Post Tenebras Lux* (London: Weardale Press, 1929)

Margaret Hill (née Keynes), *An Approach to Old Age and its Problems* (London: Oliver & Boyd, 1961)

Florence Ada Keynes, *Gathering Up the Threads: A Study in Family Biography* (Cambridge: W Heffer, 1950)

Geoffrey Keynes, *The Gates of Memory* (Oxford: Oxford University Press, 1981)

John Maynard Keynes, *The Economic Consequences of the Peace* (London: 1919)

Margaret Keynes, *The Problem of Boy Labour in Cambridge* (Cambridge: Bowes and Bowes, 1911)

Margaret Keynes (nèe Darwin), *A House by the River: Newnham Grange to Darwin College* (Cambridge: privately printed, 1984)

Dan H. Lawrence (ed.), *Bernard Shaw: Collected Letters 1911–1925* (London: Max Reinhardt, 1985)

Henrietta Leslie, *More Ha'Pence than Kicks: Being Some Thing Remembered* (London: MacDonald & Co, 1942)

Frederick Myers, *Human Personality and its Survival of Bodily Death* (London, New York, Bombay: 1907)

Winifred Peck, *A Little Learning: Or a Victorian Childhood* (London: Faber & Faber, 1952)

Emmeline Pethick-Lawrence, *My Part in a Changing World* (Victor Gollanz, 1938)

Gwen Raverat, *Period Piece: A Cambridge Childhood* (London: Faber & Faber, 1960)

Mary Reed Bobbitt, *With Dearest Love to All: The Life and Letters of Lady Jebb* (Chicago: Henry Regnery, 1960)

Lina Richter, *Family Life in Germany under the Blockade* (National Labour Press, 1905)

Secondary Source Books

The 1989 UN Convention on the Rights of the Child (Save the Children)

Carole Angier, *Margaret Hill* (privately published, 1978)

Noel Annan, *The Dons: Eccentrics and Geniuses* (London: Harper Collins, 1999)

Lucy Bland, *Banishing the Beast: English Feminism and Sexual Morality 1885–1914* (London: Penguin, 1995)

Elizabeth Bradburn, *Margaret Macmillan: Portrait of a Pioneer* (London: Routledge, 1989)

Ann Braude, *Radical Spirits: Spiritualism and Women's Rights in Nineteenth Century America* (Bloomington, Indianapolis: Indiana University Press, 1989)

Neville Brown, *Dissenting Forbears: The Maternal Ancestors of J.M. Keynes* (Chichester: Phillimore, 1988)

Gertrude Bussey and Margaret Tims, *Pioneers for Peace: WILPF 1915–1965* (Oxford: Alden Press, 1980)

E. Clason, *Save the Children and Children's Rights in a Historical Perspective 1919–1994* (International Save the Children Alliance, 1994)

Chr. A.R. Christophersen, *Fridtjof Nansen: A Life in the Service of Science and Humanity* (UN High Commission for Refugees and Norwegian Refugee Council, 1961)

Richard Dawkins, *The God Delusion* (London: Bantam, 2006)

Phyllis Deane, *The Life and Times of J. Neville Keynes: A Beacon in a Tempest* (Cheltenham: Edward Elgar, 2001)

Bjørn Egge, *Fridtjof Nansen's Struggle for Human Rights and Human Dignity* (UNOG, 1994)

Geoffrey Finlayson, *Citizen, State, and Social Welfare in Britain 1830–1990* (Oxford: Clarendon Press, 1994)

Catherine Foster, *Women for All Seasons: The Story of the Women's International League for Peace and Freedom* (London: University of Georgia Press, 1989)

Michael Freeden, *The New Liberalism: An Ideology of Social Reform* (Oxford: Oxford University Press, 1984)

Kathleen Freeman, *If Any Man Build: The History of Save the Children* (London: Hodder & Stoughton, 1965)

Michael Freeman, *The Moral Status of Children: Essays on the Rights of the Child* (The Hague: Kluwer Law International, 1997)

Michael Freeman, 'Laws, Conventions, Rights', in *The Moral Status of Children: Essays on the Rights of the Child* (The Hague: Martinus Nijkoff, 1997)

Edward Fuller, *She Championed Children: The Story of Eglantyne Jebb* (London: Save the Children, 1956)

Anne Hamlin, *Pioneers of the Past* (Cambridge: Newnham College, 2001)

Tony Harrison, *Fram* (London: Faber & Faber, 2008)

Roy Harrod, *The Life of John Maynard Keynes* (London: Macmillan, 1963)

Jenny Hazelgrove, *Spiritualism and British Society Between the Wars* (Manchester: Manchester University Press, 2000)

Harry Hendrick, *Child Welfare: Historical Dimensions, Contemporary Debate* (Bristol: Policy Press, 2003)

Richard Holmes, *Footsteps: Adventures of a Romantic Biographer* (London: Flamingo, 1995)

Michael Holroyd, *Bernard Shaw: Volume 3, 1918–1950, The Lure of Fantasy* (London: Penguin, 1993)

Georgina Howell, *Daughter of the Desert: The Remarkable Life of Gertrude Bell* (London: Macmillan, 2006)

Martin Hoyles and Phil Evans, *The Politics of Childhood* (London: Journeyman, 1989)

Stephen Humphries, *Hooligans or Rebels: An Oral History of Working Class Childhood and Youth, 1889–1939* (Oxford: Blackwell, 1981)

Roland Huntford, *Nansen: The Explorer as Hero* (London: Abacus, 2001)

Jules Kosky, *Top of the Hill: A History of Hill Homes* (London: Hill Homes, 1994)

Seth Koven, *Slumming: Sexual and Social Politics in Victorian London* (Princeton and Oxford: Princeton University Press, 2004)

Jane Lewis, *Women in England 1870–1950: Sexual Divisions and Social Change* (Hemel Hempstead: Wheatsheaf, 1984)

Jane Lewis (ed.), *The Voluntary Sector, the State and Social Work in Britain: Charity Organisation Society/Family Welfare Association Since 1869* (Aldershot: Edward Elgar, 1995)

B.H. Liddell Hart, *History of the First World War* (Trowbridge & Esher: Redwood Burn, 1979)

Norman and Jeanne MacKenzie (eds.), *The Diaries of Beatrice Webb* (Virago, 2000)

Sir Arthur Marshall, *The Marshall Story: A Century of Wheels and Wings* (Sparkford: Patrick Stephens, 1994)

R.G. Martin, *Save the Child: The Story of Eglantyne Jebb* (London: Lutterworth Press, 1969)

J.M.H. Moll, 'Sir James Berry', in *Presidents of the Royal Society of Medicine: Illustrated Profiles 1805–1996 Dr William Saunders to Sir Donald Harrison* (Royal Society of Medicine Press, 1996)

Caroline Moorhead, *Dunant's Dream: War, Switzerland and the History of the Red Cross* (London: Harper Collins, 1999)

Sarah Musgrove (ed.), *Children's Rights: Reality or Rhetoric? The UN Convention on the Rights of the Child: The First Ten Years* (London: International Save the Children Alliance, 1999)

David Newsom (ed.), *On the Edge of Paradise: A.C. Benson: The Diarist* (London: John Murray, 1980)

Colin Nicholson, *The Longman Companion to the First World War* (Longman, 2001)

Alex Owen, *The Darkened Room: Women, Power, and Spiritualism in Late Victorian England* (Chicago, London: Chicago University Press, 1989)

John F. Pollard and Geoffrey Chapman, *The Unknown Pope: Benedict XV (1914–1922) and the Pursuit of Peace* (London, New York: Continuum, 2005)

Roy Porter, *Flesh in the Age of Reason* (London: Allen Lane, 2003)

J.W. Robertson Scott, *The Story of the Women's Institutes Movement in England and Wales and Scotland* (Idbury, Kingham: The Village Press, 1925)

Michael E. Rose, *The Relief of Poverty 1834–1914* (London: Macmillan, 1974)

Sheldon Rothblatt, *The Revolution of the Dons: Cambridge and Society in Victorian England* (Cambridge: Cambridge University Press, 1968)

Save the Children, *Child Rights: A Second Chance* (London: International Save the Children Alliance, 2001)

Robert Skidelsky, *John Maynard Keynes, Volume One: Hopes Betrayed 1883–1920* (London: Macmillan, 1983)

Robert Skidelsky, *Henry Sidgwick, 1838–1900* (Cambridge: Newnham College, 1988)

Robert Skidelsky, *John Maynard Keynes 1883–1946: Economist, Philosopher, Statesman* (London: Macmillan, 2003)

Susan Sontag, *Regarding the Pain of Others* (New York: Picador, 2003)

Frances Spalding, *Gwen Raverat: Friends, Family and Affections* (London: The Harvill Press, 2001)

Anne Summers, *Female Lives, Moral States: Women, Religion and Public Life in Britain 1800–1930* (Newbury: Threshold Press, 2000)

Claire Tomalin, *Thomas Hardy: The Time-Torn Man* (London: Penguin, 2006)

Martha Vicinus, *Independent Women: Work and Community for Single Women 1850–1920* (Chicago: The University of Chicago Press, 1985)

Andrew Vincent and Raymond Plant, *Philosophy, Politics and Citizenship: The Life and Thought of British Idealists* (Oxford: Basil Blackwell, 1984)

L. Patrick Wilkinson, *A Century of King's 1873–1972* (Cambridge: King's College, 1980)

Francesca Wilson, *Rebel Daughter of a Country House: The Life of Eglantyne Jebb, Founder of the Save the Children Fund* (London: George Allen and Unwin, 1967)

Anne Wiltsher, *Most Dangerous Women: Feminist Campaigners of the Great War* (London: Pandora, 1985)

Joseph Wood Krutch (ed.), Henry Thoreau, *Walden and Other Writings* (London: Bantam, 1981)

Patrick Wright, *Iron Curtain: From Stage to Cold War* (Oxford: Oxford University Press, 2007)

Dictionary of National Biography (Oxford: Oxford University Press, 1990)

Press and Journal Articles

Anne Anderson, 'Victorian High Society and Social Duty: the Promotion of "Recreative Learning and Voluntary Teaching"', *History of Education*, 31(4): 311–334 (2002)

Kofi Annan, 'Foreword', *The Progress of Nations 2000* (UNICEF, 2000)

Joanna Bourke, 'Women and Employment on the Home Front During World War One', www.bbc.co.uk/history/war/wwone/women_employment (July 2004)

Kate Bradley, 'The Child's Guardian? Children's Charities and the Shaping of Attitudes towards Child Abuse and Child Protection, 1908–1948', Social History Society conference (2007)

Ben Buxton, 'Dorothy Buxton's Long Crusade for Social Justice', *Cambridge* (journal of the Cambridge Society), 50: 74–77 (2002)

Mark Freeman, 'The Provincial Social Survey in Edwardian England', *Historical Research*, 75(187): 79–89 (2002)

Sonja Grover, 'On Recognising Children's Universal Rights: What Needs to Change in the CRC?' *International Journal of Children's Rights*, 12: 259–271 (2004)

Michael King, 'Children's Rights as Communication: Reflections on Autopoietic Theory and the UN Convention', *Modern Law Review*, 57(3): 385–401 (1994)

Seth Koven, 'Dr Barnardo's "Artistic Fictions": Photography, Sexuality, and the Ragged Child in Victorian London', *Radical History Review*, 69(Autumn): 6–45 (1997)

Linda Mahood, 'Feminists, Politics and Children's Charity: The Formation of the Save the Children Fund', *Voluntary Action*, 5(1): 71–88 (2002)

Linda Mahood, 'Elementary Teaching as Toil: The Diary and Letters of Miss Eglantyne Jebb, a Gentlewoman Schoolmistress', *History of Education*, 35(3): 321–343 (2006)

Linda Mahood, 'Eglantyne Jebb: Remembering, Representing and Writing a Rebel Daughter', *Women's History Review*, 17(1): 1–20 (2008)

Dominique Marshall, 'The Construction of Children as an Object of International Relations: The Declaration of Children's Rights and the Child Welfare Committee of the League of Nations, 1900–1924', *International Journal of Children's Rights*, 7(2): 103–148 (1999)

Dominique Marshall, 'Humanitarian Sympathy for Children in Times of War', in James Marten (ed.) *Children and War: A Historical Anthology* (London, New York: New York University Press, 2003)

Dominique Marshall, 'Children's Rights in Imperial Political Cultures: Missionary and Humanitarian Contributions to the Conference on the African Child of 1931', *International Journal of Children's Rights*, 12(3): 273–318 (2004)

Reggie Norton, 'Benedict XV and the Save the Children Fund', *The Month* (July 1995)

Vanessa Pupavac, 'Misanthropy Without Borders: The International Children's Rights Regime', *Disasters*, 25(2): 95–112 (2001)

Polly Toynbee, 'We Need to Start a Social Revolution by Putting Children First', *Guardian Unlimited* (19 October 2007)

Richard Van Vleck, 'The Electronic Reactions of Albert Abrams', *American Artifacts: Scientific Medical and Mechanical Antiques*, 39

Catherine Wynne, 'Arthur Conan Doyle and Psychic Photographs', *History of Photography*, 22: 385–392 (1998)

Slavoj Žižek, 'Against Human Rights', *New Left Review*, 34: 115–131 (2005)

Websites

www.britannica.com

www.everychildmatters.gov.uk/strategy/childrenscommissioner

www.parliament.uk/parliamentary_publications_and_archives

www.savethechildren.org

www.unhchr.ch

www.unicef.org

Index

Aberdeen, Lady 305
acting 22-3, 35
admirers 36-7
Ador, Gustave 277, 308, 350
advertising campaign 263–4
Agricultural Organisation Society
    (AOS) 176–7, 195, 342
Albert Hall Famine Meeting 243–5
American Relief Administration
    (ARA) 248, 288, 294, 350, 352
Anderson, Mosa 212, 215-16, 225,
    227, 255
'Answers' 51
appearance 37, 100, 257–9, 335
articles 167, 203, 299
Asquith, HH 111
Austria 232, 236-37, 240, 251, 271,
    285, 341, 345, 349
Ayscough, John 9–10, 19

Baha'i movement 297
Balkans 140–67, 174–5
Bannerman, Sir Henry Campbell 102
'Barbarous Balkans, The' 167
Benson, Arthur 76, 87,103,170, 344
Bentinck, Lady Norah 253, 348
BER (Boys Employment Register)
    119–20, 121–3
Berry, Sir James 207, 320, 344
Besant, Walter 24
Bethnal Green settlement 46–7

blockade, British economic 218–19,
    223, 224, 225, 226–7, 229,
    230-31
Blomfield, Lady Sara 297, 325
Bodkin, Sir Archibald 241–2
Book of Dreams 186
books 14–15, 29, 34, 44, 45
Brailsford, Henry Noel 244
Briarland Recorder, The 17
Brittain, Vera, 53, 193
Brooke, Rupert 117, 129, 215
Bun, Aunt *see* Jebb, Louisa (Aunt Bun)
Buxton, Charles Roden 82–3, 90,
    101, 102-03, 228, 281–2, 339,
    340, 341, 342
    and the Balkans 141, 142, 165–7
    election candidate 111, 112, 113
    First World War 196–7, 215
    and the League of Nations 308, 311
    in Russia 287–8
Buxton, David 216, 217
Buxton, Dorothy Frances (née Jebb)
    4, 13, 32, 71, 92–3, 112–3, 118,
    192–3, 203, 280
    in Cambridge 96
    and Charles 82, 83, 90, 101
    childhood 17, 18, 21, 26, 29, 38
    children 110–11
    clothes 258
    Fight the Famine Council 227,
    228, 231

Buxton, Dorothy Frances (cont.):
  Gamul's death 38-9, 40, 41
  in memory of Eglantyne 328, 329
  with the MRF 164
  Save the Children Fund 245–6,
    247–8, 250, 286-7, 270, 347
  spiritualism 170, 180
  war work 196, 197–8, 208, 209,
    211–3, 216–20, 225–6
Buxton, Eglantyne Roden 110, 217,
  274, 323, 340
Buxton, Noel 83, 141, 142, 165–7,
  196, 228
Buxton, Victoria 82, 89–90, 142–3,
  253, 341, 355

Cambridge 71, 72–4, 96, 105, 106
Cambridge: A Brief Study in Social
  Questions 105–8, 109
Cambridge Magazine 214, 216, 219–21
'Cambridge Register of Social and
  Philanthropic Agencies, The'
  109–10
Campbell-Bannerman, Sir Henry 102
Carrie, Aunt see Jebb, Caroline
Catholic Apostolic Church 48
Catholic churches 267, 269–70,
  275–6
Cavell, Edith 242-43, 346
Cecil, Lord Robert 255
censorship 210–11, 212–13
charities digest 100–1, 104–8, 109–10
Charter for Children 301, 304–8
childhood 9, 15-18, 21-3, 26
children 52–3, 58, 60–2, 65–7, 68–9,
  107, 272
  starving 231, 232, 236, 237–9, 240,
    247–9, 250–1
Children's Charter 306–8, 311–113
Christianity 175–6, 273–4, 297–8

Christmas at The Lyth 22–3
churches 48, 267–70, 275–6
Churchill, Winston 165, 223, 229
citizenship 106–7
climbing 125–7, 178, 301
clothes 257–9
Confessions of a Kleptomaniac 206
Conversations with the Dead 178, 181,
  182, 185–6
correspondence with Margaret Keynes
  115–6, 123–5, 127–8, 129–31,
  132–3,136–7
COS (Charities Organisation Society)
  12, 95–6, 97–8, 265
Courtenay, Lady Kathleen (Kate) 227,
  255
Cows for Vienna 260–1, 271

dancing 22, 36
Darwin, Gwen see Raverat, Gwen
Davidson, Archbishop Randall 267,
  269, 291
'Dawn of a New Era' 299
death
  belief 185
  desire 201
  Eglantyne's 325–6
debating 34–5
'Declaration of the Rights of the
  Child' 306–8, 311
Defence of the Realm Act (DORA)
  210, 241
depressions 62–3, 320
Dimsdale, Elsie 83, 86, 87, 88, 338
Dimsdale, Marcus Southwell 74–82,
  83–4, 85–7, 338
Dmitrovich, Captain 152–3, 158
dogs, named after Eglantyne 328–9
drama 22–3, 35
drawings 3–4, 18, 331

dreams 186–7
Dunant, Henri 276, 278, 350

Economic Consequences of the Peace, The
  (Maynard Keynes) 225
education 53–6, 64
  Eglantyne's 28–37, 43–51
Egypt 49–50
Elgström, Anna Lenah 281
Eliot, George, 13–14, 73, 121, 279
Elkin, Winnie 256–7, 261
Ellis, Marion 228–9
Em *see* Ussher, Em (Emily)
Encyclical 267
Experimenting with Dreams 187
extra-curriculum activities 34–6

Fabian Society 96
faith 48–49, 63, 173–5, 204, 273–4,
  297–8, 324
Family Life in Germany Under the
  Blockade (Richter) 266
famine in Russia 287–94
'Farewell to Jack' 79
Ferrière, Dr Frédéric 219, 238, 277
Ferrière, Suzanne 277–8, 279–80, 310
Fight the Famine Council 227–31,
  233, 235, 239, 241, 253, 347
films about famine 292
First World War 171, 190–1, 192–5,
  203–4, 209–23
friendships 43–4
Fry, Joan 240
Fry, Margery 34
fundraising 73–4, 162–3, 252–7,
  259–67, 269–72, 328
funeral 325–6

Galsworthy, John 265
General Congress on Child Welfare
  313

Geneva 276, 278–9
Germany
  British attitude 211–12, 223–4
  grants 285–6
  starvation 238–9
Gilmore, Emily (Aunt Nony) 9, 39
Gilmore, James 59–60
Golden, Lewis 255, 262
Gould, Barbara Ayrton 234–5, 240–1
Gracechurch (Ayscough) 9–10
Grant, Duncan 129, 340
Greece 294
grief at Gamul's death 39–40

Hanbury, Lady Violet 253
'Handcuffed' 259–60
handwriting 331–2
Hardy, Thomas 215, 220, 265
Harrison, Jane 88, 99, 170, 215, 338
health 62–3, 70, 110, 120–1, 162
  Dorothy's 217, 321
  thyroid disorder 199–202, 204–5,
    207, 280, 317–19, 320–2, 324–5,
    343–44, 355
health resorts 124–5
Hill, Archibald Vivian (AV) 131–4,
  135, 136, 140–1, 190, 199
Hill, Mary Eglantyne (Polly) 136–37
history at Oxford 33–4
Hobhouse, Emily 101, 111, 285, 286,
  351
Hodges, Katherine 145, 146, 148,
  152, 160, 194
Holgate, Maud 44, 50, 89, 94, 177,
  179–80, 184, 187
holidays 23, 49–50, 70–1, 126–7,
  177–8
Holmes, Richard 6, 168, 341
Home Arts and Industries Association,
  The 9, 24–5

homosexuality 137, 138
Hoover, Herbert, 228, 236, 288
House of the Soul, The (Underhill) 182
human rights 300–1, 302–16
Hungary 312

illness 62–3, 70, 110, 120–1, 162
    Dorothy's 217
    thyroid disorder 199–202, 204–5,
        207, 280, 317–19, 320–2, 324–5
International Committee of Women
    for Permanent Peace 197–8
International Council for Women
    305, 306
International Save the Children
    Alliance 298, 335
internationalism 274–7, 308

James, Uncle *see* Gilmore, James
Jebb, Arthur 9–12, 13–14, 22, 26–7,
    29, 38, 53, 335
Jebb, Caroline 7, 25, 72–4, 80, 88,
    135, 170, 337, 353
Jebb, Dick 13, 28, 30, 36, 74, 89, 111,
    169, 341, 343
Jebb, Dorothy *see* Buxton, Dorothy
    Frances
Jebb, Eglantyne 13, 25–6, 90
    acting 22–3, 35
    admirers 36–7
    appearance 37, 100, 257–9, 335
    articles 167, 203, 299
    charities digest 100–1, 104–6
    childhood 9, 15–18, 21–3, 26
    climbing 125–7, 178, 301
    clothes 257–9
    correspondence with Margaret
        Keynes 115–6, 123–5, 127–8,
        129–31, 132–3, 136–7
    dancing 22, 36

death 325–6
debating 34–5
depressions 62–3, 320
and Dorothy 207–8
drama 22–3, 35
drawings 3–4, 18, 331
dreams 186–7
education 28–37, 43–51
essay 174, 175–6
faith 48-49, 63, 173-5, 204, 273-4,
    297–8, 324
friendships 43–4
fundraising 73–4, 162–3, 252–7,
    259–67, 269–72, 328
funeral 325–6
health 62–3, 70, 110, 120–1, 162
holidays 23, 49–50, 70–1, 126–7,
    177–8
journals 186–7
mountain climbing 126–7, 178,
    301
novels 26, 110, 206
obituaries 5-6, 329-30
plays 22–3, 323
poems 16, 17, 33–4, 51, 79, 80–1,
    104–5, 226, 259, 322–3, 327, 328
politics 101–3, 113
riding 79-82
romance 74–9, 81–2, 83–4, 87
rowing 35–6
rule-breaking 32, 273
Save the Children Fund 246–8,
    254, 274
sketches 18, 35, 48, 331
spiritualism 42, 169–74, 178–89
sports 35–6
stories 9, 15, 16–17, 18, 323
suicidal thoughts 83, 319
teaching 53–4, 55–9, 60–2, 63, 64
thyroid disorder 199–202, 204–5,

207, 280, 317–9, 320–2, 324–5,
343-4, 355
Jebb, Eglantyne Louisa *see* Jebb, Tye
Jebb, Em (Emily) *see* Ussher, Em
(Emily)
Jebb, Gamul 13, 14, 18, 29, 39, 41,
42–3
death 37–8
and natural sciences 21–2
Jebb, Gem 56, 64, 176, 202–3, 254,
325, 329, 337
Jebb, Lill (Louisa) *see* Wilkins, Lill
Jebb, Lionel 7–8, 115, 282
Jebb, Louisa (Aunt Bun) 9, 10, 18–20,
21, 29–30, 62, 71, 258, 320
Jebb, Sir Richard Claverhouse 54–5,
71, 72–3, 103, 118, 205
Jebb, Tye 9, 11–12, 13, 18, 19–20,
23–5, 37-38, 70, 124, 135
death 319, 320
move to Cambridge 71
and mysticism 172
and religion 38, 48
Jerome, Jerome K. 220–1, 265
jingoism 209, 211–12, 223–4
Jones, Frieda 46, 47, 81–2, 121, 175,
176, 331, 344
journals 186–7

Kastler, Heddie 16, 191, 344
Kempe, Dorothy 31, 36, 43–4, 46,
65, 89
Keynes, Florence 96, 99–101, 112,
116, 118, 132, 140, 174, 199
Keynes, Geoffrey 100, 117, 129
Keynes, John Maynard 100, 103, 117,
122, 128, 133–4, 136, 199, 222,
228, 263, 340
at Versailles 224, 225, 226–7
Keynes, Margaret 87, 100, 108, 111,

116, 117, 118–19, 128–9, 225,
340
and the BER, 120, 121–3
and Eglantyne 115-6, 123–4,
126–7, 130–1, 132, 133–8,
173–4, 200, 254, 325
in the First World War 198–9

Lady Margaret Hall (LMH) 30–5,
43–6, 49, 50–1
land girls 195
'Last Message, A' 327
League of Nations 274, 276, 289, 290,
296, 308–11, 354
Leslie, Henrietta 215, 255, 261,
262–3, 266–7, 280, 285, 301, 325
liberalism 103, 304
liberation of women 193–4, 197–8
libraries 11, 14-15, 34, 52, 57, 109, 296
literature 14–15, 18, 22, 44
Lloyd George, David 112, 165, 212,
223, 224, 230, 256
love
for Marcus 74–82, 83–4, 87
for Margaret 126–8, 129–31,
132–3, 134–8, 183–4
Lyth, The 7–8, 14, 21, 22, 71

MacDonald, Ramsay 5, 196, 219–20,
274, 311, 330
Macedonia 141–3, 144, 159–60,
247
MacKenzie, William 278, 301, 321,
325, 327–8
MacMillan, Margaret 64, 65, 228
McQueen, Nurse 160
*Manual of Prayers for Private Use during
the General Election* 113
Mark, Mr 153, 154, 155, 156
Marlborough 59, 60

marriages 83, 88–9, 90
Marshall, Alfred 45, 96
Marshall, Mary Paley 97, 98–9, 119,
    339
Masterman, Charles 102, 141, 142
maternalism 66–8
media 209–14, 215, 217–21, 227,
    235–6, 263–4, 291–2
memorials 328–9
Mewes, George 292
Middleton, Jim 283
Milroy, Lilias 37, 43, 44
'Mischief Pot, The' 16–17
Monastir 159–60
Mosley, Lady Cynthia 256, 348
motherhood 52, 67–8
mountain climbing 126–7, 178, 301
MRF (Macedonian Relief Fund) 140,
    141, 143, 145, 149–50, 153–4,
    159, 160
MRF report 155–6
Munro, Hector 236–7, 267–9, 346
Murray, Gilbert 215, 220, 228
mysticism 48–9, 172–3

Nansen, Fridtjof 289–90, 292–3, 302,
    352
National Schools 46, 55–6
newspapers 209–14, 215, 217–21,
    227, 235–6, 263–4, 291–2
Nony, Aunt see Gilmore, Emily (Aunt
    Nony)
'Notes from the Foreign Press' 213
novels 26, 110, 206

obituaries 5–6, 329-30
Ogden, Charles Kay 214–15, 222–3,
    344
Oxford University 28–9, 30–7, 43–6,
    47–9, 50–1

Oxford Women's Inter-Collegiate
    Debating Society 34–5

pacifism 192–4, 209, 213–14, 215
Parmoor, Lord 227–9, 345
Pearson, Miss 31
Peck, Winifred 45
Peckham, Mr 149, 150–2
Pethwick-Lawrence, Emmeline 234,
    252
Philipps, Elsbeth (Elsie) see Dimsdale,
    Elsie
philosophy 45
photography 250–1, 292
Pilkington, Colonel Henry Lionel
    177, 178, 179, 180–3, 184–6,
    187–8
plays 22–3, 323
Plough, The 176–7, 178
poems 16, 17, 33–4, 51, 69, 79, 80–1,
    104-5, 226, 259, 322–3, 327, 328
    by John Galsworthy 265
'Poems of Old Age' 322–3
politics 101–3, 113
Pope Benedict XV 229, 267–9, 275
possessions at death 327, 356
Post Tenebras Lux 328
PR (public relations) 242–3, 250–1
prejudice 56–7
press 209–14, 215, 217–21, 227,
    235–6, 263–4, 291–2
Preston, Mildred 43
Princess Anne, Her Royal Highness The
    Princess Royal ix–x, 328–9, 356
propaganda against Germany 209,
    211–12, 223–4
prosecution for distributing leaflets
    240–2
psychic experiences 41–2, 169–74,
    178–89

psychology 179
public speaking 280, 281–2
Pullen, Miss 61

Raverat, Gwen (née Darwin) 73, 75,
   129, 254, 339
reading 14–15, 18, 44, 45
Real Enemy, The 322
Rebel, The 26
Rebel Daughter of a Country House
   (Wilson) 4
Red Cross 145, 161, 219, 237–8, 239,
   248, 276–7, 282, 350
refugees 150, 159, 162, 199, 239, 289,
   294
relief agencies 237–8, 239, 277, 282–4
religion 48, 273–4
responsibility, individual versus
   collective 182
Richard, Uncle *see* Jebb, Richard
   Claverhouse
riding 18, 79–82
rights of children 300–1, 302–16,
   352-3
Ring Fence, The 46, 81–2, 121, 176,
   181, 356
Roman Catholic churches 267,
   269–70, 275–6
romance 74–9, 81–2, 83–4, 87
rowing 35–6
Royden, Maude, 34, 196, 255, 336
rule-breaking 32, 273
Russell, Bertrand 101, 111, 196, 215
Russell, Dora 214
Russia, famine 287–94, 351

Salvation Army 248, 282
Save the Children Fund 1-2, 5, 176,
   233, 242, 245–9, 252–7, 259–72,
   274, 279, 282–3

child welfare programmes 295–7
children's rights 305–8, 311–12
criticism from the press 291–2
funds for Russia 293–4
and Nansen 289–90
prioritising funds 284–7
Save the Children Fund International
   Union 276–7, 279, 282,
   284, 286, 287, 290, 295–6,
   298–9
SCF *see* Save the Children Fund
schools 53, 55, 57, 59, 60–1
Scottish Highlands 205–7
seclusion 205–7
Serbia 147, 148, 151–2, 165
settlements 46–7
Shakespeare readings 22
Sharp, Evelyn 198, 241–2
Shaw, George Bernard 141, 215, 221,
   265–7, 349
Shropshire 23, 70
Sidgwick, Henry 45
Sidgwick, Nora 170
sketches 18, 35, 48, 331
Slemmer, Carrie *see* Jebb, Caroline
Smillie, Robert 244–5, 261
Smith, Canon Reginald 38
Smuts, General 220, 224
snobbery 56–7
Snowden, Ethel 196, 230, 240, 255,
   270-271, 272
Snowden, Philip 196, 213, 218
social issues 23–4, 93–114
social novels 26, 206
Society of Friends 197, 212, 239–40,
   248, 282, 284
Soul's Roadbook, The 174, 175–6
spiritualism 42, 169–74, 178–89
sports 35–6
starvation 218–19, 232, 236, 237–8

'starving baby' leaflets 232–3, 234, 240–1
Stockwell Teacher Training College 56–8
stories 9, 15, 16–17, 18, 323
suffrage 101-2, 106, 303
   women's 111–12, 116
suicidal thoughts 83, 319
supranationalism 274–7, 297, 308

Taksim, Hassan 166
Talbot, Mary 31, 44, 75
teaching 53–4, 55–9, 60–2, 63, 64
Thoreau, Henry 44, 258
thyroid disorder 199–202, 204–5, 207, 280, 317–9, 320–2, 324–5, 343-4, 355
'To My History Lecturer' 33
Toynbee, Charlotte 55, 56, 96, 110, 207
Trail of the Black and Tans, The (Ussher) 195–6
translations 209, 213–14, 215, 217–23, 227
Turkey 144
Tydraw 23

unconscious mind 179
Underhill, Evelyn 182, 341
Union of Democratic Control (UDC) 196, 215, 235
Union Internationale de Secours aux Enfants see Save the Children Fund International Union
United Nations Convention on the Rights of the Child (UNCRC) 2, 301, 313–5, 354
university 28–9, 30–7, 43–6, 47–9, 50–1
Ussher, Em (Emily) 8, 17–18, 20, 21, 28, 29, 38–9, 41, 48, 169, 327, 342

birth 12
last days with Eglantyne 324–5
marriage 71, 89
novel 195–6

Vadjkai, Julie Eve, 295
Vienna 237, 260–1, 271, 296

Walden (Thoreau) 44
Wales 23
war
   Balkan conflict 140, 144, 149–50, 155, 156, 158, 159
   First World War 165, 190–52
War and The Balkans, The (Charles and Noel Buxton) 166
Weardale, Lord 255, 293, 319
Webb, Beatrice 66, 89, 101, 111, 209, 223–4, 228, 233–4
white flame, the 280, 329
White Flame, The (Dorothy Buxton) 4
'Who Makes War' 203–4
Wilkins, Lill (Louisa) 21, 28, 29–30, 48, 71, 90, 169, 176, 195, 203, 321, 336, 338, 342
   birth 12–13
   clothes 258
   travels 89–90
women, liberation 193–4, 197–8
Women's Institute 95, 342
Women's International League for Peace and Freedom (WILPF) 198, 227, 228, 276, 345
Women's Land Army 195
women's suffrage 111–12
Woodrow, Wilson 229, 248, 308, 346
Wordsworth, Elizabeth 30–1, 96
Wordsworth, Ruth 31, 36, 43, 50, 202, 323–3

Eglantyne's lack of maternal feelings
   65, 67
Eglantyne's public speaking 281
Eglantyne and Save the Children
   Fund 249–50, 261, 271
Eglantyne and spiritualism 171–2,
   179

Eglantyne and spirituality 259
   holiday with Eglantyne 110
World's Children 296, 299

xenophobia 212, 223–4

Z, Mr 154, 156-7